Postmenopausal Osteoporosis

Hormones and Other Therapies

CONTROVERSIAL ISSUES IN CLIMACTERIC MEDICINE SERIES

Postmenopausal Osteoporosis

Hormones and Other Therapies

Edited by

A. R. Genazzani

Past President of the International Menopause Society
and
Chairman of the Division of Obstetrics and Gynecology
University of Pisa, Italy

Published under the auspices of the
International Menopause Society

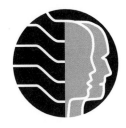

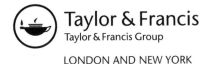

Taylor & Francis
Taylor & Francis Group

LONDON AND NEW YORK

First published in the United Kingdom in 2006
by Taylor & Francis,
an imprint of the Taylor & Francis Group,
2 Park Square, Milton Park
Abingdon, Oxon OX14 4RN, UK

Tel.:   +44 (0) 20 7017 6000
Fax.:   +44 (0) 20 7017 6699
E-mail: info.medicine@tandf.co.uk
Website: http://www.tandf.co.uk/medicine

British Library Cataloguing in Publication Data

Data available on application

Library of Congress Cataloging-in-Publication Data

Data available on application

ISBN10: 1-84214-311-5
ISBN13: 9-78-1-84214-311-7

Distributed in North and South America by

Taylor & Francis
2000 NW Corporate Blvd
Boca Raton, FL 33431, USA

Within Continental USA
Tel.: 800 272 7737; Fax.: 800 374 3401
Outside Continental USA
Tel.: 561 994 0555; Fax.: 561 361 6018
E-mail: orders@crcpress.com

Distributed in the rest of the world by
Thomson Publishing Services
Cheriton House
North Way
Andover, Hampshire SP10 5BE, UK
Tel.: +44 (0) 1264 332424
E-mail: salesorder.tandf@thomsonpublishingservices.co.uk

The image on the cover has been reproduced with the kind permission of Professor Alan Boyde, Queen Mary, University of London UK

Composition by Parthenon Publishing
Printed and bound by Antony Rowe Ltd., Chippenham, Wiltshire, UK

Contents

List of contributors

D. Agnusdei
Medical Fellow – Osteoporosis, Europe and
  Latin America
Eli Lilly and Company
Lilly Italia, SpA
Via Gramsci 731
50019 Sesto Fiorentino
Florence
Italy

F. Albani
Department of Obstetrics and Gynecology
Policlinico S. Matteo
University of Pavia
Piazzale Golgi 2
27100 Pavia
Italy

J. M. Alt
Solvay Pharmaceuticals
Hans-Böckler-Allee 20
30173 Hannover
Germany

L. Bacciottini
Department of Internal Medicine
University of Florence
Viale G. Pieraccini 6
50139 Florence
Italy

G. I. Baroncelli
Endocrine Unit
Division of Pediatrics
Department of Reproductive Medicine and
  Pediatrics
University of Pisa
Pisa
Italy

E. Bartolini
Department of Internal Medicine
University of Florence
Viale G. Pieraccini 6
50139 Florence
Italy

C. E. Bogado
Clinical Research Department
Instituto de Investigaciones Metabolicas
and
USAL University
Buenos Aires
Argentina

M. L. Brandi
Department of Internal Medicine
University of Florence
Viale G. Pieraccini 6
50139 Florence
Italy

E. Canalis
Department of Research
Saint Francis Hospital and Medical Center
Hartford, CT 06105
USA
and
The University of Connecticut School of
  Medicine
Farmington, CT 06030
USA

A. M. Carossino
Department of Internal Medicine
University of Florence
Viale G. Pieraccini 6
50139 Florence
Italy

F. Cetani
Department of Endocrinology and Metabolism
University of Pisa
Via Paradisa 2
56124 Pisa
Italy

C. Christiansen
Center for Clinical and Basic Research
Ballerup Byvej 222
Ballerup
Denmark

R. Civitelli
Division of Bone and Mineral Diseases
Washington University School of Medicine
216 S. Kingshighway Blvd
St. Louis, MO 63110
USA

V. Deregowski
Department of Research
Saint Francis Hospital and Medical Center
Hartford, CT 06105
USA

S. Detaddei
Department of Obstetrics and Gynecology
Policlinico S. Matteo
University of Pavia
Piazzale Golgi 2
27100 Pavia
Italy

A. Diez-Pérez
Autonomous University of Barcelona
Department of Internal Medicine
Hospital del Mar
P. Maritim 25-29
08002 Barcelona
Spain

V. Edusa
Department of Obstetrics, Gynecology and
  Reproductive Sciences
Center for Research in Reproductive Biology
and
The Yale Center for Musculoskeletal Disorders
Yale University
333 Cedar St, FMB 331
New Haven, CT 06520
USA

B. Ettinger
Clinical Professor of Medicine
University of California
156 Lombard Street #13
San Francisco, CA
USA

A. Fadiel
Department of Obstetrics, Gynecology and
  Reproductive Sciences
Center for Research in Reproductive Biology
and
The Yale Center for Musculoskeletal Disorders
Yale University
333 Cedar St, FMB 331
New Haven, CT 06520
USA

A. Falchetti
Department of Internal Medicine
University of Florence
Viale G. Pieraccini 6
50139 Florence
Italy

F. Ferdeghini
Department of Obstetrics and Gynecology
Policlinico S. Matteo
University of Pavia
Piazzale Golgi 2
27100 Pavia
Italy

M. Gambacciani
Department of Obstetrics and Gynecology
University of Pisa
Via Roma 67
56100 Pisa
Italy

E. Gazzerro
Department of Research
Saint Francis Hospital and Medical Center
Hartford, CT 06105
USA
and
The University of Connecticut School of
  Medicine
Farmington, CT 06030
USA

H. K. Genant
Professor Emeritus
University of California
San Francisco
USA
and
Chairman, Board of Directors
Synarc, Inc

A. R. Genazzani
Department of Obstetrics and Gynecology
University of Pisa
Via Roma 67
56100 Pisa
Italy

L. Gennari
Department of Internal Medicine
Endocrine-Metabolic Sciences and Biochemistry
University of Siena
Viale Bracci 1
53100 Siena
Italy

D. Goltzman
Department of Medicine
McGill University
Montreal
Canada

J. Haapalahti
Orion Diagnostica R&D
Oulu
Finland

P. Hadji
Philipps University Marburg
Department of Gynecology and Obstetrics
Head of the Department of Endocrinology,
  Osteoporosis and Reproductive Medicine
Pilgrimstein 3
35037 Marburg
Germany

J. Heikkinen
Deaconess Institute of Oulu
Oulu
Finland

K. Henriksen
Nordic Bioscience
Herlev Hovedgade 207
Herlev
Denmark

E. Horner
Chelsea and Westminster Hospital
London
UK

Y. Jiang
Osteoporosis and Arthritis Research Group
University of California
San Francisco
USA

J. A. Kanis
WHO Collaborating Centre for Metabolic Bone
  Disease
University of Sheffield
Sheffield S10 2RX
UK

M. A. Karsdal
Nordic Bioscience
Herlev Hovedgade 207
Herlev
Denmark

J. S. Lee
Fellow in Endocrinology
Division of Endocrinology and Metabolism
University of California
156 Lombard Street #13
San Francisco, CA
USA

M. R. McClung
Oregon Osteoporosis Center
5050 NE Hoyt, Suite 651
Portland, OR 97213
USA

C. Marcocci
Department of Endocrinology and Metabolism
University of Pisa
Via Paradisa 2
56124 Pisa
Italy

G. Martini
Department of Internal Medicine
Endocrine-Metabolic Sciences and Biochemistry
University of Siena
Viale Bracci 1
53100 Siena
Italy

D. Merlotti
Department of Internal Medicine
Endocrine-Metabolic Sciences and Biochemistry
University of Siena
Viale Bracci 1
53100 Siena
Italy

F. Naftolin
Department of Obstetrics, Gynecology and
  Reproductive Sciences
Center for Research in Reproductive Biology
and
The Yale Center for Musculoskeletal Disorders
Yale University
333 Cedar St, FMB 331
New Haven, CT 06520
USA

R. E. Nappi
Department of Obstetrics and Gynecology
Policlinico S. Matteo
University of Pavia
Piazzale Golgi 2
27100 Pavia
Italy

R. Nuti
Department of Internal Medicine
Endocrine-Metabolic Sciences and Biochemistry
University of Siena
Viale Bracci 1
53100 Siena
Italy

A. Ornati
Department of Obstetrics and Gynecology
Policlinico S. Matteo
University of Pavia
Piazzale Golgi 2
27100 Pavia
Italy

S. Ortolani
Center for Metabolic Bone Disease
Istituto Auxologico Italiano
Divisione di Endocrinologia
Via Ariosto 13
20145 Milan
Italy

B. Pampaloni
Department of Internal Medicine
University of Florence
Viale G. Pieraccini 6
50139 Florence
Italy

S. E. Papapoulos
Department of Endocrinology & Metabolic
  Diseases
Leiden University Medical Centre
Albinusdreef 2
2333 ZA Leiden
The Netherlands

R. C. Pereira
Department of Research
Saint Francis Hospital and Medical Center
Hartford, CT 06105
USA

A. Pinchera
Department of Endocrinology and Metabolism
University of Pisa
Via Paradisa 2
56124 Pisa
Italy

F. Polatti
Department of Obstetrics and Gynecology
Policlinico S. Matteo
University of Pavia
Piazzale Golgi 2
27100 Pavia
Italy

S. H. Ralston
Professor of Medicine and Bone Metabolism
University of Aberdeen Medical School
Institute of Medical Sciences
University of Aberdeen
Aberdeen AB25 2ZD
UK

D. M. Reid
Professor of Rheumatology
University of Aberdeen
Medical School
Foresterhill
Aberdeen AB25 2ZD
UK

R. Rizzoli
Division of Bone Diseases [WHO Collaborating
  Center for Osteoporosis Prevention]
Department of Rehabilitation and Geriatrics
University Hospital of Geneva
CH 1211 Geneva 14
Switzerland

J. Ryan
Mapi Values Ltd
Adelphi Mill
Bollington
Cheshire SK10 5JB
UK

G. Saggese
Endocrine Unit
Division of Pediatrics
Department of Reproductive Medicine and
  Pediatrics
University of Pisa
Pisa
Italy

N. A. Sims
St. Vincent's Hospital
University of Melbourne
Melbourne
Victoria
Australia

A. Sommacal
Department of Obstetrics and Gynecology
Policlinico S. Matteo
University of Pavia
Piazzale Golgi 2
27100 Pavia
Italy

J. Studd
Professor of Gynaecology
Chelsea and Westminster Hospital
London
UK

D. W. Sturdee
Department of Obstetrics and Gynaecology
Solihull Hospital
Solihull B91 2JL
UK

L. B. Tankó
Center for Clinical and Basic Research
Ballerup Byvej 222
Ballerup
Denmark

O. Tuncalp
Department of Obstetrics, Gynecology and
  Reproductive Sciences
Center for Research in Reproductive Biology
and
The Yale Center for Musculoskeletal Disorders
Yale University
333 Cedar St, FMB 331
New Haven, CT 06520
USA

W. H. Utian
Gynecologist, The Cleveland Clinic
President Rapid Medical Research
Professor Emeritus, Case University, Cleveland,
 Ohio
Executive Director, The North American
 Menopause Society
5900 Landerbrook Drive, Suite 195
Mayfield Heights, OH 44124
USA

A. Verza
Department of Obstetrics and Gynecology
Policlinico S. Matteo
University of Pavia
Piazzale Golgi 2
27100 Pavia
Italy

E. Vignali
Department of Endocrinology and Metabolism
University of Pisa
Via Paradisa 2
56124 Pisa
Italy

J. Wactawski-Wende
Department of Social and Preventive Medicine
School of Public Health and Health Professions
University at Buffalo
Buffalo, NY 14221
USA

A. D. Woolf
Department of Rheumatology
Royal Cornwall Hospital
Peninsula Medical School
Universities of Exeter and Plymouth
Truro TR1 3LJ
UK

Y. Zöllner
Solvay Pharmaceuticals
Hans-Böckler-Allee 20
30173 Hannover
Germany

Preface

The International Menopause Society (IMS) is a society with a world-wide responsibility, and the primary aim of the IMS is to support basic and clinical research in climacteric medicine and, on this basis, sustain global good medical practice. Many questions have been raised in recent times on menopause, hormone replacement and other therapies. For these reasons, on behalf of the IMS, we have organized workshops called 'Controversial Issues in Climacteric Medicine', gathering internationally recognized experts from all around the world to discuss and debate with the aim of elucidating the up-to-date consensus on the management of specific issues of climacteric medicine. Previous workshops have covered different issues regarding cardiovascular disease, the brain, and cancer. Recently, in November 2004 in Pisa, we organized a workshop on postmenopausal osteoporosis and the therapeutic options.

Why osteoporosis? The reasons are epidemiological and pathophysiological: the vast majority of subjects suffering form osteoporosis are postmenopausal women, who develop the risk of fragility fractures. Therefore, the IMS has to be deeply involved in studies and investigations regarding osteoporosis and to take the responsibility to educate and inform about osteoporosis diagnosis and treatment. The successful detection, prevention and treatment of osteoporosis are a rather recent challenge of modern medicine. Estrogen deficiency plays a pivotal role in determining the etiology of the most common form of osteoporosis: postmenopausal osteoporosis. Established treatments are available, preventive strategies are accessible. However, osteoporosis is even now underdiagnosed and undertreated. In our Workshop, different issues were covered, from epidemiology to the controversies on measurements of bone mineral density and their value in diagnosing osteoporosis and in assessing the risk of fracture. Concerning the issue of treatment, the most relevant, hormone replacement, and all the different options were covered and carefully discussed.

We would like this opportunity to express our appreciation and gratitude to all the speakers and moderators for their hard work in the long days of our Workshop and their devoted efforts in writing and reviewing the different chapters of this book. Thanks to their hard work, we hope to strengthen awareness in the medical community and particularly among gynecologists, supporting the physicians in providing proper counselling for the prevention of osteoporosis and osteoporotic fractures, which currently severely affect up to 40% of women over the age of 50 years.

A. R. Genazzani
Past President of the IMS

Magnitude and impact of osteoporosis and fractures

1

C. Marcocci, F. Cetani, E. Vignali and A. Pinchera

INTRODUCTION

Osteoporosis is currently defined as a skeletal disorder characterized by compromised bone strength predisposing a person to an increased risk of fracture[1]. Bone strength primarily reflects the integration of bone quality and bone density. Bone quality refers to architecture, turnover, damage accumulation and mineralization. Bone density is expressed as grams of mineral per area or volume, and in a given individual is determined by peak bone mass and amount of bone loss. A fracture occurs when a failure-inducing force such as trauma is applied to osteoporotic bone. Thus, osteoporosis is a significant risk factor for fracture, and a distinction between risk factors that affect bone metabolism and the risk factors for fracture must be made.

Historically, osteoporosis and its sequelae were recognized over 150 years ago, when it was observed that hip fractures might result from an age-related reduction in bone mass or quality. However, the term osteoporosis entered medical parlance in France and Germany in the 19th century, where it was coined as a histological description for aged human bone, emphasizing the apparent porosity of the tissue. The histological term subsequently evolved to discriminate this condition from that of osteomalacia, and came to mean bone present in reduced quantity, with normal mineralization.

Osteoporosis has clinical and public-health importance, and osteoporotic fractures are one of the most common causes of disability and a major contributor to medical-care costs in many regions of the world. Indeed, for white women, the one-in-six lifetime risk of sustaining a hip fracture is greater than the one-in-nine risk of developing breast cancer[2,3]. The social burden of fractures will increase throughout the world as the population ages. In this chapter we summarize the epidemiology of osteoporosis and osteoporotic-related fractures and determine the impact that this condition has on society.

Clinically, osteoporosis is recognized by the occurrence of characteristic low-trauma fractures, so that any clinically meaningful definition of osteoporosis must include fracture. The main advantage of a fracture-based definition is that this is a discrete event that can be diagnosed using a simple algorithm. The obvious disadvantage with this definition is that diagnosis will be exceptionally delayed in a disease where currently prevention is the optimum treatment. This has led to present-day attempts to use bone mass, as assessed by non-invasive densitometric techniques, to predict future risk of fracture.

There is a well-established relationship between bone mineral density (BMD) and the ability of bone to withstand forces, such that 75–90% of the variance in bone strength is related to BMD. Advances in medical technology have developed highly accurate and reproducible methods of measuring BMD, with minimal radiation exposure, so that they are ideal for diagnosis and monitoring in osteoporosis. Using BMD, prospective studies have shown that the risk of osteoporotic fracture increases continuously and progressively as BMD declines.

MAGNITUDE OF THE PROBLEM

How many people suffer from osteoporosis? It is clear that the answer to this question will depend on whether osteoporosis is defined on the basis of low bone mass or whether the emphasis, instead, is on osteoporosis-related fractures.

Low bone mass is analogous to high blood pressure in terms of its relationship to stroke, and the risk of fracture increases when bone density declines, just as the risk of stroke increases when blood pressure rises. However, not all strokes occur in hypertensive subjects, and fragility fractures may occur in the absence of low bone mass, although low bone mass is one of the most strongly established risks of osteoporotic fractures. Bone loss commonly occurs as men and women age; however, an individual who does not reach the peak of bone mass during childhood and adolescence may develop osteoporosis without the occurrence of accelerated bone loss. Hence, suboptimal bone growth in childhood and adolescence is as important as later bone loss in the development of osteoporosis.

Currently, there is no accurate measure of overall bone strength. Bone mineral density as reported above is frequently used as a proxy measure, and accounts for approximately 70% of bone strength. An expert panel of the World Health Organization (WHO) recently proposed diagnostic criteria for osteoporosis based on bone density, considering osteoporosis to be present when BMD levels in white women are more than 2.5 standard deviations (SDs) below the young normal mean[4]. Women with a history of one or more fragility fractures are deemed to have severe ('established') osteoporosis. Low bone mass ('osteopenia') is defined by BMD levels more than 1 SD below the young normal mean, but less than 2.5 SD below. It is not clear how to apply this diagnostic criterion to men and children, or across ethnic groups. Because of the difficulty of accurate measurement and standardization between instruments and sites, controversy exists among experts regarding the continuous use of this diagnostic criterion.

Most data on the prevalence of osteoporosis derive from the Third National Health and Nutrition Examination Survey (NHANES III), a large sample of the United States population. As assessed at the femoral neck, 20% of postmenopausal white women have osteoporosis[5]. No criteria for osteoporosis have been established for non-white women, but 10% of Hispanic women and 5% of African-American women have femoral neck BMD values more than 2.5 SD below the young normal mean for white women. Using the same cut-off value, osteoporosis prevalence rates for white, Hispanic and African-American men aged 50 years and over are 4, 2 and 3%, respectively[5]. However, these differences are related to overestimation of areal BMD (g/cm^2) in individuals with larger skeletons[6]. When bone size is taken into account, differences in bone density between men and women[7,8] and between women of difference races are reduced[9–11].

Osteoporosis is a systemic disease, and a greater proportion of the population is seen to be affected when more skeletal sites are assessed. Most white women under the age of 50 years have normal bone density, but, with advancing age, the proportion with osteoporosis increases dramatically. Among women aged 80 years and over, for example, only 3% have normal bone density at the hip, spine and forearm, while 27% have osteopenia at one skeletal site or another, and 70% have osteoporosis. As judged from these data, about 54% of postmenopausal white women in the United States have osteopenia and another 30% have osteoporosis[12].

The alternative approach to define the magnitude of osteoporosis is to assess the frequency of fragility fractures. There are no data regarding the prevalence of distal forearm fracture. The prevalence of hip fracture has been estimated at 5% for women at the age of 65 years and over and at 0.6% for all ages[13]. Most available information relates to vertebral fractures. In the European Vertebral Osteoporosis Study, 15 570 women and men were selected from population registers in 36 European Centers and evaluated according to a standardized protocol. The overall prevalence of vertebral fracture depends upon the method used for their evaluation. Using a morphometric approach, the overall prevalence of deformity was about 12% in both men and women, but the increase in prevalence with age was steeper among women. Thus, the frequency of deformities in women aged 50–54 years was 5%, rising to 24% at age 75–79 years, while the prevalence rose from 10% among men aged 50–54 years to 18% at age 75–79 years[14–17].

Using fracture incidence rates from the United States, the estimated lifetime risk of a hip fracture is 17% in white women and 6% in white men[18,19]. This compares with risks of 16 and 5% for clinically diagnosed vertebral fractures and 16 and 2% for distal forearm fractures in white women and men, respectively. The lifetime risk of any of the three fractures is 40% for women and 13% for men from age 50 years onward[18].

EPIDEMIOLOGY OF FRACTURES

Fracture incidence in the community is bimodal, with peaks in youth and in the very elderly[2]. In young people, fractures of the long bones predominate, often following substantial trauma, and the incidence is greater in young men than in young women. Above the age of 35 years, overall incidence in women increases and the female rates become twice those in men[20]. In the United States, about 70% of all fractures in subjects aged 45 years or over have been attributed to osteoporosis. In this chapter, we concentrate on fractures of the hip and spine because they arise frequently and have been the most intensively studied.

Hip fractures

Hip fractures are strongly related to low BMD, and have become the international barometer of osteoporosis, cause more disability and cost more to repair than other types of osteoporotic fracture. They are almost always treated in hospital, and are therefore easier to count and compare from country to country. Hip fracture incidence rates increase exponentially with age in both women and men in most regions of the world[21]. This rise in fracture risk results from an age-related decrease in BMD at the proximal femur, as *in vivo* surrogate for bone fragility, and an age-related increase in falls, which are responsible for at least 90% of all hip fractures[22].

The incidence of hip fracture differs between populations. Thus, age-adjusted incidence rates are higher among white women in Scandinavia than in women of comparable age in North America or Oceania[21], whereas rates vary more

than seven-fold in European countries[23,24]. Similar variation is seen in the USA, with higher rates recorded in the south-east than in the north or west of the continent[25]. Rates of hip fracture are also higher in urban than in rural areas of the same country[26], suggesting that factors related to urbanization, such as decreased physical activity and conversion from softer ground to hardwood, tile, concrete and asphalt surfaces, could contribute to an increased risk of hip fracture.

In the USA and Europe, the incidence of hip fractures in women is twice that seen in men at any age, because women have a lower BMD. Furthermore, women live longer than men, and hence more than three-quarters of all hip fractures occur in women. Worldwide, the risk of hip fracture varies more in women than in men, i.e. the rates in men and women are similar in low-risk populations, particularly those of Asian or African heritage. This variation cannot be explained by race-specific variation in bone density, and might be due to the larger bone size with a greater mechanical strength[27], a lower risk of falling or other factors[28]. Important causes of hip fracture in men are diseases associated with secondary osteoporosis and falling[29].

Like other complex chronic diseases, e.g. osteoarthritis and atherosclerosis, the pathogenesis of hip fractures is multifactorial, and no single factor (bone loss or falls) can completely account for their occurrence. Thus, hip fractures are strongly associated with BMD in the proximal femur, but there are also many clinical predictors of hip fracture risk that are independent of bone density. A set of potential risk factors for hip fracture was assessed in the Study of Osteoporotic Fractures, a prospective study of 9516 white and Asian-American women (Table 1). Hip fracture incidence was 17 times greater among 15% of the women who had five or more of the risk factors, exclusive of bone density, compared with 47% of the women who had two risk factors or fewer. However, the women with five risk factors had an even greater risk of hip fracture if their bone density Z score was in the lowest tertile. The majority of hip fractures in both sexes follow a fall from standing height or less in individuals with reduced bone strength[23]. Over a lifetime, bone density at the femoral neck declines by an

Table 1 Main risk factors for hip fracture with and without adjustment for previous fractures and calcaneal bone mineral density (BMD) in 9516 white women. Values are expressed as relative risk (95% confidence interval). Modified from reference 31

Risk factor	Base model	Adjusted for fractures and BMD
Age (per 5 years)	1.5 (1.3–1.7)	1.4 (1.2–1.6)
Increase in weight since age 25 years (per 20%)	0.6 (0.5–0.7)	0.8 (0.6–0.9)
Height at age 25 years (per 6 cm)	1.2 (1.1–1.4)	1.3 (1.2–1.5)
Current use of long-acting benzodiazepine (vs. not)	1.6 (1.1–2.4)	1.6 (1.1–2.4)
Previous hyperthyroidism (vs. none)	1.8 (1.2–2.6)	1.7 (1.2–2.5)
Current caffeine intake	1.3 (1.0–1.5)	1.2 (1.0–1.5)
History of maternal hip fracture (vs. none)	2.0 (1.4–2.9)	1.8 (1.2–2.7)
Current use of anticonvulsant drugs (vs. not)	2.8 (1.2–6.3)	2.0 (0.8–4.9)
Inability to rise from chair	2.1 (1.3–3.2)	1.7 (1.1–2.7)

estimated 58% in women. For each 1 SD decline in BMD, there is a 2.0–3.6-fold increase in the age-adjusted risk of fracture. Simultaneously there is a dramatic increase in the likelihood of falling, from about one in five women aged 40–49 years to nearly half of women aged 85 years or older. The pathophysiology of falling is complex, but only 1% of falls lead to hip fracture. This is because the amount of force delivered to the proximal femur depends on various protective responses and on the orientation of the faller.

In Europe, the number of individuals aged 65 years and older is expected to increase from about 68 million in 1990 to more than 133 million in 2050, whereas in Asia the number will grow from 145 million to 894 million; this demographic trend alone could cause the number of hip fractures worldwide to increase from an estimated 1.7 million in 1990 to a projected 6.3 million in 2050, with most of the world's future hip fractures happening in Asia[31].

Vertebral fractures

The epidemiology of vertebral fracture is less well established than that of hip fracture, because there is not an accepted definition of vertebral fracture and because a substantial proportion of them escape clinical diagnosis.

Indeed, only about one-third of all vertebral deformities come to medical attention, and less than 10% necessitate admission to hospital. Even when there is a vertebral fracture on the radiograph, it is often not mentioned by the radiologist, is rarely noted in the medical records of the patient and does not always prompt appropriate treatment. The recognition of a vertebral fracture, even if asymptomatic, is important, because its presence may initiate a vicious circle characterized by back pain, immobilization, increased rate of bone loss, BMD reduction and, therefore, increased rate of further osteoporotic fractures.

Vertebral fractures are defined either by morphometric criteria or by qualitative assessment. For morphometric evaluation, the anterior, middle and posterior heights are measured, and various methods have been proposed based upon absolute reduction in height or reduction compared with height in a reference population.

The severity of vertebral fractures can be defined according to the method proposed by Genant, who defines a fracture as mild, moderate or severe according to the percentage of height reduction[32]. Severe vertebral deformities alone produce symptoms that lead to diagnosis, and the incidence of these vertebral fractures rises rapidly with age in both sexes. After about age 60 years, women in the USA and Europe have about a two-fold to three-fold greater incidence of vertebral fractures than do men. The results of most studies indicate that the prevalence of vertebral fractures in men is similar to, or even greater than that in women aged 50–60 years, probably due to a higher frequency of traumatic vertebral fractures among young and middle-aged men.

When comparable methods and definitions have been used in studies[32,33], the prevalence of vertebral fractures has been more similar across regions, compared with that seen for hip fractures (Table 2).

Thus despite their lower hip fracture rates, vertebral fracture prevalence among women in Hiroshima is 20–80% greater than for white women in Rochester, Minnesota, USA[34]. Similarly, the risk of vertebral fractures among postmenopausal women in Beijing is only about 25% lower than that noted in Rochester, even though the incidence of hip fractures in Beijing is just an eighth of that in women from Rochester.

About 25% of vertebral fractures are due to falls, and most are precipitated by activities of daily life. The majority of fractures are due instead to the compressive loading associated with lifting, changing positions and so on, or are discovered incidentally. The compressive strength of a vertebral body is partly determined by BMD, and each SD decrease in lumbar spine BMD is associated with about a two-fold increase in spine fracture risk[35]. The most frequent vertebral levels involved are T8 and T12/L1. The occurrence of one vertebral fracture, even an asymptomatic one detected incidentally on a routine radiograph, increases the likelihood of additional fractures by at least four-fold. This increased risk is independent of bone density, and hence vertebral fractures that arise with minimum trauma signal an underlying bone fragility that is not measured by densitometry.

Efforts to identify other risk factors can best be described as inconsistent. Age, history of fracture, history of osteoporosis, decreased height and physical activity were associated with vertebral fractures in men and women in the European Vertebral Osteoporosis Study[36], but three of these are manifestations of vertebral osteoporosis *per se*. In men, cigarette smoking, consumption of alcoholic beverages, secondary osteoporosis and a history of trauma, tuberculosis or peptic ulcer were risk factors for vertebral fracture, whereas obesity was protective. Other risk factors that have been reported for vertebral fractures in women include late menarche, early menopause,

Table 2 Population-based studies of the prevalence of vertebral fracture in women aged 50 years or older in several locations around the world. Modified from reference 31

Age (years)	Europe	Minnesota	Hiroshima	Beijing
50–54	11.5	4.7	5.4	4.9
55–59	14.6	5.8	4.1	—
60–64	16.8	6.3	4.9	16.2
65–69	23.5	13.2	8.2	—
70–74	27.2	15	24.8	19
75–79	34.8	22.2	36.8	—
80–84	—	50.8	42.9	36.6
≥ 85	—	50.8	25.0	—

short duration of fertility, low consumption of cheese and yogurt, low physical activity and family history of hip fracture, whereas use of oral contraceptives and alcohol consumption reduce the risk[36–38].

Distal forearm fractures

Distal forearm fractures almost always follow a fall on the outstretched arm. They display a different pattern of incidence compared with that of hip or vertebral fractures. In white women, incidence rates increase linearly from age 40 to 65 years, and then stabilize for reasons that remain obscure but may relate to a change in the pattern of falling with advancing age, so that elderly women with slower gait and impaired neuromuscular coordination are more likely to fall on their wrist[39,40]. Alternatively, the plateau in incidence may be due to reversal of the cortical porosity that develops in the distal forearm around the time of the menopause. In addition, compared with hip fracture, a greater proportion of distal forearm fractures occur outdoors, and a winter peak in incidence has been associated with periods of icy weather[41]. In men, the incidence of distal forearm fractures remains relatively constant and low between ages 20 and 80 years. Consequently, the majority of such fractures occur in women, and the age-adjusted female to male ratio of 4 : 1 is more marked than for hip or vertebral fractures. Nonetheless, the incidence of distal forearm fracture varies from one geographic area to another, generally in parallel with hip fracture incidence rates.

Other fractures

Incidence rates for fractures of the proximal tibia, pelvis, distal femur and proximal humerus also increase with age in elderly women and, to a lesser extent, in aging men[20]. About 75% or more of all proximal humerus fractures are due to falls, and are more frequent in frail women with poor neuromuscular function. Moderate trauma also accounts for the majority of isolated pelvic fractures and occurs among persons aged 35 years or older, and nearly 70% are in women. Severe trauma is associated with most multiple pelvis and acetabular fractures.

Distal femur fractures also have some of the characteristics of an age-related fracture[42]. The incidence of fractures of the femur shaft in Stockholm is greater in women than in men after 65 years; most fractures in this age group are due to falls or severe trauma. Moderate trauma, however, accounts for half of all distal femur fractures in Rochester, and this subgroup of cases exhibit age-related increases in incidence among both men and women like those seen for hip fractures. Proximal tibia fractures have been classified as 'composite' fractures, with peaks in incidence among the young and the old. About 40% of these fractures are due to severe trauma and a quarter are due to falls. Incidence rates are highest in adolescent boys, but age-adjusted incidence rates are 30% greater among women. In elderly women, a low BMD increases the risk of leg fractures.

IMPACT OF OSTEOPOROTIC FRACTURES

The adverse outcomes of osteoporotic fractures fall into three broad categories: mortality, morbidity and cost.

Mortality

The effect of fractures on survival appears to differ with the type of fracture. Hip fractures are the most serious, leading to an overall reduction in survival of 10–20%. The risk of death is greatest immediately after fracture (within the first 6 months and diminishing with time)[42]. Few of these deaths can be attributed to the hip fracture *per se*; most are due instead to chronic illnesses that lead to both the fracture and the patient's ultimate demise. Mortality differs, however, by age and sex. In one population-based study, a relative survival of 92% was found for white hip-fracture subjects under 75 years of age, compared with only 83% for those aged 75 years and over. Despite their greater average age at the time of fracture, survival is better among women[42]. This sex difference appears to arise from the greater frequency of other chronic diseases among men who sustain hip fractures. Thus, most deaths appear to be due to serious coexisting illnesses and not to acute complications of the fracture. By contrast, there is no excess mortality among patients who sustain a distal forearm fracture. Vertebral fractures, however, have a raised mortality rate that extends well beyond the first year after the fracture[43]. Some authors[44] reported that women with vertebral fractures had enhanced risk of death due to pulmonary and cardiovascular disease, but the impaired survival may be due to poor health or other underlying conditions that carry an increased risk of death.

Morbidity

The major consequences of vertebral fracture are kyphosis, back pain and height loss. Many fractures arise without pain. Women with vertebral deformities, incidentally found in routine radiographs of populations, are more likely to have chronic back pain and functional difficulties, as well as future fractures, suggesting that current medical practice misses most real vertebral fractures. New compression fracture causes acute symptoms that resolve over weeks or months[45]. A more prolonged clinical course affects a proportion of patients who experience chronic pain while standing and during physical stress, particularly bending.

Hip fractures necessitate hospitalization, and in 1985 the average length of hospital stay in

England and Wales was 30 days, meaning that 3500 National Health Service hospital beds were occupied daily. While these patients are at high risk of acute complications, such as pressure sores, pneumonia and urinary tract infections, the most important long-term outcome is impairment in the ability to walk. About one-fifth of patients are non-ambulatory even before fracture, but of those able to walk, half cannot walk independently afterward[46]. Finally, about 30% of patients with hip fracture may become totally dependent, and the risk of institutionalization is great[47].

About 20% of all patients with distal forearm fractures are hospitalized, and they account for some 50 000 hospital admissions and over 400 000 physician visits in the United States each year. Only 16% of forearm fractures occurring in women aged 45–54 years required in-patient care, compared with 76% of those in women aged 85 years. Nearly half of all patients report only fair or poor functional outcomes at 6 months following a distal forearm fracture.

Economic cost

Fractures in the United States may cost as much as $20 billion per year, with hip fractures accounting for over a third of the total[48]. The greater expense is for in-patient medical services and nursing-home care. The direct cost includes an estimated 547 000 hospitalizations and 4.6 million hospital-bed days for the care of osteoporotic fractures in the United States in 1995[49]. In England, hip fracture alone uses one-fifth of all orthopedic beds, at a direct cost of £850 million per year in 1999[50]. In Switzerland, however, osteoporotic fractures account for more hospital-bed days than myocardial infarction and stroke. In France, an estimated 56 000 hip fractures annually cost about FF 3.5 billion.

Future projection

The financial and health-related costs of osteoporosis can only rise in future generations. Life expectancy is increasing around the globe, and the number of elderly individuals is rising in every geographic region. The estimated 322 million individuals in the world aged 65 years or over at present is expected to reach 1555 million by the year 2050[51]. Using current estimates for hip fracture incidence from various parts of the world, it can be calculated that about half of all hip fractures among elderly people in 1990 took place in Europe and North America. By 2050, the rapid aging of the Asian and Latin American populations will result in the European and North American contribution falling to only 25%, with over half of all hip fractures occurring in Asia[52]. It is clear, therefore, that osteoporosis will become a global problem over the next half century and that measures are urgently required to avert this trend.

The increase in hip fracture incidence seen in some countries will worsen these projections even after adjustment for growth in the elderly population. An increase of only 1% in the age-adjusted incidence rate each year might cause the estimated number of hip fractures in 2050 to reach 8.1 million. On the basis of current trends, hip fractures might increase in the United Kingdom from 46 000 in 1985 to 117 000 in 2016[52]. In Australia, they could rise from 10 150 in 1986 to 18 550 in 2011, with a doubling in the cost of care in constant dollars from $38 to $69 million annually.

Incidence rates for fractures at other skeletal sites have also risen during the past half century. It might reflect the influence of some increasingly prevalent risk factor for osteoporosis or falling. Another explanation is increasing frailty among the elderly population, especially since many of the disorders contributing to frailty are also associated with osteoporosis and the risk of falling. Finally, the trends could arise from a cohort phenomenon, i.e. some adverse influence that acted at an earlier time is now manifesting as a rising fracture incidence in successive generations. For example, it has been speculated that the increase in adult height during this century led to a secular trend toward longer hip axis length, which may increase the risk of hip fracture. However, analysis of data from the Oxford Record Linkage Study revealed a declining incidence of hip fracture in more recent birth cohorts[53]. This is confirmed in a recent survey in southern England, where fracture rates increased in the elderly between 1978 and 1995, but were tending to decrease among people under 70 years of age.

Incidence rates for fractures at other skeletal sites have also risen during the past half century. Studies from Malmö, Sweden, have suggested age-specific secular increases for distal forearm, ankle, proximal humeral and vertebral fractures. The observation for vertebral fractures is particularly important, as it points to an increasing prevalence of osteoporosis, rather than falling, as a general explanation for these trends. Recent data from the northern United States confirmed increases in the incidence of clinically diagnosed vertebral fractures among postmenopausal women until the early 1960s, with a plateau in rates thereafter. As with the Swedish data, these rate changes paralleled those observed for hip fractures in the same population. In Tables 3 and 4 are shown the projections for the number of hip fractures throughout Europe and worldwide, respectively among both men and women.

Table 3 European projections for hip fracture

	Number of hip fractures ($\times 10^3$)	
Year	Men	Women
2000	88	326
2020	139	456
2050	230	742

Table 4 Worldwide projections for hip fracture

	Number of hip fractures* ($\times 10^3$)	
Year	Men	Women
1990	0.3	0.3
2000	0.4	1.1
2025	0.8	1.8
2050	1.4	3.1

*Stable incidence

CONCLUSIONS

Osteoporosis is a complex, multifactorial chronic disorder in which a variety of pathophysiologic mechanisms lead to a progressive reduction in bone strength and an increased risk of fracture. Whether the disease is defined by low bone mass or by the occurrence of specific fractures, osteoporosis is clearly a common condition. Thus, a third of postmenopausal white women in the United States can be expected to have osteoporosis in the lumbar spine, proximal femur or mid-radius at any point in time, while the lifetime risk of a hip, spine or distal forearm fracture from age 50 years onward in this group approaches 40%. Osteoporotic fractures are an important cause of disability and medical costs worldwide. An understanding of the epidemiology of these fractures could help to focus efforts on prediction of fractures in those at greatest risk. Those countries with high fracture risk might be able to reduce fractures by the aggressive implementation of programs to assess and treat high-risk individuals, whereas areas with limited medical resources and a lower incidence of disabling osteoporotic fractures might need guidelines that are much more selective about screening and the use of drug therapies.

References

1. NHI Consensus Development Panel on Osteoporosis Prevention, Diagnosis, and Therapy. Osteoporosis prevention, diagnosis, and therapy. *J Am Med Assoc* 2001; 285: 785–95

2. Melton LJ III. Who has osteoporosis? A conflict between clinical and public health perspectives. *J Bone Miner Res* 2000; 15: 2309–14

3. Seely DG, Browner WS, Nevitt MC, et al. Which fractures are associated with low appendicular bone mass in elderly women? *Ann Intern Med* 1991; 115: 837–42

4. World Health Organization. Assessment of fracture risk and its application to screening for postmenopausal osteoporosis. Geneva: WHO, 1994

5. Looker AC, Orwoll ES, Johnston CR, et al. Prevalence of low femoral bone density in older U.S. adults from NHANES III. *J Bone Miner Res* 1997; 12: 1761–8

6. Seeman E. Growth in bone mass and size: are racial and gender differences in bone mineral density more apparent than real? *J Clin Endocrinol Metab* 1998; 83: 1414–19

7. Faulkner RA, McCulloch RG, Fyke SL, et al. Comparison of areal and estimated volumetric bone mineral density values between older men and women. *Osteoporo Int* 1995; 5: 271–5

8. Melton LJ III, Atkinson EJ, O'Connor MK, et al. Bone density and fracture risk in men. *J Bone Miner Res* 1998, 13: 1915–23

9. Marcus R, Greendale G, Blunt BA, et al. Correlates of bone mineral density in the postmenopausal estrogen/progestin interventions trials. *J Bone Miner Res* 1994; 1467: 76

10. Cundy T, Cornish J, Evans MC, et al. Sources of interracial variation in bone mineral density. *J Bone Miner Res* 10; 368: 73

11. Bhudhikanov GS, Wang MC, Eckert K, et al. Differences in bone mineral in young Asian and Caucasian Americans may reflect differences in bone size. *J Bone Miner Res* 1996; 11: 1545–56

12. Melton LJ III. How many women have osteoporosis now? *J Bone Miner Res* 1995; 10: 175–7

13. Melton LJ III, Therneau TM, Larson DR. Long-term trends in hip fracture prevalence: The influence of hip fracture incidence and survival. *Osteoporos Int* 1998; 8: 68–74

14. Jensen GF, Christiansen C, Boesen J, et al. Epidemiology of postmenopausal spinal and long bone fractures. A unifying approach to postmenopausal osteoporosis. *Clin Orthop* 1982; 166: 75–81

15. Ettinger B, Black DM, Nevitt MC, et al. The study of Osteoporotic Fractures Research Group, contribution of vertebral deformities to chronic back pain and disability. *J Bone Miner Res* 1992; 7: 449–56

16. Melton LJ III, Lane AW, Cooper C, et al. Prevalence and incidence of vertebral deformities. *Osteoporos Int* 1993; 3: 113–19

17. Jones G, White C, Nguyen T, et al. Prevalent vertebral deformities: relationship to bone mineral density and spinal osteophytosis in elderly men and women. *Osteoporos Int* 1996; 6: 233–9

18. Melton LJ III, Chrischilles EA, Cooper C, et al. How many women have osteoporosis? *J Bone Miner Res* 1992; 7: 1005–10

19. Garraway WM, Stauffer RN, Kurland LT, et al. Limb fractures in a defined population. I. Frequency and distribution. *Mayo Clin Proc* 1979; 54: 701–7

20. Donaldson LJ, Cook A, Thomson RG. Incidence of fractures in a geographically defined population. *J Epidemiol Community Health* 1990; 44: 241–4

21. Melton LJ III, Cooper C. Magnitude and impact of osteoporosis and fractures. In Marcus R, Feldman D, Kelsey J, eds. *Osteoporosis*, 2nd edn. San Diego: *Academic Press* 2001; 1: 1557–67

22. Youm T, Koval KJ, Kummer FJ, et al. Do all hip fractures result from a fall? *Am J Orthop* 1999; 28: 190–4

23. Johnell O, Gullberg B, Allander E. The apparent incidence of hip fracture in Europe: a study of national register sources. *Osteoporos Int* 1992; 2: 298–302

24. Effors I, Allander E, Kanis JA, et al. The variable incidence of hip fracture in southern Europe: the Medos Study. *Osteoporos Int* 1994; 5: 253–63

25. Jacobsen SJ, Goldberg J, Miles TP, et al. Regional variation in the incidence of hip fracture: US white women aged 65 years and older. *J Am Med Assoc* 1990; 264: 500–2

26. Gardsell P, Hohnell O, Nilsson BE, et al. Bone mass in an urban and a rural population: a comparative, population based study in southern Sweden. *J Bone Miner Res* 1991; 12: 311–18

27. Einborn TA. Bone strength: the bottom line. *Calcif Tissue Int* 2001; 12: 595–604

28. Villa ML, Nelson L, Nelson D. Race, ethnicity and osteoporosis. In Marcus R, Feldman D, Kelsey J, eds. *Osteoporosis*, 2nd edn. San Diego: Academic Press, 2001; 1: 1569–84

29. Poor G, Atkinson EJ, O'Fallon WM, et al. Predictors of hip fractures in elderly men. *J Bone Miner Res* 1995; 10: 1900–7

30. Cummings SR, Melton LJ III. Epidemiology and outcomes of osteoporotic fractures. *Lancet* 2002; 359: 1761–7

31. Cooper C, Campion G, Melton LJ III. Hip fractures in the elderly: a world-wide projection. *Osteoporos Int* 1997; 7: 407–13

32. O'Neill TW, Felsenberg D, Varlow J, et al. The prevalence of vertebral deformity in European men and women: the European Vertebral Osteoporosis Study. *J Bone Miner Res* 1996; 11: 1010–18

33. Davies KM, Stegman MR, Heancy RP, et al. Prevalence and severity of vertebral fracture: the Saunders County Bone Quality Study. *Osteoporos Int* 1996; 6: 160–5

34. Ross PD, Fujiwara S, Huang C, et al. Vertebral fracure prevalence in women in Hiroshima compared to Caucasian or Japanese in the US. *Int J Epidemiol* 1995; 24: 1171–7

35. Marshall D, Jonell O, Wedel H. Meta-analysis of how well measures of bone mineral density predict occurrence of osteoporotic fractures. *Br Med J* 1996; 312: 1254–9

36. Janott J, Hallner D, Pfeiffer A, et al. Risk factors of osteoporosis: results of EVOS in Germany. *Scand J Rheumatol* 1996; 25 (Suppl 103): 123

37. Navez Diaz M, O'Neill TW, Silman AJ. The influence of alcohol consumption on the risk of vertebral deformity. *Osteoporos Int* 1997; 7: 65–71

38. O'Neill TW, Silman AJ, Naves Diaz M, et al. Influence of hormonal and reproductive factors on the risk of vertebral deformity in European women. *Osteoporos Int* 1997; 7: 72–8

39. Graafmans WC, Ooms ME, Bezemer D, et al. Different risk profiles for hip fractures and distal forearm fractures: a prospective study. *Osteoporos Int* 1996; 6: 427–31

40. Kelsey JL, Browner WS, Seeley DG, et al. Risk factors, falls, and fracture of the distal forearm in Manchester, UK. *Am J Epidemiol* 1992; 135: 477–89

41. Jacobsen SJ, Sargent DJ, Atkinson EJ. Contribution of weather to the seasonability of distal forearm fractures: a population-based study in Rochester, Minnesota. *Osteoporos Int* 1999; 9: 254–9

42. Melton LJ III. Epidemiology of fractures. In Riggs BI, Melton LJ III, eds. *Osteoporosis: Etiology, Diagnosis and Management*. New York: Raven Press, 1988: 133–54

43. Kanis JA, Oden A, Johnell O, et al. Excess mortality after hospitalization for vertebral fracture. *Osteoporos Int* 2004; 15: 108–11

44. Kado DM, Browner WS, Pressman AR, et al. Mortality following fractures in older women: a prospective study. *Arch Intern Med* 1999; 159: 1215–20

45. Ross PD, Davis JW, Epstein RS, et al. Pain and disability associated with new vertebral fractures and other spinal conditions. *J Clin Epidemiol* 1994; 47: 231–9

46. Melton LJ III. Excess mortality following vertebral fracture. *J Am Geriatr Soc* 2000; 48: 338–9

47. Bonar SK, Tinetti ME, Speechley M, et al. Factors associated with short- versus long-term skilled nursing facility placement among community-living hip fracture patients. *J Am Geriatr Soc* 1990; 38: 1139–44

48. Praemer A, Furner S, Rice DP. Musculoskeletal conditions in the United States. Park Ridge: American Academy of Orthopedic Surgeons, 1992

49. Ray NF, Chan JK, Thamer M, et al. Medical expenditures for the treatment of osteoporotic fractures in the United States in 1995: report from the National Osteoporosis Foundation. *J Bone Miner Res* 1997; 12: 24–35

50. Royal College of Physicians. Guidelines for the prevention and treatment of osteoporosis. London: Royal College of Physicians, 1999

51. Cooper C, Campion G, Melton LJ III. Hip fracture in the elderly: a worldwide projection. *Osteoporos Int* 1992; 2: 285–9

52. Hoffemberg R, James OFW, Brocklehurst ID, et al. Fractures neck of femur: prevention and management. Summary and recommendations of a report of the Royal College of Physicians. *J R Coll Phys London* 1989; 23: 8–12

53. Evans JG, Seagroatt V, Goldacre MJ, et al. Secular trends in proximal femoral fracture. Oxford Record Linkage Study area and England 1968–86. *Epidemiol Community Health* 1997; 51: 424–9

Impact of osteoporosis on quality of life and quality of life on osteoporosis: rationale and methodology for accurate assessment

2

W. H. Utian

INTRODUCTION

Quality of life (QOL) is increasingly being recognized as a key outcome measure of quality of health-care. There is considerable evidence that the complications of osteoporosis will have a negative impact on QOL. However, less well recognized, QOL will actually have an impact on osteoporosis. To explain this fact, it is necessary that the construct 'QOL' be more clearly articulated. The term QOL is still far too loosely defined, more often a cliché rather than the precise instrument it really should be.

Quality of life is an issue that has important implications for both patients and the health professionals who provide medical care to them[1]. How individuals perceive quality of life depends on many factors and affects all aspects of functioning as well as satisfaction with the health-care received. A patient's perception of quality of life may be critical for adherence to a prescribed plan of health-care. If a patient believes that a treatment will decrease distress or will decrease distress in the future, she may be more likely to adhere to that treatment regimen. Similarly, if a treatment prescribed by a physician causes distressing side-effects or if a patient worries that the treatment will cause harm, the patient may be less likely to comply with the plan of care[2]. It would therefore be beneficial for health-care providers to be able to measure this perception accurately and incorporate it into care plans in order to meet their health-care needs.

DEFINITIONS

Perceived quality of life is difficult to define and measure, because there is no universal agreement on what it is and how it can be quantified. Objective measurements of health status do not describe the patient's own sense of overall life satisfaction. Quality of life may be defined as a reflection of a person's beliefs about functioning and achievement in various aspects of life. From a behavioral perspective, it can be viewed as a spectrum that ranges from perceived distress at one end to the absence of distress and a sense of well-being at the other. From a medical perspective, quality of life is defined in the domains of physical and psychological functioning. 'Health-related' quality of life can be conceptualized as patients' perception of their physical, cognitive and mental health as well as their social circumstances[3].

Traditionally, medicine has used concrete biomedical measurements to assess quality of life. Although these outcome measures are essential to determining a patient's health status, they are not the whole picture, and do not always accurately reflect the patient's global sense of well-being. Many factors must be examined when assessing quality of life, including somatic, psychological and cognitive symptoms, sexual functioning and social/life circumstances.

Somatic symptoms usually have a significant impact on perceived quality of life, and it is very important that any quality of life assessment accurately identifies and measures somatic symptoms. Nonetheless, while health status is a domain that may be critical to an individual's quality of life, it must be emphasized that the multidimensional construct of quality of life is actually independent of health status. Rather, it is a subjective appraisal of life satisfaction. For example, one person may objectively be experiencing debilitating and/or painful symptoms but perceive their life as having excellent quality, while another person may be symptom-free but perceive their life to have poor quality. Therefore, the construct of quality of life may more accurately refer to a 'sense of well-being' that is impacted on by the experience of symptoms but not solely determined by them. Indeed, the World Health Organization (WHO) has emphasized that QOL should be perceived as being greater than disease or infirmity[4].

In essence, then, a clear distinction needs to be made between health-related QOL (HRQOL) and global or overall QOL. With this background, it is worth considering the broad groups of instruments that have been developed and could be applied to the evaluation of QOL in osteoporosis.

INSTRUMENTS FOR DETERMINING QUALITY OF LIFE IN OSTEOPOROSIS

Osteoporosis itself is not a diagnosis impacting on QOL because it is a silent disease. The complications thereof, essentially fractures, are what will drive the impact on QOL through symptomatic and functional sequelae. Measuring QOL in osteoporosis would therefore be of value for the following reasons[5]:

(1) To assess therapeutic trade-offs;

(2) To compare safety and efficacy of different interventions;

(3) To compare the relative burden of different diseases;

(4) To assess the cost-effectiveness of different interventions.

Given the broad objectives, the varying definitions of QOL and the global sense of well-being

versus health-related perception of QOL, it should come as no surprise that several instruments are currently available that measure generic, performance- and disease-targeted factors[6], and global QOL.

The following are examples[6].

Generic

Generic instruments really measure functional ability that can be related to a medical problem, for example by using an instrument to quantify level of function, and then applying that measure of ability to function against a measure of vertebral compression fractures.

Functional Status Index[7]   This is an example of such an instrument. Thus, for example, Lyles and colleagues utilized this instrument to measure functional ability and then to illustrate the negative impact of osteoporotic vertebral compression factors on the ability to function normally[8].

Functional status

Short form (SF)-36[9]   This is a widely employed generic symptom profile instrument used to measure HRQOL. Another widely used example is the Nottingham Health Profile (NHP)[10]. Instruments such as these are of value to assess co-morbidity and disease burden when evaluating osteoporosis, that is, they are measures of HRQOL.

Osteoporosis-targeted instruments

Several osteoporosis-specific health-related QOL instruments have been developed, of which the following are examples:

(1) *Osteoporosis Patient Assessment Questionnaire (OPAQ)*[11]   This is a self-report instrument.

(2) *QOL Questionnaire of the European Foundation for Osteoporosis (QUALEFFO)*[12]   This is a questionnaire, translated into multiple languages, intended for use in clinical trials on vertebral fractures.

(3) *Osteoporosis Target QOL Survey Instrument for Use in the Community (OPTQOL)*[13] Translated into several languages and culturally adapted, the instrument allows cross-cultural studies of the community impact of osteoporosis.

(4) *Osteoporosis QOL Questionnaire (OQLQ)*[14] The original 30-question OQLQ has been reduced to a mini-OQLQ of ten questions. This is an interviewer-based questionnaire of value in patients with back pain, and is useful in clinical settings.

(5) *The Short Quality of Life Questionnaire* This instrument was developed through equating items from two existing instruments, the OQLQ and the QUALEFFO[15]. This is another attempt at developing a shorter questionnaire for use in clinical practice. It still requires further validation.

Global quality of life

Finally, there are instruments being developed to measure global sense of well-being in specific populations. The *Utian Quality of Life Scale (UQOL)* is a measure of global QOL in women aged 45–65 and serves as one example[16].

Conclusion

To achieve the best assessment of overall QOL in osteoporosis, a combination of instruments may be necessary. These should include measures of overall self-perception of health, function, impact of the disease on independence, and global sense of well-being.

IMPACT OF OSTEOPOROSIS ON QUALITY OF LIFE

Long-term outcomes of osteoporosis including fracture rates, physical changes such as kyphosis and pain are well documented. It is only with the recent development of instruments such as those outlined above that the psychological effects, social consequences and overall impact on quality of life are becoming known. The following are examples of such new information:

(1) Decreased health-related QOL was demonstrated utilizing the QUALEFFO and NHP[17] to be related to the number of vertebral fractures and not bone density.

(2) In the Multiple Outcomes of Raloxifene Evaluation (MORE) Study, utilization of OPAQ helped to determine that the effect of prevalent vertebral fractures was dependent on the location within the spine, and was strongest in the lumbar region (L1–L4). Incident vertebral fractures significantly decreased OPAQ scores on physical function, emotional status, clinical symptoms and overall HRQOL[18].

(3) The OPTQOL questionnaire was used in a community setting, confirming that the negative impact of osteoporosis on QOL seems to be more related to the physical manifestations of osteoporosis than to bone density levels[19].

Not all studies have been confirmatory in differentiating a QOL impact between patients with or without subclinical fractures. For example, a study utilizing the QUALEFFO showed no overall difference, despite some QOL impairments in patients with subclinical fractures[20]. This negative study could of course reflect the discriminating power, or lack thereof, of the instrument itself.

Vertebral and hip fractures have been demonstrated to have a considerably greater and prolonged impact on HRQOL than have forearm and humerus fractures. This study ultimately utilized only a symptom profile (SF-36) and extrapolated the QOL impact[21]. In a study using the mini-OQLQ, QOL was noted to be decreased in patients who sustained incident vertebral and non-vertebral fractures[22].

IMPACT OF QUALITY OF LIFE ON OSTEOPOROSIS

Even less well defined than the impact of osteoporosis on global QOL is the reverse. Few attempts have been made to determine the impact of global QOL on compliance/adherence with drug therapies, exercise programs or fracture outcomes. What has become manifestly obvious is that persistence or adherence to therapeutic regimens is poor, and attempts are being made to determine the reasons for this situation.

The enigma of patients understanding the impact of poor compliance with treatment for a known condition yet not continuing medication has been well reviewed[23]. More specifically, early discontinuation of treatment for osteoporosis also remains poorly explained. It is clear that treatment side-effects need to be minimized, and that patients should be educated about the problem[24]. Nonetheless, that would not adequately address the issue of poor adherence to therapy.

One effective approach has been to monitor patients more closely and to present information on response to therapy on an ongoing basis[25]. This still does not explain a relationship between global QOL and treatment adherence.

CONCLUSIONS

There is a need for recognition of the impact of osteoporosis-related factors on global QOL as well as an understanding of the reverse, namely, QOL on the outcome of osteoporosis-related factors. Understanding both sides of the coin would assist health-care providers to appreciate more fully the importance of prevention and treatment. Moreover, a clearer understanding of these factors may well drive better adherence to and persistence with treatments for osteoporosis.

To achieve this goal, well-validated instruments to measure both health-related QOL and global QOL must be further enhanced and utilized. Examples of existing instruments have been reviewed. Multiple other advantages exist in using such tools, including assessing therapeutic trade-offs in randomized trials, comparing the overall benefit of different interventions, and the cost-effectiveness of such treatments.

At this time, there is little evidence to guide the choice of one instrument or system over another for assessing their relevance, superiority, cost-effectiveness of interventions or overall impact on health-outcome measures. Further research is urgently needed to characterize these associations.

References

1. Utian WH, Janata JW, Kingsberg SA, et al. Determinants and quantifications of quality of life after the menopause: the Utian Menopause Quality of Life Score. In Aso T, Yanaihara T, Fujimoto S, eds. *Menopause at the Millennium*. Carnforth, UK: Parthenon Publishing, 2000; 141–4

2. Mansfield PK, Voda AM. Hormone use among middle-aged women: results of a three-year study. *Menopause* 1994; 1: 99–108

3. Wiklund I, Karlberg J. Evaluation of quality of life in clinical trials: selecting qualify-of-life measures. *Controlled Clin Trials* 1991; 12 (Suppl): 204S–16S

4. World Health Organization. Constitution of the World Health Organization, Switzerland (Basic Documents), 1947. Geneva: WHO, 1947

5. Greenedale GA, Silverman SL, Hays RD, et al. Health-related quality of life in osteoporosis clinical trials [Editorial]. *Calcif Tissue Int* 1993; 53: 75–7

6. Silverman SL, Cranney A. Quality of life measurement in osteoporosis. *J Rheumatol* 1997; 24: 1218–21

7. Jette AM, Deniston OL. Interobserver reliability of a functional status instrument. *J Chron Dis* 1978; 31: 573–80

8. Lyles KW, Gold DT, Shipp KM, et al. Association of osteoporotic vertebral compression fractures with impaired functional status. *Am J Med* 1993; 94: 595–601

9. Ware JE, Sherbourne CD. The MOS 36-item short form health survey (SF-36) conceptual framework and item selection. *Med Care* 1992; 30: 473–83

10. Bergner M, Bobbit RA, Kressel S, et al. The Sickness Impact Profile: conceptual formulation

and methodology for the development of a health status measure. *Int J Health Serv* 1976; 6: 393–415

11. Silverman SL, Mason J, Greenwald M. The Osteoporosis Assessment Questionnaire (OPAQ): a reliable and valid self-assessment measure of quality of life in osteoporosis. *J Bone Miner Res* 1994; 8: 343

12. Lips P, Cooper C, Agnusdei D, et al. Quality of life as outcome in the treatment of osteoporosis; the development of a questionnaire for quality of life by the European Foundation for Osteoporosis. *Osteoporos Int* 1997; 7: 36–8

13. Chandler JM, Martin AR, Girman C, et al. Reliability of an osteoporosis-targeted quality of life survey instrument for the use in the community: OPTQOL. *Osteoporos Int* 1998; 8: 127–35

14. Cook DJ, Guyatt GH, Adach JD, et al. Development and validation of the mini-osteoporosis quality of life questionnaire (OQLQ) in osteoporotic women with back pain due to vertebral fractures. Osteoporosis Quality of Life Study Group. *Osteoporos Rheumatol* 1999; 10: 207–13

15. Badio X, Prieto L, Roset M, et al. Development of a short osteoporosis quality of life questionnaire by equating items from two existing instruments. *J Clin Epidemiol* 2002; 55: 32–40

16. Utian WH, Janata JW, Kingsberg SA, et al. The Utian Quality of Life (UQOL) Scale: development and validation of an instrument to quantify quality of life through and beyond menopause. *Menopause* 2002; 9: 402–10

17. Oleksik A, Lips P, Dawson A, et al. Health-related quality of life in postmenopausal women with low BMD with or without prevalent vertebral fractures. *J Bone Miner Res* 2000; 15: 1384–92

18. Silverman SL, Minshall ME, Shen W, et al. The relationship of health-related quality of life to prevalent and incident vertebral fractures in postmenopausal women with osteoporosis: results from the Multiple Outcomes of Raloxifene Evaluation Study. *Arthritis Rheum* 2001; 44: 2611–19

19. Martin AR, Sornay-Rendu E, Chandler JM, et al. The impact of osteoporosis on quality of life: the OFELY Cohort. *Bone* 2002; 31: 32–6

20. Romagnoli E, Carnevale V, Notroni I, et al. Quality of life in ambulatory postmenopausal women: the impact of reduced bone mineral density and subclinical vertebral fractures. *Osteoporos Int* 2004; 15: 975–80

21. Hallberg I, Rosenqvist AM, Kartous L, et al. Health-related quality of life after osteoporotic fractures. *Osteoporos Int* 2004; 15: 834–41

22. Adachi JD, Ionnidis G, Olszynski WP, et al. The impact of incident vertebral and non-vertebral fractures and health-related quality of life in postmenopausal women. *BMC Musculoskelet Disord* 2002; 3: 11–16

23. Cramer JA. Partial medical compliance: the enigma in poor medical outcomes. *Am J Managed Care* 1995; 1: 167–74

24. Tosteson AN, Grove MR, Hammond CS, et al. Early discontinuation of treatment for osteoporosis. *Am J Med* 2003; 115: 209–16

25. Clowes JA, Peel NF, Eastell R. The impact of monitoring or adherence and persistence with anti-resorptive treatment for postmenopausal osteoporosis: a randomized controlled trial. *J Clin Endocrinol Metab* 2004; 89: 1117–23

Novel signals determining skeletal cell fate and function

3

E. Canalis, V. Deregowski, R. C. Pereira and E. Gazzerro

Skeletal cells and their environment determine bone mass. Cells of the osteoblastic lineage and signals that determine their replication and differentiation to mature osteoblasts, and signals determining the apoptosis of mature osteoblasts and osteocytes, define the cell population that regulates bone formation. Cells of the osteoclastic lineage and signals that determine their recruitment, genesis, function and death define the cell population that regulates bone resorption. Consequently, bone remodeling is determined by two cell populations and the signals affecting their fate and function. These signals are systemic and local, and include hormones and growth factors. Recent research has focused on local signals, including cell-to-cell interactions, their downstream events and their impact on the fate and function of cells of the osteoblastic lineage.

Skeletal cells synthesize a number of growth factors (Table 1)[1,2]. Some, such as fibroblast growth factor (FGF) and platelet-derived growth factor (PDGF), are mostly mitogens, whereas other factors, such as insulin-like growth factors (IGFs), enhance the differentiated function of the osteoblast[2,3]. It is important to note that, whereas IGFs enhance the expression of the osteoblastic phenotype, they do not direct the differentiation of mesenchymal cells toward osteoblasts (Table 2)[3,4]. In contrast, bone morphogenetic proteins (BMPs) induce the differentiation of cells of the osteoblastic lineage into mature cells that express the osteoblastic phenotype, and also enhance the function of the osteoblast (Table 3)[5]. Most BMPs are structurally related and belong to the transforming growth factor β (TGFβ) superfamily of peptides[6]. IGFs and BMPs act as autocrine factors that determine

Table 1   Skeletal growth factors

Platelet-derived growth factor (PDGF) A and B
Fibroblast growth factor (FGF) 1 and 2
Transforming growth factor β (TGFβ) 1, 2 and 3
Insulin-like growth factor (IGF)-I and -II
Bone morphogenetic protein (BMP) 2, 4 and 6
Other cytokines and growth factors

Table 2   Skeletal effects of insulin-like growth factor (IGF)

Increase osteoblastic function
    increase collagen expression
    increase bone formation
Decrease osteoblastic apoptosis
Increase remodeling

Table 3   Skeletal actions of bone morphogenetic proteins (BMPs)

Modest mitogens
Induce differentiation of mesenchymal cells toward
  osteoblasts
Enhance osteoblastic function

osteoblast function, and play a critical role in the maintenance of bone integrity. The activity of IGFs and BMPs needs to be tightly regulated, and this occurs by local feedback mechanisms, specific binding proteins and the modulation of their signal transduction pathways by extracellular and intracellular signals. Dysregulation of growth factor activity can have serious skeletal consequences, and humans with excessive expression of BMP 4 have fibrodysplasia ossificans progressiva, whereas overexpression of BMP antagonists causes osteopenia in the mouse[5,7]. Gain-of- and loss-of-function mutations of low-density lipoprotein receptor-related protein 5 (LRP5), a coreceptor for Wnt signaling, result in a respective increase and decrease in bone mass[8,9].

The effects of BMPs can be modulated by a group of extracellular and intracellular proteins that limit BMP action. BMP antagonists are expressed by skeletal cells, and their presumed role is to temper BMP activity in target tissues. BMP antagonists are not specifically expressed in skeletal cells. Extracellular BMP antagonists are believed to prevent BMP signaling by binding BMPs, therefore precluding their binding to specific cell-surface receptors[5]. Upon binding to their specific receptors, BMPs signal through the activation of Smad 1/5/8 and the mitogen-activated protein kinase pathways[5]. The overexpression of extracellular BMP antagonists has been used to determine the autocrine role of BMPs in various cell systems, since the null mutation of most BMPs results in embryonic lethality. Noggin, one of the better characterized BMP antagonists, is a secreted glycoprotein with a molecular mass of 64 kDa, that binds BMPs specifically and not other members of the TGFβ family of peptides[10,11]. Mice overexpressing noggin under the control of the osteocalcin promoter develop skeletal fragility, indicating that noggin has a detrimental effect in bone by binding skeletal BMPs[12]. Homozygous null mutations of the *noggin* gene in the mouse result in serious developmental abnormalities, joint lesions, axial skeletal defects and embryonic lethality[13]. These observations indicate the need for a fine balance between the expression of local BMPs and their antagonists. The importance of adequate noggin expression is confirmed by human studies demonstrating that heterozygous null mutations of the *noggin* gene result in multiple joint lesions[14]. Transgenic mice overexpressing noggin develop osteopenia and fractures. Total bone mineral density (BMD) is reduced and histomorphometric analysis reveals a decrease in cancellous bone volume of 70%, secondary to decreased osteoblastic function. To determine whether BMPs also have an effect on stromal cell differentiation, we compared the maturation and cellular function of stromal and osteoblastic cells from noggin transgenic mice as well as cell lines in which noggin was constitutively expressed. Stromal cells overexpressing noggin did not differentiate into mature osteoblasts, indicating that BMPs are essential for osteoblastic function and differentiation[15].

The Wnt family of secreted glycoproteins, like BMPs, play a critical role in development, cell fate and skeletal cell differentiation, and abnormal Wnt signaling is implicated in osteoporosis and osteopetrosis[8,9,16,17]. In the absence of Wnt proteins, Axin, adenomatous polyposis coli, β-catenin, glycogen-synthase kinase-3β (GSK-3β), and other proteins form a complex in which β-catenin is phosphorylated by GSK-3β leading to β-catenin degradation. The binding of Wnt proteins to their specific Frizzled transmembrane receptors and to the coreceptors LRP5 and -6 leads to inhibition of GSK-3β and to the stabilization of β-catenin[16,17]. This allows for β-catenin nuclear translocation and its association with members of the lymphoid enhancer-binding factor/T cell-specific factor (LEF/TCF) family of transcription factors and the transcriptional regulation of target genes. The Wnt/β-catenin signaling pathway is central to osteogenesis and bone formation, and Wnt and BMPs have similar and related effects. The mechanisms of this relationship have not been established, but LRP5 is induced by BMP 2, and TGFβ and Wnt signaling pathways converge at the level of LEF[8,18]. Recent clinical findings demonstrating changes in bone mass in gain- and loss-of-function LRP5 mutations confirm the role of Wnt in skeletal physiology. Wnt interacts with other signals determining cell fate, and its interactions with the Notch signaling pathway are of particular relevance to osteoblastic cell fate.

Notch 1, -2, -3 and -4 are closely related, conserved transmembrane receptors that mediate cell-to-cell interactions controlling cell fate decisions[19]. Notch genes have an extracellular and an intracellular domain, and their ligands Delta 1–4, and Serrate/Jagged 1 and -2, are single-pass transmembrane proteins which, following binding, induce the proteolytic cleavage of Notch, leading to the release of the Notch intracellular domain (NotchIC) and its translocation to the nucleus[20]. There, it complexes with the CSL family of DNA-binding proteins, the primary transcriptional mediators of Notch signaling. In mammals, the CSL nuclear protein is C-promoter binding factor 1 (CBF1), or recombinational signal binding protein of the Jκ immunoglobulin (Ig) gene (RBP-Jκ). Notch signaling independent of CBF1/RBP-Jκ also occurs, and Notch can form a complex with Deltex and related genes[21].

Notch1 and -2 and their ligands, Delta1 and Jagged1, are expressed by osteoblasts, whereas Notch3 and -4 are not[22]. Activated Notch1 receptors prevent osteoblast differentiation and chondrocyte maturation, resulting in shorter skeletal elements that lack ossification[23]. The constitutive overexpression of Notch1IC in stromal and osteoblastic cells impairs osteoblastic maturation and favors adipogenesis (Table 4)[24]. It is of interest that Notch1 and Wnt have opposite effects on cell differentiation, since Wnt signaling inhibits adipogenesis and it has the potential to induce osteoblastic differentiation. Recently, we demonstrated that the constitutive overexpression of Notch1IC in stromal cells opposes Wnt/β-catenin signaling[24]. Wnt–Notch interactions may occur at multiple levels, including the binding of Notch by Wnt and by molecules implicated in the implementation of Wnt signaling, and by enzymes involved in the phosphorylation and activation/deactivation of both signaling pathways.

Homozygous null mutations of the *Notch1* and -2 and *cbf1/rbp-Jκ* genes result in serious developmental abnormalities and embryonic lethality[25,26]. The phenotypic lethality has not permitted the definition of Notch1 function in

Table 4 Skeletal actions of Notch

Notch1 blocks osteoblastogenesis

Notch1 opposes Wnt/β-catenin signaling

Notch1 does not alter bone morphogenetic
  protein (BMP) signaling

---

adult bone *in vivo*. However, there are a number of observations substantiating the physiological and clinical importance of Notch in the skeleton. *Jagged2* mutants in the mouse exhibit marked defects in limb and craniofacial development, syndactylism and cleft palate, and *delta3* mutations cause vertebral and rib deformities[27,28]. Frame-shift mutations leading to loss of function of the *jagged1* gene in humans cause Alagille syndrome, an autosomal dominant disorder characterized by defects in multiple organs including the skeleton, where butterfly vertebrae and craniosynostosis are found[29]. Mutations of the ligand *Delta3* are linked to a developmental defect of the axial skeleton called spondylocostal dysostosis[30]. The observations indicate that Notch1 is a novel regulator of skeletal metabolism.

The CCAAT-enhancer-binding proteins (C/EBPs) are a family of transcription factors that regulate cell differentiation[31]. To date, six C/EBPs have been characterized, α, β, δ, γ, ε and ζ. The C/EBP proteins contain a highly conserved DNA-binding domain and a leucine zipper dimerization domain, and can form homo- and heterodimers that bind to similar sequence motifs. C/EBPs are expressed in multiple cell types, including osteoblasts and adipocytes, and some are critical for adipocyte differentiation and maturation[32,33]. It is important to note that C/EBPs also play a central role in the regulation of IGF-I transcription and can interact with other transcriptional activators, including runt-related transcription factor-2 (Runx-2), and as a consequence, activate osteocalcin transcription[34]. Glucocorticoids induce adipogenesis, and enhance the expression of C/EBP β and δ in osteoblasts, and we demonstrated that these two transcription factors play a role in the downregulation of IGF-I transcription by glucocorticoids[35]. Because C/EBP β and δ are essential for adipogenesis, and cortisol shifts cellular differentiation away from osteoblasts, the findings suggested that C/EBP β and δ play a role in directing mesenchymal cells away from the osteoblastic and toward the adipocytic pathway.

C/EBP ζ, more often termed C/EBP homologous protein (CHOP), or growth arrest and DNA damage-inducible gene (GADD) 153, is a member of the C/EBP family of transcription

Table 5 Actions of CCAAT-enhancer-binding protein (C/EBP) homologous protein (CHOP)

Mediates endoplasmic reticulum stress-induced apoptosis

Forms dimers with classic C/EBPs acting as dominant negative

Blocks adipogenesis

Enhances osteoblastogenesis by sensitizing bone morphogenetic protein (BMP)/Smad and Wnt/β-catenin signaling

---

factors, with unique roles in cell proliferation, differentiation and apoptosis (Table 5)[36]. CHOP heterodimerizes with other C/EBPs, but does not bind to classic C/EBP consensus DNA sequences. In ST-2 murine stromal cells, the levels of CHOP transcripts rise as the cells differentiate toward osteoblasts, and recently we demonstrated that overexpression of CHOP accelerates osteoblastic differentiation, enhancing the effect of BMP and sensitizing the BMP/Smad signaling pathway in osteoblastic cells[37]. CHOP overexpression also suppressed adipogenesis, suggesting that there may be a trade between osteoblastogenesis and adipogenesis. The role of CHOP in skeletal function was confirmed by recent studies from our group demonstrating that *chop*-null mutations lead to impaired osteoblastic function *in vivo*. The *chop*-null skeletal phenotype is similar to the phenotype of *atf 4*-null mice, and ATF 4 enhances the transcription of CHOP[38]. *Atf 4*-null mice exhibit osteopenia due to decreased bone formation[39].

In conclusion, results from recent investigations demonstrate the existence of novel extracellular and intracellular signals that determine the fate and function of cells of the osteoblastic lineage. Often these signals regulate BMP/Smad and Wnt/β-catenin signal transduction, either by sensitizing or opposing their activities in cells of the osteoblastic lineage.

ACKNOWLEDGMENTS

This work was supported by grants from the National Institutes of Health, AR21707, DK42424 and DK45227, and fellowship awards by the Arthritis Foundation.

References

1. Margolis RN, Canalis E, Partridge NC. Anabolic hormones in bone: basic research and therapeutic potential. *J Clin Endocrinol Metab* 1996; 81: 2872–7

2. Delany AM, Canalis E. Growth factors and bone. In LeRoith D, Bondy C, eds. *Growth Factors and Cytokines in Health and Disease*. Greenwich, CT: JAI Press, 1997; 3A: 127–55

3. Zhao G, Monier-Faugere MC, Langub MC, et al. Targeted overexpression of insulin-like growth factor I to osteoblasts of transgenic mice: increased trabecular bone volume without increased osteoblast proliferation. *Endocrinology* 2000; 141: 2674–82

4. Thomas T, Gori F, Spelsberg TC, et al. Response of bipotential human marrow stromal cells to insulin-like growth factors: effect on binding protein production, proliferation, and commitment to osteoblasts and adipocytes. *Endocrinology* 1999; 140: 5036–44

5. Canalis E, Economides AE, Gazzerro E. Bone morphogenetic proteins, their antagonists and the skeleton. *Endocr Rev* 2003; 24: 218–35

6. Schmitt JM, Hwang K, Winn SR, et al. Bone morphogenetic proteins: an update on basic biology and clinical relevance. *J Orthop Res* 1999; 17: 269–78

7. Shafritz AB, Shore EM, Gannon FH, et al. Overexpression of an osteogenic morphogen in fibrodysplasia ossificans progressiva. *N Engl J Med* 1996; 335: 555–61

8. Gong Y, Slee RB, Fukai N, et al. LDL receptor-related protein 5 (LRP5) affects bone accrual and eye development. *Cell* 2001; 107: 513–23

9. Boyden LM, Mao J, Belsky J, et al. High bone density due to a mutation in LDL-receptor-related protein 5. *N Engl J Med* 2002; 346: 1513–21

10. Smith WC, Harland RM. Expression cloning of noggin, a new dorsalizing factor localized to the Spemann organizer in xenopus embryos. *Cell* 1992; 70: 829–40

11. Valenzuela DM, Economides AN, Rojas E, et al. Identification of mammalian noggin and its expression in the adult nervous system. *J Neurosci* 1995; 15: 6077–84

12. Devlin RD, Du Z, Pereira RC, et al. Skeletal overexpression of noggin results in osteopenia and reduced bone formation. *Endocrinology* 2003; 144: 1972–8

13. Brunet LJ, McMahon JA, McMahon AP, et al. Noggin, cartilage morphogenesis, and joint formation in the mammalian skeleton. *Science* 1998; 280: 1455–7

14. Gong Y, Krakow D, Marcelino J, et al. Heterozygous mutations in the gene encoding noggin affect human joint morphogenesis. *Nature Genet* 1999; 21: 302–4

15. Gazzerro E, Du Z, Devlin RD, et al. Noggin arrests stromal cell differentiation *in vitro*. *Bone* 2003; 32: 111–19

16. Dale TC. Signal transduction by the Wnt family of ligands. *Biochem J* 1998; 329: 209–23

17. Gumbiner BM. Propagation and localization of Wnt signaling. *Curr Opin Genet Dev* 1998; 8: 430–5

18. Nishita M, Hashimoto MK, Ogata S, et al. Interaction between Wnt and TGF-β signalling pathways during formation of Spemann's organizer. *Nature (London)* 2000; 403: 781–4

19. Mumm JS, Kopan R. Notch signaling: from the outside in. *Dev Biol* 2000; 228: 151–65

20. Schroeter EH, Kisslinger JA, Kopan R. Notch-1 signalling requires ligand-induced proteolytic release of intracellular domain. *Nature (London)* 1998; 393: 382–6

21. Yamamoto N, Yamamoto S, Inagaki F, et al. Role of Deltex-1 as a transcriptional regulator downstream of the Notch receptor. *J Biol Chem* 2001; 276: 45031–40

22. Pereira RMR, Delany AM, Durant D, et al. Cortisol regulates the expression of Notch in osteoblasts. *J Cell Biochem* 2002; 85: 252–8

23. Crowe R, Zikherman J, Niswander L. Delta-1 negatively regulates the transition from prehypertrophic to hypertrophic chondrocytes during cartilage formation. *Development* 1999; 126: 987–98

24. Sciaudone M, Gazzerro E, Priest L, et al. *Notch 1* impairs osteoblastic cell differentiation. *Endocrinology* 2003; 144: 5631–9

25. Swiatek PJ, Lindsell CE, del Amo F, et al. *Notch1* is essential for postimplantation development in mice. *Genes Dev* 1994; 8: 707–19

26. Oka C, Nakano T, Wakeham A, et al. Disruption of the mouse *RBP-Jκ* gene results in early embryonic death. *Development* 1995; 121: 3291–301

27. Kusumi K, Sun ES, Kerrebrock AW, et al. The mouse pudgy mutation disrupts *Delta* homologue DII3 and initiation of early somite boundaries. *Nature Genet* 1998; 19: 274–8

28. Sidow A, Bulotsky MS, Kerrebrock AW, et al. *Serrate2* is disrupted in the mouse limb-development mutant *syndactylism*. *Nature (London)* 1997; 389: 722–5

29. Li L, Krantz ID, Deng Y, et al. Alagille syndrome is caused by mutations in human *Jagged1*, which encodes a ligand for Notch1. *Nature Genet* 1997; 16: 243–51

30. Bulman MP, Kusumi K, Frayling TM, et al. Mutations in the human delta homologue, DLL3, cause axial skeletal defects in spondylocostal dysostosis. *Nature Genet* 2000; 24: 438–41

31. Hanson RW. Biological role of the isoforms of C/EBP minireview series. *J Biol Chem* 1998; 273: 28543

32. Lee YH, Sauer B, Johnson PF, et al. Disruption of the c/ebpα gene in adult mouse liver. *Mol Cell Biol* 1997; 17: 6014–22

33. Tanaka T, Yoshida N, Kishimoto T, et al. Defective adipocyte differentiation in mice lacking the C/EBPβ and/or C/EBPδ gene. *Eur Med Biol Org J* 1997; 16: 7432–43

34. Gutierrez S, Javed A, Tennant DK, et al. CCAAT/enhancer-binding proteins (C/EBP) β and δ activate osteocalcin gene transcription and synergize with runx2 at the C/EBP element to regulate bone-specific expression. *J Biol Chem* 2002; 277: 1316–23

35. Delany AM, Durant D, Canalis E. Glucocorticoid suppression of IGF I transcription in osteoblasts. *Mol Endocrinol* 2001; 15: 1781–9

36. Ron D, Habener JF. CHOP, a novel developmentally regulated nuclear protein that dimerizes with transcription factors C/EBP and LAP and functions as a dominant-negative inhibitor of gene transcription. *Genes Dev* 1992; 6: 439–53

37. Pereira RC, Delany AM, Canalis E. CCAAT/enhancer binding protein homologous protein (CHOP) induces osteoblastic differentiation. *Endocrinology* 2004; 145: 1952–60

38. Ron D. Translational control in the endoplasmic reticulum stress response. *J Clin Invest* 2002; 110: 1383–8

39. Yang X, Matsuda K, Bialek P, et al. ATF4 is a substrate of RSK2 and an essential regulator of osteoblast biology: implication for Coffin–Lowry syndrome. *Cell* 2004; 117: 387–98

Sex steroid hormones and bone formation   4

R. Civitelli

INTRODUCTION

Estrogen replacement therapy (HRT) has been used for over 30 years as the main therapeutic approach for prevention of postmenopausal bone loss. Estrogens as well as androgenic hormones are inhibitors of bone resorption, and, although the exact action of these steroid hormones on osteoclastogenesis is still not completely clear, it has been assumed that the major target cells are cells of the osteoclastic lineage. Therefore, the concept that estrogen may affect the osteoblast arm of the bone remodeling cycle is still controversial. A major limitation to *in vitro* studies is that there is large species variability in response to sex steroids. For example, estrogen can result in bone-anabolic effects in rodents, but not in humans. Therefore, some of the findings obtained in rodents will have to be considered with caution when extrapolating to human biology.

Although estrogen can affect cells of the osteoclastic lineage at multiple points during their differentiation program, thus modulating bone resorption (reviewed in references 1 and 2), several lines of evidence indicate that sex steroids can also regulate the function of cells of the osteoblastic lineage. For example, estrogen receptors are present in osteoblasts, and effects on cell proliferation, expression of osteoblastic genes and cell death (apoptosis) have all been described in *in vitro* models of osteoblast differentiation (reviewed in references 3 and 4). Furthermore, loss of sex steroids leads to increased bone formation in addition to increased bone resorption, and, although this may represent an indirect effect due to the coupling of the bone remodeling cycle, data are emerging suggesting that estrogen may also directly modulate bone formation (Figure 1).

SEX STEROIDS AND OSTEOBLAST DIFFERENTIATION

While *in vitro* studies pointed to a potential effect of estrogen in modulating osteoblast function, only an *in vivo* setting would establish whether a direct action of sex steroids on osteoblasts is relevant for estrogen modulation of bone mass and, most important, for the mechanism of estrogen-dependent bone loss. Bone loss following ovariectomy (OVX) or orchiectomy (ORX) in rats or mice is widely used to model the consequences of estrogen or androgen failure on bone homeostasis. However, the increase in bone resorption that follows gonadal removal complicates the detection of direct effects of estrogen on osteoblasts. The ensuing increase in bone formation may be an indirect consequence of bone turnover activation. Important advances in this area have been made by one group of investigators who focused on a particular mouse model, the senescence accelerated mouse (SAMP-6), which is thought to reproduce many of the changes that occur in aging in a shorter than natural time-frame. In particular, this mouse model develops what can be called an age-induced bone loss characterized by decreased bone turnover, associated with decreased osteoblastogenesis[5].

To understand whether sex hormones do indeed target cells of the osteoblastic lineage in the context of decreased osteoblastogenesis, Jilka and co-workers assessed the osteogenic potential of bone marrow cells derived from OVX or ORX SAMP-6 mice[5]. The bone marrow of adult animals contains both hematopoietic and mesenchymal stem cells, undifferentiated cells that give rise to multiple lineages (chondro-osteoblasts, adipocytes, myocytes), and are able to self-renew, i.e. produce daughter cells with the same multilineage potential (Figure 2). The

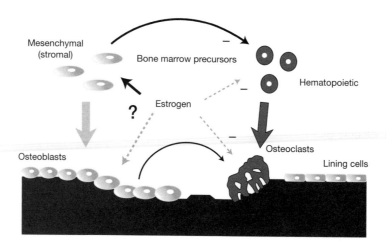

Figure 1 Estrogen modulation of bone cells. Osteoblasts and osteoclasts derive from mesenchymal/stromal and hematopoietic precursors, respectively. Estrogen inhibits osteoclast differentiation and function via different interacting molecular mechanisms, thus suppressing bone resorption. They also affect the bone formation arm of the remodeling cycle, although the site of estrogen interaction with the osteoblast lineage is still not totally clear

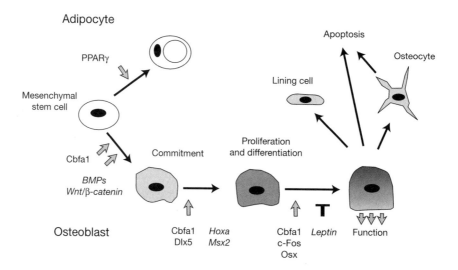

Figure 2 Model of osteoblast differentiation. Osteoblasts derive from mesenchymal stem cells residing in the bone marrow of adult bone. These cells can also give rise to adipocytes (and myoblasts during skeletal development), under the influence of extracellular cues (growth factors, cytokines, mechanical signals as well as direct cell–cell contact). Committed osteoblasts undergo several steps to acquire the ability to synthesize bone matrix and mineralize it. These steps are modulated by time- and phase-specific up- and down-regulation of transcription factors, either stimulators or repressors (only a few are indicated). After the bone formation cycle is completed, osteoblasts can either undergo programmed cell death (apoptosis), or remain on the bone surface (lining cells), or become encased within the bone as osteocytes. PPARg, peroxisome proliferator-activated receptor g; BMPs, bone morphogenetic proteins

number of undifferentiated progenitors can be measured by determining the number of cells in the bone marrow that are able to produce single cell colonies, when seeded at low density, i.e. colony-forming units-fibroblast (CFU-F). Although, typically, CFU-Fs are defined as just colonies forming from single bone marrow cells without particular phenotypic features, Jilka and colleagues used alkaline phosphatase staining to identify these cells[5]. Ultimately, interpretation is more important than definition, and indeed alkaline phosphatase-positive CFU-Fs do contain osteoprogenitor cells, even though not all of them will commit to osteogenesis. Therefore, in their system, CFU-F represents the number of osteoprogenitors present in marrow at the time of isolation. In a similar fashion, colonies that produce mineralized matrix when grown in mineralizing medium, CFU-osteoblast (CFU-OB), represent bone marrow cells that are able to differentiate fully to bone-forming osteoblasts. Therefore, they are thought to represent committed osteoprogenitors. CFU-OBs are contained in CFU-Fs, representing only a fraction of these cells. Thus, by counting the number of CFU-Fs or CFU-OBs, one can determine the osteogenic potentials of the bone marrow.

Within the first months of life, the osteogenic potential of SAMP-6 mice is similar to that of normal animals. However, after 4 months of age, when the skeleton reaches maturity, the number of CFU-Fs and CFU-OBs markedly decreases in SAMP-6 mice, reflecting decreased osteogenic potential at both the osteoprogenitor and committed precursor levels. As expected, the number of osteoclasts is also sharply decreased in bone marrow cells of these mice, although the number of osteoclast precursors, assessed as CFU-granulocyte-macrophage, is normal. Therefore, the osteoclastogenic defect in these animals is not due to lack of precursors but to a defective progression toward fully differentiated osteoclasts[5]. Since the most important osteoclastogenic signals are provided by cells of the osteoblastic lineage, the authors asked whether this osteoclastogenic defect might be secondary to an osteoblast defect. Interestingly, when bone marrow cells from SAMP-6 mice were co-cultured with calvaria cells derived from normal mice, the osteoclastogenic defect was completely corrected, and osteoclasts were produced in normal numbers. Consequently, the decreased osteoclastogenesis in this model of defective osteoblastogenesis is almost entirely secondary to a failure of osteoblastic cells to support osteoclastogenesis.

These observations were rapidly extended to estrogen- and androgen-dependent modulation of osteoclastogenesis, and almost identical results were obtained in SAMP-6 mice after orchiectomy. Similar to what was observed following OVX in females, testes removal in SAMP-6 males did not trigger the expected increase in osteoclastogenesis, or in bone marrow osteogenic precursors, indicating that the defective support of osteoclasts by osteoblastic cells is sex hormone-aspecific. The decreased osteogenic and osteoclastogenic potential in gonadectomized SAMP-6 bone marrow was also correlated with decreased bone formation and resorption parameters on bone histology[6]. Thus, SAMP-6 mice do not exhibit increased activation frequency following ovariectomy, in agreement with the failure to develop increased osteoclastogenesis in vitro after OVX. More important, these animals, which are already osteopenic at 4 months of age, do not experience the rapid bone loss occurring in normal mice upon OVX or ORX. Therefore, at least in this model of osteoblastogenic bone marrow defect, the ability of sex hormones to modulate osteoclast differentiation seems to be entirely dependent upon cells of the osteoblastic lineage, supporting the notion that simulation of bone resorption by sex steroid hormones is mediated by an effect on cells of the osteoblastic lineage[6].

To demonstrate this premise further, Jilka and co-workers simultaneously measured osteoblastogenesis and osteoclastogenesis in mice after OVX. In these studies, they proved that, following ovarian removal, there is a concomitant increase in CFU-Fs, CFU-OBs and osteoclasts in the bone marrow[7]. This increase is maximal about 30 days after surgery, and the effect tends to wane approximately 70–80 days thereafter. The timing of these changes was tightly correlated with rapid loss of histologically determined cancellous bone volume. Subsequently, the investigators repeated the OVX experiment in animals which were then treated with the bisphosphonate, alendronate. Interestingly, while treatment with alendronate completely repressed bone resorption and decreased both osteoclast number and CFU-OBs in sham-operated animals, it only partially prevented the increase of both osteoblastogenic and osteoclastogenic cells after OVX[7]. When calculated as percentage changes relative to non-OVX mice, both osteoclast number and CFU-OBs increased in OVX, alendronate-treated animals to a similar extent to that in placebo-treated animals. These results provide further evidence to the premise that osteoclastogenesis stimulated by loss of ovarian function does not depend on cell-autonomous, estrogen-dependent regulation of osteoclast formation or activity, but is an indirect consequence of estrogen effects on bone marrow osteoblastogenesis[7].

Therefore, this series of studies in SAMP-6 mice demonstrated that, in a condition in which the bone marrow fails to increase osteoclasts in response to gonadectomy, there is also failure to mount an osteoblastogenic response. In addition, attenuated activation of osteoblastogenesis after gonadectomy parallels reduced osteoclastogenesis, and this attenuated response occurs after gonadectomy in both genders. Thus, the suppressive effect of sex hormones on bone marrow stromal/osteoblastic cells seems to be cell-autonomous.

SEX HORMONES ACT AT EARLY STEP OF OSTEOBLASTOGENESIS

The body of work described above on the gonadectomy model of sex steroid hormone failure indicates that estrogen and androgen inhibit the function and/or differentiation of osteoblasts. The next important issue was to determine which steps of the osteoblast differentiation program sex steroid hormones alter. Osteoblasts are derived from mesenchymal stem cells, which, under the influence of extracellular cues, can undergo early commitment to become chondroosteogenic, and, as their differentiation progresses, tissue-specific genes are activated until these committed cells become fully functioning, matrix-secreting and mineralizing osteoblasts.

This complex, multistep process is orchestrated by activation of specific transcriptional factors[8–10]. Therefore, there are several points at which sex hormones may interact with this system (Figure 2).

In a series of elegant studies, Di Gregorio and co-workers demonstrated that the CFU-OB cells are committed precursors which retain the ability of self-renewal. As already noted, self-renewal is a feature of stem cells which allows them to produce daughter cells and yet maintain multipotentiality. When these authors cultured secondary colonies from cells taken from colonies that were generated from freshly isolated bone marrow progenitors, they were able to reproduce exactly the same type and number of secondary colonies starting from either CFU-F or CFU-OB cells[11]. Thus, both CFU-Fs and CFU-OBs are capable of self-renewal, and therefore they both represent cells at relatively early stages in the osteoblastic differentiation program. This by itself is an important discovery. More to the point of the present review, *in vivo* treatment of mice with estradiol dose-dependently suppressed CFU-OB self-renewal, obtained by counting the number of CFU-OBs produced by secondary cultures, with 10^{-9} mol/l being the least effective dose. Furthermore, the effect of estrogen was completely prevented, *in vitro*, either in the presence of a competitive estrogen receptor inhibitor (ICI 182 780), or when estrogen receptor-α (ERα)-deficient cells were used[11], demonstrating that attenuation of CFU-OB formation by estrogen administration is entirely dependent on ERα.

This series of studies demonstrated that the antiosteogenic effect of estrogen occurs early in the osteoblast differentiation program, before progenitor cells become committed to osteogenesis and are still capable of self-renewal, a phase defined by these transit-amplifying progenitors. Cells in this phase represent 85% of CFU-OBs, and the stage immediately before osteoblast commitment[11]. Therefore, inhibition of osteoprogenitor self-renewal represents a key mechanism of the antibone remodeling effect of sex steroids (Figure 3).

These seminal data provided critical information that furthered our understanding of how sex steroids modulate bone remodeling. However,

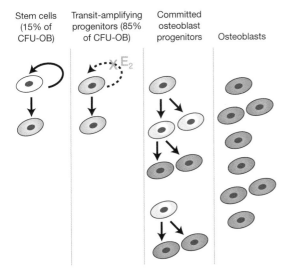

Stem cells (15% of CFU-OB) Transit-amplifying progenitors (85% of CFU-OB) Committed osteoblast progenitors Osteoblasts

Figure 3 Estrogen modulation of osteoblastogenesis. Mesenchymal stem cells are able to self-renew (produce like daughter cells) and give rise to different lineages. Before commitment to osteogenesis, osteoblast progenitors undergo an intermediate phase, during which they are still capable of self-renewal (transit amplifying progenitors). Estrogen (17β-estradiol, E2) inhibits self-renewal of these progenitor cells, thus limiting the number of cells undergoing osteoblast commitment. CFU-OB, colony-forming units-osteoblast. Modified with permission from reference 11

they also left a number of open questions. First, while the results clearly point to a critical role of osteoblasts in mediating the effect of estrogen on bone turnover, estrogen undoubtedly has direct effects on the osteoclast lineage. Therefore, the relative roles of these multiple effects of estrogen on bone cells remain to be elucidated, also in light of species differences in hormone response. The second major question is whether reduced osteoclastogenesis is really entirely dependent upon a reduced number of osteoblasts or down-regulation of osteoclastogenic factors, in particular the receptor activator of nuclear factor kappa B (NFκB) (RANK)–RANK ligand–osteoprotegerin system. Finally, we still need to understand the molecular mechanisms of estrogen-dependent inhibition of bone marrow progenitor self-renewal.

Recent data begin to shed some light on at least some of these critical issues. For example, using a gene array approach to identify differentially expressed genes by osteoblasts derived from bones of estrogen-treated rats, von Stechow and co-workers demonstrated that estrogen treatment increased mRNA expression of many genes, including parathyroid hormone receptor 1, RANK and RANK ligand[12]. Interestingly, among the genes up-regulated by estrogen in a model in which high-dose estrogen induces bone-anabolic effects, 65 genes were found to be up-regulated by parathyroid hormone as well, also a bone-anabolic agent. As is typical in these types of studies, substantial additional work is required to sort further through the many genes regulated by estrogen when used *in vivo*, but these results already provide initial, useful information that can be applied to understand how estrogen modulates osteoblastogenesis at the molecular level.

SEX HORMONES REGULATION OF OSTEOBLAST APOPTOSIS

The same group of investigators explored another potential point of interaction between sex hormones, further downstream in the osteoblast differentiation program. Based on *in vitro* data, it had been hypothesized that the profound bone erosion of cancellous bone after estrogen removal is related to removal of the stimulatory effect of estrogen on osteoclast programmed cell death, or apoptosis[13]. Regulation of cell life-span is a critical regulatory point; considering the relatively high renewal rate of bone-forming cells, even small changes in osteoblast life-span may have substantial long-term consequences. By direct *in vivo* assessment of apoptosis in osteoblasts, Jilka and co-workers were able to demonstrate that the prevalence of apoptotic osteoblasts at a specific point in time in adult mice is 0.6%[14]. Although this prevalence may seem extremely low, assuming that the active life-span of an osteoblast is approximately 12 days, one can calculate that the fraction of all osteoblasts undergoing apoptosis is 60–80%. This figure would be consistent with the generally held belief that, after one remodeling cycle, only a minority of osteoblasts survive, either as lining cells on the bone surface or within the bone matrix as osteocytes. Therefore, it is reasonable to conclude that most osteoblasts eventually will die by apoptosis. Therefore, interference with this process would greatly affect the number of active osteoblasts that are present in bone at a certain time.

Work led by Jilka, Kousteni and Manolagas demonstrated that OVX or ORX in mice sharply increases the number of apoptotic osteoblasts, from less than 1% to approximately 15% prevalence. Once again, this effect was sex hormone-aspecific and it was seen on both osteoblasts and osteocytes, although the increased apoptosis in osteocytes was substantially lower than in osteoblasts[15]. Further analysis of apoptosis in calvaria cell cultures demonstrated that treatment with either estradiol or the non-aromatizable androgen, dihydrotestosterone, dose-dependently prevented apoptosis induced by etoposide. Elegant molecular, structure–function studies also demonstrated that the antiapoptotic effect of estrogen was dependent on the presence of ERα, as was its effect on osteoblastogenesis. However, unlike the latter effect, inhibition of apoptosis did not require ERα transcriptional activity. This novel, tantalizing result was obtained by ERα mutational analysis, demonstrating that prevention of etoposide-induced apoptosis by estrogen was not detected when the ERα was forced to localize exclusively in the nucleus. However, estrogen prevented apoptosis when mutated forms of ERα lacking a nuclear localization signal were present on the cell surface[15]. This striking finding not only pointed to an unexpected mechanism for the antiapoptotic effect of estrogen, but also disclosed an alternative function of ERα, independent of its transcriptional activity and nuclear localization.

THE ANTIAPOPTOTIC EFFECT OF ESTROGEN IS VIA 'NON-GENOTROPIC' MECHANISMS

Follow-up studies demonstrated that estrogen can activate signaling cascades, in particular the extracellular signal-regulated kinase (ERK), phosphatidylinositol 3-kinase (PI3K) and c-Jun N-terminal kinase (JNK) pathways, all present at the cell membrane and all typically activated by membrane-bound, peptide hormone receptors, and reverse changes in kinase activity induced by OVX[15]. Therefore, survival signals generated by estrogen do not require nuclear localization but activation of membrane signaling cascades. Based on these observations, the author proposed a model of 'non-genotropic' effects of estrogen, specifically mediating antiapoptotic signals. Based on these results, estrogen action on target cells is much more complex than previously thought. In addition to the classic binding to ERα (and ERβ in certain tissues) and activation of gene transcription for estrogen response elements in promoters of target genes, sex hormones can also bind cell-surface receptors, activating signaling cascades converging onto regulation of cell survival genes (Figure 4). It is still unclear whether the cell-surface receptor binding estrogen is the same ERα that localizes to the cell membrane, or whether there is a different cell-surface receptor, perhaps similar in structure to the pentahelix class of membrane receptors, that can be modulated by sex steroids and activate the kinase cascade linked to cell survival signals. Clarifying this novel mode of estrogen action will be important not only for estrogen regulation of bone metabolism but also for understanding the biologic role of sex hormones and their receptors.

Other non-conventional modes of estrogen signaling are beginning to emerge. A recent study by McCarthy and co-workers demonstrates that estrogen-ligated ERα can bind Runx2, the earliest and most specific osteoblast transcriptional factor[17]. The ERα–Runx2 complex can in turn bind to Runx2 response elements in osteoblast-specific genes to effect transcriptional regulation. At the same time, ERα–Runx2 binding may subtract active ERα from the conventional estrogen response element (ERE)-dependent responses, which control non-tissue-specific actions of estrogen, for example, the cell division cycle. Therefore, Runx2 may serve to integrate estrogen activity on osteoblast gene transcription, modulating the estrogen effect in a tissue-specific fashion[17].

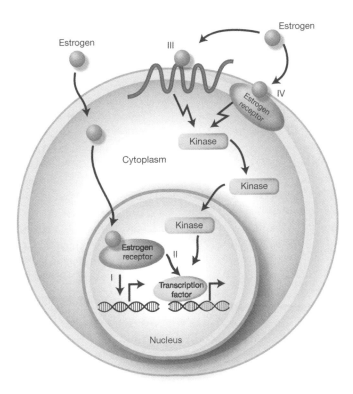

Figure 4 Modes of estrogen action on target cells. In the classic mechanism, estrogen, a steroid hormone, enters the cell through the plasma membrane and binds to nuclear estrogen receptors to effect gene transcription via estrogen response elements. In the proposed alternative 'non-genotropic' mechanism, estrogen binds surface receptors, either the same estrogen receptors localized to the surface, or novel, yet unidentified, surface receptors linked to kinase cascades. These ultimately alter gene transcription via mechanisms independent of estrogen response elements. Modified with permission from reference 15

Thus, modulation of osteoblast survival is a second critical point at which estrogen interferes with osteoblast function and bone formation. However, these data remain controversial. First of all, the *in vitro* systems in which most of the data are obtained do not take into account the complexity of the bone marrow microenvironment. It is easy to envision that many local factors may also regulate osteoblast apoptosis, and whether estrogen is a key element in such a complex system remains to be determined. Second, less than 20% of osteoblasts or osteocytes undergo apoptosis after estrogen withdrawal. Although this change may be of relevance considering the life-span of these cells, it still remains a relatively modest effect overall. In summary, the discovery that estrogen affects the osteoblast arm of the remodeling cycle in addition to the osteoclast lineage is by itself a notion of considerable importance in understanding the biologic role of sex hormones in bone homeostasis, although the contribution of this action to the development of estrogen-dependent bone loss still remains to be fully elucidated.

References

1. Zaidi M, Blair HC, Moonga BS, et al. Osteoclastogenesis, bone resorption, and osteoclast-based therapeutics. *J Bone Miner Res* 2003; 18: 599–609

2. Riggs BL. The mechanisms of estrogen regulation of bone resorption. *J Clin Invest* 2000; 106: 1203–4

3. Migliaccio S, Marino M. Estrogens and estrogen receptors: new actors in the plot of transcriptional regulation of genomic responses. *Calcif Tissue Int* 2003; 72: 181–2

4. Manolagas SC, Kousteni S, Jilka RL. Sex steroids and bone. *Recent Prog Horm Res* 2002; 57: 385–409

5. Jilka RL, Weinstein RS, Takahashi K, et al. Linkage of decreased bone mass with impaired osteoblastogenesis in a murine model of accelerated senescence. *J Clin Invest* 1996; 97: 1732–40

6. Weinstein RS, Jilka RL, Parfitt AM, Manolagas SC. The effects of androgen deficiency on murine bone remodeling and bone mineral density are mediated via cells of the osteoblastic lineage. *Endocrinology* 1997; 138: 4013–21

7. Jilka RL, Takahashi K, Munshi M, et al. Loss of estrogen upregulates osteoblastogenesis in the murine bone marrow. Evidence for autonomy from factors released during bone resorption. *J Clin Invest* 1998; 101: 1942–50

8. Karsenty G, Wagner EF. Reaching a genetic and molecular understanding of skeletal development. *Dev Cell* 2002; 2: 389–406

9. Franceschi RT. The developmental control of osteoblast-specific gene expression: role of specific transcription factors and the extracellular matrix environment. *Crit Rev Oral Biol Med* 1999; 10: 40–57

10. Lian JB, Stein GS. The temporal and spatial subnuclear organization of skeletal gene regulatory machinery: integrating multiple levels of transcriptional control. *Calcif Tissue Int* 2003; 72: 631–7

11. Di Gregorio GB, Yamamoto M, Ali AA, et al. Attenuation of the self-renewal of transit-amplifying osteoblast progenitors in the murine bone marrow by 17 beta-estradiol. *J Clin Invest* 2001; 107: 803–12

12. von Stechow D, Zurakowski D, Pettit AR, et al. Differential transcriptional effects of PTH and estrogen during anabolic bone formation. *J Cell Biochem* 2004; 93: 476–90

13. Hughes DE, Dai A, Tiffee JC, et al. Estrogen promotes apoptosis of murine osteoclasts mediated by TGF-β. *Nat Med* 1996; 2: 1132–6

14. Jilka RL, Weinstein RS, Bellido T, et al. Osteoblast programmed cell death (apoptosis): modulation by growth factors and cytokines. *J Bone Miner Res* 1998; 13: 793–802

15. Kousteni S, Bellido T, Plotkin LI, et al. Nongenotropic, sex-nonspecific signaling through the estrogen or androgen receptors: dissociation from transcriptional activity. *Cell* 2001; 104: 719–30

16. Lorenzo J. A new hypothesis for how sex steroid hormones regulate bone mass. *J Clin Invest* 2003; 111: 1641–3

17. McCarthy TL, Chang WZ, Liu Y, Centrella M. Runx2 integrates estrogen activity in osteoblasts. *J Biol Chem* 2003; 278: 43121–9

The effect of sex steroids on osteoclast function

5

K. Henriksen, N. A. Sims, L. B. Tankó and M. A. Karsdal

INTRODUCTION

Estrogen deficiency arising after the menopause or upon surgical removal of the ovaries leads to accelerated bone loss and promotes the development of postmenopausal osteoporosis in approximately one-third of the female population[1]. The primary consequence of the relative lack of estrogen is an increase in bone resorption, which can be attributed to marked increases in both the number and resorptive activity of osteoclasts[2]. Although bone formation also shows a notable increase upon the propagation of estrogen deficiency, the rise in resorption exceeds the increase in formation, the net changes leading to loss of bone mass. While bone resorption is carried out by osteoclasts, the paths by which estrogen exerts its inhibitory effects on these cells are still under debate. Although osteoclasts possess estrogen receptors and thus can be direct targets of estrogen action, a considerable part of the effect is believed to be indirect and mediated by osteoblasts and various cells of the immune system[3]. Research attempting the clarification of how estrogen acts on bone metabolism includes: the direct effects of sex steroids on osteoclasts investigated in simple *in vitro* systems; the impact of sex steroid receptor deficiency on osteoclastic function and skeletal homeostasis using data from estrogen and androgen receptor knock-out mice; and finally the *in vivo* effects of sex steroids on bone turnover assessed in various clinical settings. The current review combines these three major approaches to bring forward the present understanding of the action of sex steroids on osteoclast function and overall bone turnover.

THE SEX STEROIDS AND THEIR RECEPTORS IN GENERAL

Sex steroids combine with sex steroid receptors and function as ligand-gated transcription factors[4]. Sex steroid receptors contain two major domains: the ligand-binding domain and the DNA-binding domain[4]. After binding of the sex steroid to its receptor, either a hetero- or a homodimer is formed, and specific gene expression is induced[5,6]. This specific gene expression is most likely tissue-specific, and depends on specific cofactors expressed in the individual cells[4].

Sex steroids are all cholesterol derivatives, which can, via enzymatic processing in various tissues, transform to progesterone, testosterone or estradiol. Testosterone can irreversibly be converted to estradiol by the enzyme aromatase[7,8], illustrating that sex steroids are interconnected, some serving as precursors for others[4].

The effects of sex steroids are complex and mediated through various receptors. To date, five different receptors have been identified: estrogen receptors alpha (ERα) and beta (ERβ), the androgen receptor (AR) and progesterone receptors A and B[4]. A word of note should be given regarding the estrogen-related receptors α, β and γ, which share high resemblance with the estrogen receptors, but do not bind estrogen as natural ligands[5,6,9].

In addition to the classical genomic effects of estrogen, emerging evidence suggests nongenomic effects of estrogen receptors[4]. In particular, mitogen-activated protein kinases (MAPKs) p44/42 in combination with the non-receptor tyrosine kinase pp60*src* are reported to be important in this context[10,11].

Collectively, numerous receptors and pathways mediate the effects of sex steroids, which also illustrate the complexity of the interactions between sex steroids and bone. The following review attempts to ease the understanding of these complex processes, combining three areas of expertise: *in vitro*, *in vivo*, and clinical investigations.

ESTROGEN RECEPTORS ON OSTEOCLASTS

The identification of sex steroid receptors was an essential step in investigating the direct effects of sex steroids on osteoclasts and their precursors. Studies addressing the role of estrogen receptors, ERα and ERβ, in bone metabolism have yielded somewhat contradictory results. Both ERα and ERβ are present in most bone cells, yet there are differences in expression densities of the cortical and trabecular compartments. ERα expression seems to dominate in cortical, whereas ERβ is the most prominent component in trabecular bone[12]. The first observation suggesting direct effects of estrogen on osteoclasts was the identification of estrogen receptors on avian osteoclasts[13]. Both estrogen receptors have now been identified in cells of the osteoclast lineage[14]. ERβ was detected in both precursors and mature osteoclasts[15-18]. Most investigators found ERα in preosteoclasts only[19], yet[20,21] some groups located these receptors in mature osteoclasts as well[22-24]. A potential explanation for these apparently contradictory findings rests in the relatively low expression rate of ERα in mature osteoclasts, being close to the detection limit of the methods used (see discussion by Vanderschueren and colleagues[14]). The intracellular localization of the ERβ is still a controversial issue, some suggesting nuclear localization[12], and others advocating cytoplasmic localization[18]. The estrogen-related receptor α (ERRα) is also expressed by osteoclasts, and seems to play a role in bone turnover. Nevertheless, since estrogen is not a natural ligand of this receptor, we refrain from discussing it further in this review[25]. Collectively, both estrogen receptors are present in mature osteoclasts and their precursors, implying that some of the regulatory effects of estrogen are likely mediated by direct action on osteoclasts.

ESTROGEN EFFECTS ON OSTEOCLASTS AND THEIR PRECURSORS

Estrogen has been shown to exert direct anti-osteoclastic effects at several stages of osteoclastic differentiation and function. For simplicity, we have separated the osteoclastic life-span into the following categories:

(1) Differentiation/osteoclastogenesis;

(2) Resorption/activity;

(3) Apoptosis.

Differentiation of osteoclasts is a complex process involving commitment of cells of the monocyte lineage to differentiate into osteoclast precursors, and then fusion of the osteoclast precursors into mature bone-resorbing osteoclasts. A direct effect of estrogen on osteoclast differentiation was found by two independent groups[26,27], both demonstrating that estrogen can directly inhibit the formation of multinucleated osteoclasts by suppression of the receptor activator of nuclear factor-kappa B (NFκB) ligand (RANKL)-induced c-*Jun* activation in precursor cells. Estrogen was also shown to reduce basal c-*Jun* N-terminal kinase (JNK) activity, but not NFκB activity, resulting in lowered formation of c-*Jun*/c-*Fos* and *JunD*/c-*Fos* heterodimers. The latter results in lowered secretion of the pro-osteoclastic cytokine tumor necrosis factor α (TNFα), evoking reduced formation of mature osteoclasts, probably by lowering the number of precursors that can differentiate into osteoclasts[28]. Furthermore, estrogen was found to inhibit osteoclastic differentiation in a human system[19]. The same study also showed that the inhibitory role of estrogen on osteoclast differentiation is likely mediated via the ERα. Finally, it was recently demonstrated that estrogen treatment of differentiating osteoclasts leads to down-regulation of the β3-integrin[29], which is essential for normal resorptive function of the osteoclasts[30]. We have studied the effect of estrogen on the differentiation of CD14+ isolated human monocytes into osteoclasts, and our unpublished data support a negative regulatory function of estrogen in osteoclastogenesis in this system as well.

Initial evidence that estrogen has a direct impact on mature osteoclasts was shown by Oursler and her colleagues[13,31] when they found that estrogen binds to a receptor on osteoclasts and can inhibit bone resorption. Further study led to the revelation that the effects of estrogen on mature osteoclasts can actually be divided into two categories: an effect on the release and function of lysosomal enzymes, and an effect on ion channels/pumps present in the osteoclasts. The Oursler group has shown that both the activity and the production of the lysosomal enzymes are down-regulated by estrogen[32,33], possibly explaining the reduction in resorption by the down-regulation of cathepsin K and tartrate-resistant acid phosphatase (TRAP), which have both been shown to participate in the bone resorption process[34–37]. Furthermore, they showed that the tyrosine kinase pp60src is also involved in the regulation of lysosomal enzyme secretion, and that this process is negatively regulated by estrogen[38]. Further supporting a direct effect of estrogen on osteoclastic secretion of lysosomal enzymes, a study by Parikka and colleagues[39] recently showed that estrogen probably reduces cathepsin K action in osteoclasts, although whether it is by down-regulation of expression or by inhibiting its activity is not yet known. However, estrogen thereby affects the degradation of the organic matrix of bone. Finally, estrogen regulates secretion of transforming growth factor β (TGFβ) by osteoclasts, and it has been speculated that this is the mechanism by which lysosomal secretion is reduced[40]. Thus, all data point toward an important role for estrogen in directly down-regulating the resorptive activity of mature osteoclasts, involving alteration of the activity of lysosomal enzymes.

On the other hand, estrogen has also been shown to affect ion transport in osteoclasts. This seems mainly to involve the inward rectified K^+ channel at the plasma membrane of the osteoclasts, leading to depolarization of the plasma membrane[41,42], and it was speculated that this could reduce the proton secretion into the resorption lacuna and thereby inhibit resorption[43]. Whether the reduction in proton transport by estrogen[43] is relevant during the resorption process is questioned by the findings of Parikka and colleagues[39], who demonstrated that only the proteolytic processes are affected by estrogen. Thus, there are some controversies between the different studies on the effect of estrogen on mature osteoclasts, yet the common conclusion is that estrogen negatively regulates the number and activity of the osteoclasts, and loss of this direct function could potentially play a role in the pathogenesis of postmenopausal osteoporosis.

The reports describing the effects of estrogen on osteoclast apoptosis are controversial. In 1997 a group demonstrated that estrogen directly induced apoptosis in a pure culture of rabbit osteoclasts, and these effects could be blocked by the antiestrogen tamoxifen[44]. In contrast, two other publications have shown that estrogen has no apoptotic effect on osteoclasts, and that tamoxifen induces apoptosis via its non-estrogenic effects[45,46]. However, there are also reports that show that neither estrogen nor raloxifene affect the apoptosis of osteoclasts[19]. The explanation for these contradictory findings might rest in differences in species or the presence of cell types other than osteoclasts in the latter two studies. Since no systematic studies have been performed on pure human osteoclasts, e.g. human CD14+ prepared osteoclasts, addressing the effects of estrogen on apoptosis, these issues are yet to be clarified.

In conclusion, estrogen seems to have important direct effects on several stages of osteoclast differentiation and function *in vitro* (Figure 1). There are still many open questions about the direct effects, whether they are genomic or nongenomic and, most important, whether these effects also apply *in vivo*. This final question can probably only be answered by generation of cell-type-specific knock-out animals, where the estrogen receptor(s) are ablated in only a limited population of cells. To clarify the direct effects of estrogen on osteoclasts, an osteoclast-specific knock-out of the receptors would be extremely interesting, for example using the ctsk-cre transgenic mouse line[47].

ANDROGEN EFFECTS ON OSTEOCLASTS AND THEIR PRECURSORS

Direct effects of androgens on osteoclasts have received limited attention. Although androgen receptors were shown on non-human osteoclasts[48,49], immunohistochemical techniques have failed to confirm this finding in human osteoclasts[50,51]. The idea of direct effects of androgens on osteoclasts was first raised by Pederson and colleagues[48], who showed that the addition of α-dihydrotestosterone significantly reduced the ability of chicken, mouse and human osteoclasts to resorb bone, apparently by modifying the lysosomal enzyme secretion of the osteoclasts – similar to the action of estrogen[32,33]. However, it is to be emphasized that these studies were performed in mixed cell cultures that contained cells other than osteoclasts, albeit in low amounts. Thus, whether the effect is direct or not remains unclear, particularly in human cells, in which no androgen receptor has yet been identified[50,51].

More direct evidence was obtained using the murine cell line RAW264.7, which can differentiate into osteoclasts[52]. In this study, the androgen receptor was detected in RAW264.7 cells, and binding of α-dihydrotestosterone dose-dependently inhibited osteoclast formation via down-regulation of the c-*Jun* signaling pathway[52], thus mimicking the effects observed with estrogen[26,27]. The effects of androgens on osteoclasts are summarized in Figure 1.

In summary, the direct effects of androgens on osteoclasts are yet to be fully elucidated. A systematic study of a pure population of human osteoclasts and their precursors, such as the CD14+ monocytes, would greatly increase our understanding of whether androgen has any direct effect on osteoclasts, and whether it has any significant implications in bone biology.

LESSONS FROM THE ESTROGEN RECEPTOR KNOCK-OUT MOUSE

An alternative approach to the understanding of the effects of estrogen on bone turnover is to investigate the consequences of deleting the genes of estrogen receptors (knock-out models).

A global null mutation in each estrogen receptor, and estradiol treatment of ER knock-out mice, revealed that, while only ERα is required for normal bone density and bone cell activity in male mice, both ERα and ERβ are essential for the determination of bone mass and bone cell activity in female mice.

In male mice, there was neither change in trabecular or cortical bone structure, nor any change in the level of osteoblast or osteoclast numbers in the absence of ERβ. These observations indicate that ERβ is not required for normal bone metabolism or osteoclast function in male mice[53]. However, when ERα was deleted (including deletion of both ERα and ERβ), a mild osteopetrosis was observed. This was

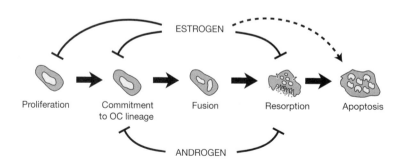

Figure 1 The direct effects of both estrogen and androgen are being investigated. However, several reports have indicated regulatory functions of the sex hormones at different stages of osteoclast development and function. OC, osteoclast

characterized by increased trabecular bone volume, reduced cortical thickness and a significant reduction in bone turnover; all bone formation and bone resorption parameters, including osteoclast number, were reduced. A low level of bone turnover in growing mice is commonly associated with increased bone mass, whereas a reduction in bone mass is associated with low bone turnover induced in adult or aged animals. Since trabecular bone arises initially from bone formation on resorbed cartilage remnants from the growth plate[54], a reduction in osteoclast numbers impairs the initial cycle of bone resorption, leaving an excess of cartilage upon which repeated cycles of slow remodeling retain a higher trabecular bone volume. This phenotype was surprising, given the increase in bone density and high level of bone turnover observed in a man with a null mutation in ERα[55]. The most striking difference between humans and mice with ERα deficiency was that circulating testosterone levels were approximately ten-fold higher than normal in the mouse[53]. Since testosterone treatment in men is known to inhibit osteoclast formation and increase bone mass[56,57], the reduced osteoclast generation and subsequent changes in bone mass observed in the absence of ERα are caused indirectly by this increase in circulating testosterone, rather than being a direct effect of ERα deletion on the osteoclast itself. Despite this complication of the knock-out phenotype, a central role for ERα in regulating bone mass in males was confirmed when it was observed that ERα[-/-] males that had been orchidectomized did not respond to estradiol treatment at doses that induced an anabolic response in wild-type littermates[58]; it is not clear from these studies whether it is an osteoclast-mediated effect that is lacking.

While only ERα appears to be essential for normal bone physiology in male mice, both ERα and ERβ play essential roles in the determination of bone mass in females. In the absence of either receptor, trabecular bone volume was significantly elevated, but in distinct ways. In the absence of ERα, bone turnover was reduced, while, in the absence of ERβ, only bone resorption was reduced[53]. Again, as in the male mice, circulating testosterone was elevated in ERα[-/-]

females, yet to a lesser extent, and there was a pronounced increase in circulating estradiol, possibly a consequence of aromatization. In the absence of ERβ alone, the bone phenotype was, however, not associated with any change in circulating sex steroids, indicating a specific inhibitory effect of ERβ deletion on osteoclast formation, and suggesting that estradiol may stimulate osteoclast formation directly via ERβ.

When both ERs were deleted, a third distinct phenotype was observed. Due to a low level of bone formation, trabecular bone volume was very low, but this was not associated with any change in circulating sex steroid levels, or any change in bone resorption. This low trabecular bone volume was comparable to that observed after ovariectomy in adult mice. Consistent with this, no reduction in trabecular bone mass or change in bone remodeling was observed after ovariectomy in ERαβ[-/-] mice, indicating that the osteoprotective effects of estradiol are mediated fully by the two estrogen receptors alone, whereas other, non-ER-mediated pathways are not required for the maintenance of normal bone mass. Furthermore, treatment of these animals with estradiol did not confer any change on bone structure or bone turnover, indicating that, in the absence of ER-mediated signaling, estradiol is unable to alter osteoblast or osteoclast differentiation.

Since removing both ERs ablated the osteoprotective effects of physiological levels of estradiol, estradiol treatment in each single knock-out can then be interpreted as revealing the effects of estradiol acting on the remaining receptor in bone. Thus, in the female ERα[-/-] mouse, any effect of estradiol must be mediated by the ERβ, and vice versa.

Indeed, in female ERβ[-/-] mice, the bone-protective response to estradiol was only slightly impaired, compared with the response of wild-type littermates treated with the same doses of estradiol, indicating that ERα, the remaining receptor, is the main mediator of estradiol effects on trabecular bone. Yet ERα is clearly not the only important receptor, as estradiol treatment of ERα[-/-] mice was able to elicit a very mild osteoprotective effect at high doses, indicating that ERβ is also able to mediate an effect of estradiol on the skeleton. Furthermore, a dose-dependent inhibition of both osteoblast and osteoclast surfaces by estradiol was observed in ERα$^{-/-}$ mice, indicating that, at lower doses, ERβ is still responsive to estradiol, and that estradiol can inhibit both osteoclast and osteoblast formation via this receptor, but not at a level that can fully protect the skeleton against ovariectomy-induced bone loss; it is not clear from these studies whether the effect of estradiol through ERβ is mediated primarily by the osteoblast or by the osteoclast lineage.

LESSONS FROM THE ANDROGEN RECEPTOR KNOCK-OUT MOUSE

The importance of estrogens in the maintenance of the adult female skeleton is well established, whereas the relative importance of estrogens versus androgens in the regulation of bone metabolism, particularly in adult males, remains unclear. Interesting observations were provided by closer analysis of orchidectomized androgen receptor knock-out (ARKO) mice. Kawano and colleagues[59] showed that inactivation of the AR in mice caused low bone mass in males but not in females. Histomorphometric analyses of 8-week-old male ARKO mice showed high bone turnover with increased bone resorption that resulted in low trabecular and cortical bone mass without affecting bone shape. Bone loss was only partially prevented by treatment with aromatizable testosterone. Non-aromatizable testosterone had no bone-protective effect in orchidectomized ARKO, indicating that testosterone has no effect on bone through either ER. Analysis of primary osteoblasts and osteoclasts revealed that a functional AR was required for the suppressive effects of androgens on osteoclastogenesis-supporting activity of osteoblasts, but not on isolated osteoclasts, a result that suggests that the effect of non-aromatized testosterone on the osteoclast is mediated by the osteoblast. Furthermore, expression of the RANKL gene, which encodes a major osteoclastogenesis inducer, was found to be up-regulated in osteoblasts from AR-deficient mice. Thus, this study provided noteworthy evidence for the concept that AR function is important for male-type bone formation and remodeling, and that its effect on the osteoclast is indirect.

Thus, the sex steroid receptor knock-outs provide evidence that the osteoprotective effects of testosterone are mediated only by the AR, and those of estradiol are mediated predominantly by ERα, and that ERβ is also able to play a role in female mice, yet not in males.

INDIRECT EFFECTS OF ESTROGEN ON OSTEOCLAST FUNCTION

Although the presence of estradiol receptors in osteoclasts argue for direct effects of estrogens, some of the modulator effects of these sex steroids is mediated via modulation of other cell types. Secretion of cytokines by stromal cells, monocytes and lymphoid cells is essential for stimulation of the differentiation of myeloid precursor cells to osteoclasts. Cytokines with direct implications for osteoclastogenesis and related bone resorption include interleukin-1 (IL-1), IL-6, IL-8, IL-11, TNFs, fibroblast growth factor (FGF), platelet-derived growth factor (PDGF), leukemia inhibitory factor (LIF), macrophage colony-stimulating factor (M-CSF) and granulocyte/macrophage colony-stimulating factor (GM-CSF).

Studies indicate that the secretion rate of many of these cytokines is largely dependent on circulating levels and bioavailability of endogenous estradiol. Circulating concentrations increase after the menopause[60–62], and can be restored by estrogen replacement therapy[63–65]. More direct evidence was obtained by Bismar and colleagues[66], who showed that aspirated bone marrow cells from the iliac crest of early-postmenopausal women (< 5 years since menopause) or those who recently discontinued hormone replacement therapy (HRT) reveal increased secretion of IL-1α, TNFα, IL-6, prostaglandin E$_2$ and GM-CSF, compared with the secretion of bone marrow cells from either premenopausal or late-postmenopausal subjects. These findings thus support the concept that this reduction in cytokine expression and a concomitant reduction in osteoclast formation is at least one component of the beneficial effects of estradiol in preventing accelerated bone resorption and consequent bone loss.

In further support, a recent study found that the pool of circulating cells expressing RANKL (marrow stromal cells, T cells, B cells) was increased in early-postmenopausal women. Furthermore, RANKL expression of these cells closely correlated with the resorption rate in these women, establishing an important role for RANKL in the pathogenesis of osteoporosis[67]. Furthermore, the authors also found that estrogen treatment significantly lowered the number of RANKL-expressing cells[67]. On the other hand, treatment with estrogen, at least in men, leads to increased osteoprotegerin (OPG) levels[68], showing an essential role for the RANKL–OPG axis in estrogen-regulated bone turnover[69].

The indirect effects of estrogen might indeed be important. As discussed, the activation of other cell types may lead to secretion of various cytokines and other messenger molecules, which in turn can influence the function of osteoclasts[3,70,71]. The cytokines that affect osteoclastogenesis or osteoclast function can be divided into antiosteoclastic and pro-osteoclastic cytokines. In general, the antiosteoclastic cytokines are up-regulated, whereas pro-osteoclastic cytokines are down-regulated by estrogen[71]. In ovariectomized animals, estrogen deficiency was shown to lead to increased levels of the pro-osteoclastic cytokines, TNFα and IL-1[72,73]. Interestingly, T cell-mediated TNFα secretion during estrogen deficiency seems to be a central player in the loss of bone, as inhibition of TNFα in ovariectomized animals seems to restore bone loss[72,74]. The pro-osteoclastic cytokine M-CSF was also shown to be up-regulated in estrogen deficiency[73,75], and might be involved in the increased pool of osteoclasts[76–78]. Furthermore, IL-6 is also up-regulated by estrogen loss, further supporting the increased osteoclastogenesis, although the effect of IL-6 may be mediated by stimulating osteoblasts to secrete pro-osteoclastic cytokines[71]. In addition, estrogen has been reported negatively to regulate inhibitors of osteoclastogenesis (OPG), in alignment with an overall negative effect on osteoclast formation and function of estrogen. Estrogen was reported to increase the expression of OPG

both *in vivo*[68] and *in vitro* in cell cultures[79–81], and thus it is likely that estrogen deficiency reduces the expression of OPG *in vivo*, thereby augmenting osteoclast activity.

Another estrogen-regulated cytokine with inhibitory impact on osteoclasts is TGFβ[70]. Estrogen up-regulates the secretion of TGFβ[82], which in turn can inhibit osteoclast differentiation[83] and bone resorption[84], and even induce osteoclast apoptosis[70,75]. Furthermore, a recent study showed that ovariectomy blunts TGFβ1 secretion in mice, and that overexpression of TGFβ1 could prevent ovariectomy-induced bone loss[85]. These observations thus demonstrate that a considerable part of the inhibitory effect of estrogen is mediated by TGFβ. TGFβ inhibits the secretion of the pro-osteoclastic cytokines TNFα and RANKL in T cells, which in turn leads to an indirect modulation of osteoclast function[85].

In summary, whether mediated through cytokines or other systems[71], estrogen suppresses osteoclast differentiation and function.

MONITORING THE REACTIVE CHANGES IN BONE RESORPTION ACCOMPANIED BY THE LACK OR REGAIN OF SEX STEROIDS

Type I collagen represents more than 90% of the organic matrix in bone. During bone resorption, some of the collagen is completely digested to its smallest units, such as free pyridinoline and deoxypyridinoline residues. However, the majority remain incompletely digested, and measurable as pyridinium cross-links. The new generation of bone resorption markers, including those measuring C- and N-terminal telopeptides of collagen type I, represent a vast improvement over the older markers in terms of specificity and sensitivity for mature bone. These currently available assays are all specific immunoassays that have been thoroughly validated for their ability to estimate bone resorption, and thus a direct measurement of osteoclast activity, which is the focus of the current review. Serum/urine levels of these markers show a correlation with histomorphometric measurements of bone resorption. Furthermore, their levels were shown to be markedly increased in various diseases characterized by increased bone turnover. Finally, their levels undergo marked decreases during treatment with antiresorptive agents both in animal models and in humans. Thus, collectively, bone resorption markers are useful surrogates of osteoclast-mediated bone resorption, and are helpful for obtaining an insight into the effects of sex steroids on bone turnover.

BONE TURNOVER AND THE MENOPAUSE: LOSS OF ESTROGEN

The most characteristic clinical situations associated with a change in bone turnover include the menarchal transition (start of ovarian estradiol production), menstrual cycles and the menopausal transition (cessation of ovarian estradiol production), which influence the circulating levels of bone resorption markers. Studies indicate that resorption markers decrease significantly following menarche[86], fluctuate in the course of the menstrual cycle[87] and increase after the menopause[88,89], which seem to support the notion that changes in circulating estradiol influence bone resorption in humans.

Studies in which documentation of ovulatory and hormonal status was accurate and detailed[90–92] indicate that reduced progesterone production resulting from shortened luteal phases does not adversely affect bone mineral density, suggesting that progesterone *per se* does not play a major role in the determination of bone turnover.

Accelerated bone loss accompanying the menopause can be restored to premenopausal levels by the use of hormone replacement therapy, which helps to prevent bone loss and osteoporotic fractures[93,94]. The greatest clinical benefits are achieved when initiating the therapy in the early years of the menopause, when accelerated bone turnover is most pronounced. When initiated in this period, even 2–3 years of treatment may provide significant long-term benefits, compared with those not receiving treatment[95].

The effect of HRT in terms of inhibiting bone turnover lasts as long as the treatment is administered. After withdrawal of estrogen, biomarkers of bone resorption increase again, followed by bone loss. Early studies with relatively short-term follow-up suggested a rebound effect of hormone withdrawal on bone loss, particularly in the first year[96,97]. This, however, is not a uniform finding[95,98]. Accelerated bone loss following withdrawal is very much a function of individual patient characteristics, and is more prevalent in lean individuals with limited endogenous resources for estradiol. These women have higher rates of bone turnover already at the initiation of therapy, making it understandable why they tend to catch up with average individuals who have not taken therapy. Overall, the years during which HRT is taken postpone the acceleration of bone loss, thereby also postponing the decline in bone mineral density to a level associated with increased risk for fractures. Collectively, HRT given for a few years should be considered for lean women with limited resources for endogenous estradiol in the early phase of their menopause, to delay rapid bone loss and thereby an increased risk for osteoporotic fractures.

To prevent the induction of endometrial cancer by long-term estrogen exposure, women with an intact uterus must take combined estradiol plus progestogen[99]. The general perception is that this supplementation does not influence the efficacy of estrogen to prevent postmenopausal bone loss or related fractures[2].

THE ROLE AND EFFECTS OF ANDROGENS IN MEN

As discussed earlier, it is still under debate whether androgens have direct implications for bone resorption. Studies undertaken in men indicate that chemical or surgical castration, as well as untreated hypogonadism, leads to accelerated bone turnover and concomitant bone loss. Despite the fact that men do not have the equivalent of the menopause and that serum total testosterone levels decrease only marginally with age[100,101], investigators found a substantial age-related decrease in bone mineral density (BMD) in both cross-sectional[102] and longitudinal[103–105] studies. Moreover, previous studies assessing the relationship between serum total testosterone levels and BMD generally found either no relationship[100,106] or even a negative association between total testosterone levels and BMD in aging men[107]. Therefore, the absence of a substantial decrease in serum total testosterone levels in aging men has led to the belief that testosterone does not play a major role in bone loss in aging men.

Smith and colleagues[108] described a male with homozygous mutations in the estrogen receptor gene who, even in the presence of normal testosterone and free testosterone levels, had unfused epiphyses and marked osteopenia, along with elevated indexes of bone turnover. Subsequently, Morishima and associates[109] and Carani and co-workers[110] reported clinical findings in two males with homozygous mutations of the aromatase gene, which is responsible for the conversion of androgens to estradiol. In both instances, BMD was significantly reduced and bone turnover markers were markedly elevated, despite normal testosterone levels. Treatment with testosterone did not restore bone metabolism in one patient, whereas treatment with estrogen markedly increased BMD in both patients.

Longitudinal studies indicate that, in contrast to the traditional belief, bioavailable estradiol, not testosterone, seems to play the key role for both acquisition of peak bone mass in young men and determination of bone loss in elderly men[105]. Szulc and colleagues[111] provided additional insights by showing that bioavailable testosterone and estradiol were positively associated with serum OPG levels, which in turn were negatively associated with biomarkers of bone resorption. Treatment with estrogen, at least in men, leads to increased OPG levels[68], also showing an essential role of the RANKL–OPG axis in estrogen-regulated bone turnover[69]. Collectively, these findings argue for critical implications of the aromatase enzyme (that converts testosterone to 17β-estradiol) in the determination of bone metabolism in males.

Regarding the relative contribution of bioavailable estradiol and testosterone to the alterations of bone turnover and consequent bone loss, the study by Falahati-Nini and co-workers[112] provides useful insights. The investigators addressed this issue directly by eliminating endogenous testosterone and estradiol production in 59 elderly men (mean age 68 years), studying them first under conditions of physiologic testosterone and estradiol replacement, and then assessing the impact on bone turnover of withdrawing both testosterone and estradiol, withdrawing only testosterone or only estradiol, or continuing both. Bone resorption markers increased significantly in the absence of both hormones and were unchanged in men receiving both hormones. According to multivariate analysis, estradiol played the major role in preventing the increase in bone resorption markers, whereas the effect of testosterone was not statistically significant. By contrast, serum osteocalcin, a bone formation marker, decreased in the absence of both hormones, and both estradiol and testosterone maintained osteocalcin levels. Thus, it seems reasonable to conclude that, in aging men, estradiol is the dominant sex steroid regulating osteoclastic bone resorption, whereas both sex steroids are important for maintaining bone formation.

KEY NOTES

(1) Sex steroids play an important role in the modulation of osteoclastic bone resorption.

(2) Loss of sex steroids leads to increased bone turnover.

(3) Estrogens are the primary determinants of bone health in both genders.

(4) The effects of estrogens are primarily mediated by the ERα in both genders.

(5) The effects of estrogens on osteoclast function are highly complex and mediated through both direct and indirect pathways.

References

1. Russell G, Mueller G, Shipman C, Croucher P. Clinical disorders of bone resorption. *Novartis Found Symp* 2001; 232: 251–67

2. Compston JE. Sex steroids and bone. *Physiol Rev* 2001; 81: 419–47

3. Riggs BL. The mechanisms of estrogen regulation of bone resorption. *J Clin Invest* 2000; 106: 1203–4

4. Monroe DG, Spelsberg TC. *Gonadal Steroids and Their Receptors*. Washington: American Society for Bone and Mineral Research, 2003: 32–8

5. Horard B, Castet A, Bardet PL, et al. Dimerization is required for transactivation by estrogen-receptor-related (ERR) orphan receptors: evidence from amphioxus ERR. *J Mol Endocrinol* 2004; 33: 493–509

6. Horard B, Vanacker JM. Estrogen receptor-related receptors: orphan receptors desperately seeking a ligand. *J Mol Endocrinol* 2003; 31: 349–57

7. Riggs BL, Khosla S, Melton LJ III. Sex steroids and the construction and conservation of the adult skeleton. *Endocr Rev* 2002; 23: 279–302

8. Khosla S, Melton LJ III, Riggs BL. Clinical review 144: estrogen and the male skeleton. *J Clin Endocrinol Metab* 2002; 87: 1443–50

9. Rollerova E, Urbancikova M. Intracellular estrogen receptors, their characterization and function [Review]. *Endocr Regul* 2000; 34: 203–18

10. Kousteni S, Han L, Chen JR, et al. Kinase-mediated regulation of common transcription factors accounts for the bone-protective effects of sex steroids. *J Clin Invest* 2003; 111: 1651–64

11. Kousteni S, Chen JR, Bellido T, et al. Reversal of bone loss in mice by nongenotropic signaling of sex steroids. *Science* 2002; 298: 843–6

12. Bord S, Horner A, Beavan S, Compston J. Estrogen receptors alpha and beta are differentially expressed in developing human bone. *J Clin Endocrinol Metab* 2001; 86: 2309–14

13. Oursler MJ, Osdoby P, Pyfferoen J, et al. Avian osteoclasts as estrogen target cells. *Proc Natl Acad Sci USA* 1991; 88: 6613–17

14. Vanderschueren D, Vandenput L, Boonen S, et al. Androgens and bone. *Endocr Rev* 2004; 25: 389–425

15. Batra GS, Hainey L, Freemont AJ, et al. Evidence for cell-specific changes with age in expression of oestrogen receptor (ER) alpha and beta in bone fractures from men and women. *J Pathol* 2003; 200: 65–73

16. Levi G, Geoffroy V, Palmisano G, de Vernejoul MC. Bones, genes and fractures: workshop on the genetics of osteoporosis: from basic to clinical research. *EMBO Rep* 2002; 3: 22–6

17. Braidman IP, Hainey L, Batra G, et al. Localization of estrogen receptor beta protein expression in adult human bone. *J Bone Miner Res* 2001; 16: 214–20

18. Vidal O, Kindblom LG, Ohlsson C. Expression and localization of estrogen receptor-beta in murine and human bone. *J Bone Miner Res* 1999; 14: 923–9

19. Ramalho AC, Couttet P, Baudoin C, et al. Estradiol and raloxifene decrease the formation of multinucleate cells in human bone marrow cultures. *Eur Cytokine Netw* 2002; 13: 39–45

20. Huang WH, Lau AT, Daniels LL, et al. Detection of estrogen receptor alpha, carbonic anhydrase II and tartrate-resistant acid phosphatase mRNAs in putative mononuclear osteoclast precursor cells of neonatal rats by fluorescence in situ hybridization. *J Mol Endocrinol* 1998; 20: 211–19

21. Kusec V, Virdi AS, Prince R, Triffitt JT. Localization of estrogen receptor-alpha in human and rabbit skeletal tissues. *J Clin Endocrinol Metab* 1998; 83: 2421–8

22. Oreffo RO, Kusec V, Virdi AS, et al. Expression of estrogen receptor-alpha in cells of the osteoclastic lineage. *Histochem Cell Biol* 1999; 111: 125–33

23. Bord S, Horner A, Beavan S, Compston J. Estrogen receptors alpha and beta are differentially expressed in developing human bone. *J Clin Endocrinol Metab* 2001; 86: 2309–14

24. Sunyer T, Lewis J, Collin-Osdoby P, Osdoby P. Estrogen's bone-protective effects may involve differential IL-1 receptor regulation in human osteoclast-like cells. *J Clin Invest* 1999; 103: 1409–18

25. Bonnelye E, Kung V, Laplace C, et al. Estrogen receptor-related receptor alpha impinges on the

estrogen axis in bone: potential function in osteoporosis. *Endocrinology* 2002; 143: 3658–70

26. Shevde NK, Bendixen AC, Dienger KM, Pike JW. Estrogens suppress RANK ligand-induced osteoclast differentiation via a stromal cell independent mechanism involving c-Jun repression. *Proc Natl Acad Sci* USA 2000; 97: 7829–34

27. Srivastava S, Toraldo G, Weitzmann MN, et al. Estrogen decreases osteoclast formation by down-regulating receptor activator of NF-kappa B ligand (RANKL)-induced JNK activation. *J Biol Chem* 2001; 276: 8836–40

28. Srivastava S, Weitzmann MN, Cenci S, et al. Estrogen decreases TNF gene expression by blocking JNK activity and the resulting production of c-Jun and JunD. *J Clin Invest* 1999; 104: 503–13

29. Saintier D, Burde MA, Rey JM, et al. 17beta-estradiol downregulates beta3-integrin expression in differentiating and mature human osteoclasts. *J Cell Physiol* 2004; 198: 269–76

30. McHugh KP, Hodivala-Dilke K, Zheng MH, et al. Mice lacking beta3 integrins are osteosclerotic because of dysfunctional osteoclasts. *J Clin Invest* 2000; 105: 433–40

31. Oursler MJ, Pederson L, Fitzpatrick L, et al. Human giant cell tumors of the bone (osteoclastomas) are estrogen target cells. *Proc Natl Acad Sci* USA 1994; 91: 5227–31

32. Oursler MJ, Pederson L, Pyfferoen J, et al. Estrogen modulation of avian osteoclast lysosomal gene expression. *Endocrinology* 1993; 132: 1373–80

33. Kremer M, Judd J, Rifkin B, et al. Estrogen modulation of osteoclast lysosomal enzyme secretion. *J Cell Biochem* 1995; 57: 271–9

34. Saftig P, Hunziker E, Wehmeyer O, et al. Impaired osteoclastic bone resorption leads to osteopetrosis in cathepsin-K-deficient mice. *Proc Natl Acad Sci* USA 1998; 95: 13453–8

35. Gowen M, Lazner F, Dodds R, et al. Cathepsin K knockout mice develop osteopetrosis due to a deficit in matrix degradation but not demineralization. *J Bone Miner Res* 1999; 14: 1654–63

36. Hayman AR, Jones SJ, Boyde A, et al. Mice lacking tartrate-resistant acid phosphatase (Acp 5) have disrupted endochondral ossification and mild osteopetrosis. *Development* 1996; 122: 3151–62

37. Hollberg K, Hultenby K, Hayman A, et al. Osteoclasts from mice deficient in tartrate-resistant acid phosphatase have altered ruffled borders and disturbed intracellular vesicular transport. *Exp Cell Res* 2002; 279: 227–38

38. Pascoe D, Oursler MJ. The Src signaling pathway regulates osteoclast lysosomal enzyme secretion and is rapidly modulated by estrogen. *J Bone Miner Res* 2001; 16: 1028–36

39. Parikka V, Lehenkari P, Sassi ML, et al. Estrogen reduces the depth of resorption pits by disturbing the organic bone matrix degradation activity of mature osteoclasts. *Endocrinology* 2001; 142: 5371–8

40. Robinson JA, Riggs BL, Spelsberg TC, Oursler MJ. Osteoclasts and transforming growth factor-beta: estrogen-mediated isoform-specific regulation of production. *Endocrinology* 1996; 137: 615–21

41. Brubaker KD, Gay CV. Depolarization of osteoclast plasma membrane potential by 17beta-estradiol. *J Bone Miner Res* 1999; 14: 1861–6

42. Okabe K, Okamoto F, Kajiya H, et al. Estrogen directly acts on osteoclasts via inhibition of inward rectifier K+ channels. *Naunyn Schmiedebergs Arch Pharmacol* 2000; 361: 610–20

43. Gay CV, Kief NL, Bekker PJ. Effect of estrogen on acidification in osteoclasts. *Biochem Biophys Res Commun* 1993; 192: 1251–9

44. Kameda T, Mano H, Yuasa T, et al. Estrogen inhibits bone resorption by directly inducing apoptosis of the bone-resorbing osteoclasts. *J Exp Med* 1997; 186: 489–95

45. Lehenkari P, Parikka V, Rautiala TJ, et al. The effects of tamoxifen and toremifene on bone cells involve changes in plasma membrane ion conductance. *J Bone Miner Res* 2003; 18: 473–81

46. Arnett TR, Lindsay R, Kilb JM, et al. Selective toxic effects of tamoxifen on osteoclasts: comparison with the effects of oestrogen. *J Endocrinol* 1996; 149: 503–8

47. Chiu WS, McManus JF, Notini AJ, et al. Transgenic mice that express Cre recombinase in osteoclasts. *Genesis* 2004; 39: 178–85

48. Pederson L, Kremer M, Judd J, et al. Androgens regulate bone resorption activity of isolated osteoclasts in vitro. *Proc Natl Acad Sci* USA 1999; 96: 505–10

49. Mizuno Y, Hosoi T, Inoue S, et al. Immunocyto-chemical identification of androgen receptor in mouse osteoclast-like multinucleated cells. *Calcif Tissue Int* 1994; 54: 325–6

50. Abu EO, Horner A, Kusec V, et al. The localiza-tion of androgen receptors in human bone. *J Clin Endocrinol Metab* 1997; 82: 3493–7

51. Noble B, Routledge J, Stevens H, et al. Andro-gen receptors in bone-forming tissue. *Horm Res* 1999; 51: 31–6

52. Huber DM, Bendixen AC, Pathrose P, et al. Androgens suppress osteoclast formation induced by RANKL and macrophage-colony stimulating factor. *Endocrinology* 2001; 142: 3800–8

53. Sims NA, Dupont S, Krust A, et al. Deletion of estrogen receptors reveals a regulatory role for estrogen receptors-beta in bone remodeling in females but not in males. *Bone* 2002; 30: 18–25

54. Sims NA, Baron R. *Bone Cells and their Function*. Philadelphia: Lippincott Williams and Wilkins, 2000: 1–16

55. Smith EP, Boyd J, Frank GR, et al. Estrogen resistance caused by a mutation in the estrogen-receptor gene in a man. *N Engl J Med* 1994; 331: 1056–61

56. Anderson FH, Francis RM, Peaston RT, Wastell HJ. Androgen supplementation in eugonadal men with osteoporosis: effects of six months' treatment on markers of bone formation and resorption. *J Bone Miner Res* 1997; 12: 472–8

57. Katznelson L, Finkelstein JS, Schoenfeld DA, et al. Increase in bone density and lean body mass during testosterone administration in men with acquired hypogonadism. *J Clin Endocrinol Metab* 1996; 81: 4358–65

58. Sims NA, Clement-Lacroix P, Minet D, et al. A functional androgen receptor is not sufficient to allow estradiol to protect bone after gonadec-tomy in estradiol receptor-deficient mice. *J Clin Invest* 2003; 111: 1319–27

59. Kawano H, Sato T, Yamada T, et al. Suppressive function of androgen receptor in bone resorp-tion. *Proc Natl Acad Sci* USA 2003; 100: 9416–21

60. Turner RT, Riggs BL, Spelsberg TC. Skeletal effects of estrogen. *Endocr Rev* 1994; 15: 275–300

61. Pacifici R. Estrogen, cytokines, and pathogenesis of postmenopausal osteoporosis. *J Bone Miner Res* 1996; 11: 1043–51

62. Manolagas SC, Jilka RL. Bone marrow, cytokines, and bone remodeling. Emerging insights into the pathophysiology of osteoporo-sis. *N Engl J Med* 1995; 332: 305–11

63. Jilka RL, Hangoc G, Girasole G, et al. Increased osteoclast development after estrogen loss: mediation by interleukin-6. *Science* 1992; 257: 88–91

64. Cosman F, Lindsay R. Selective estrogen receptor modulators: clinical spectrum. *Endocr Rev* 1999; 20: 418–34

65. Kimble RB, Vannice JL, Bloedow DC, et al. Interleukin-1 receptor antagonist decreases bone loss and bone resorption in ovariectomized rats. *J Clin Invest* 1994; 93: 1959–67

66. Bismar H, Diel I, Ziegler R, Pfeilschifter J. Increased cytokine secretion by human bone marrow cells after menopause or discontinuation of estrogen replacement. *J Clin Endocrinol Metab* 1995; 80: 3351–5

67. Eghbali-Fatourechi G, Khosla S, Sanyal A, et al. Role of RANK ligand in mediating increased bone resorption in early postmenopausal women. *J Clin Invest* 2003; 111: 1221–30

68. Khosla S, Atkinson EJ, Dunstan CR, O'Fallon WM. Effect of estrogen versus testosterone on circulating osteoprotegerin and other cytokine levels in normal elderly men. *J Clin Endocrinol Metab* 2002; 87: 1550–4

69. Hofbauer LC, Schoppet M. Clinical implications of the osteoprotegerin/RANKL/RANK system for bone and vascular diseases. *J Am Med Assoc* 2004; 292: 490–5

70. Hughes DE, Dai A, Tiffee JC, et al. Estrogen promotes apoptosis of murine osteoclasts medi-ated by TGF-beta. *Nat Med* 1996; 2: 1132–6

71. Riggs BL, Khosla S, Melton LJ III. Sex steroids and the construction and conservation of the adult skeleton. *Endocr Rev* 2002; 23: 279–302

72. Cenci S, Weitzmann MN, Roggia C, et al. Estro-gen deficiency induces bone loss by enhancing T-cell production of TNF-alpha. *J Clin Invest* 2000; 106: 1229–37

73. Kimble RB, Srivastava S, Ross FP, et al. Estrogen deficiency increases the ability of stromal cells to support murine osteoclastogenesis via an inter-

leukin-1and tumor necrosis factor-mediated stimulation of macrophage colony-stimulating factor production. *J Biol Chem* 1996; 271: 28890–7

74. Roggia C, Gao Y, Cenci S, et al. Upregulation of TNF-producing T cells in the bone marrow: a key mechanism by which estrogen deficiency induces bone loss in vivo. *Proc Natl Acad Sci* USA 2001; 98: 13960–5

75. Manolagas SC. Birth and death of bone cells: basic regulatory mechanisms and implications for the pathogenesis and treatment of osteoporosis. *Endocr Rev* 2000; 21: 115–37

76. Miyazaki T, Katagiri H, Kanegae Y, et al. Reciprocal role of ERK and NF-kappaB pathways in survival and activation of osteoclasts. *J Cell Biol* 2000; 148: 333–42

77. Fuller K, Owens JM, Jagger CJ, et al. Macrophage colony-stimulating factor stimulates survival and chemotactic behavior in isolated osteoclasts. *J Exp Med* 1993; 178: 1733–44

78. Wiktor-Jedrzejczak W, Bartocci A, Ferrante AW Jr, et al. Total absence of colony-stimulating factor 1 in the macrophage-deficient osteopetrotic (op/op) mouse. *Proc Natl Acad Sci USA* 1990; 87: 4828–32

79. Hofbauer LC, Khosla S, Dunstan CR, et al. Estrogen stimulates gene expression and protein production of osteoprotegerin in human osteoblastic cells. *Endocrinology* 1999; 140: 4367–70

80. Saika M, Inoue D, Kido S, Matsumoto T. 17beta-estradiol stimulates expression of osteoprotegerin by a mouse stromal cell line, ST-2, via estrogen receptor-alpha. *Endocrinology* 2001; 142: 2205–12

81. Bord S, Ireland DC, Beavan SR, Compston JE. The effects of estrogen on osteoprotegerin, RANKL, and estrogen receptor expression in human osteoblasts. *Bone* 2003; 32: 136–41

82. Oursler MJ, Cortese C, Keeting P, et al. Modulation of transforming growth factor-beta production in normal human osteoblast-like cells by 17 beta-estradiol and parathyroid hormone. *Endocrinology* 1991; 129: 3313–20

83. Karsdal MA, Hjorth P, Henriksen K, et al. TGF-beta controls human osteoclastogenesis through the p38 MAPK and regulation of RANK expression. *J Biol Chem* 2003; 278: 975–87

84. Heino TJ, Hentunen TA, Vaananen HK. Osteocytes inhibit osteoclastic bone resorption through transforming growth factor-beta: enhancement by estrogen. *J Cell Biochem* 2002; 85: 185–97

85. Gao Y, Qian WP, Dark K, et al. Estrogen prevents bone loss through transforming growth factor beta-signaling in T cells. *Proc Natl Acad Sci USA* 2004; 101: 16618–23

86. Cadogan J, Blumsohn A, Barker ME, Eastell R. A longitudinal study of bone gain in pubertal girls: anthropometric and biochemical correlates. *J Bone Miner* Res 1998; 13: 1602–12

87. Zittermann A, Schwarz I, Scheld K, et al. Physiologic fluctuations of serum estradiol levels influence biochemical markers of bone resorption in young women. *J Clin Endocrinol Metab* 2000; 85: 95–101

88. Rosenbrock H, Seifert-Klauss V, Kaspar S, et al. Changes of biochemical bone markers during the menopausal transition. *Clin Chem Lab Med* 2002; 40: 143–51

89. Peichl P, Griesmacher A, Pointinger P, et al. Association between female sex hormones and biochemical markers of bone turnover in peri- and postmenopausal women. *Calcif Tissue Int* 1998; 62: 388–94

90. De Souza MJ, Miller BE, Sequenzia LC, et al. Bone health is not affected by luteal phase abnormalities and decreased ovarian progesterone production in female runners. *J Clin Endocrinol Metab* 1997; 82: 2867–76

91. Hetland ML, Haarbo J, Christiansen C, Larsen T. Running induces menstrual disturbances but bone mass is unaffected, except in amenorrheic women. *Am J Med* 1993; 95: 53–60

92. Waller K, Reim J, Fenster L, et al. Bone mass and subtle abnormalities in ovulatory function in healthy women. *J Clin Endocrinol Metab* 1996; 81: 663–8

93. Christiansen C. Hormone replacement therapy and osteoporosis. *Maturitas* 1996; 23 (Suppl): S71–6

94. Delmas PD. Hormone replacement therapy in the prevention and treatment of osteoporosis. *Osteoporos Int* 1997; 7 (Suppl 1), S37

95. Bagger YZ, Tanko LB, Alexandersen P, et al. Two to three years of hormone replacement treatment in healthy women have long-term

preventive effects on bone mass and osteoporotic fractures: the PERF study. *Bone* 2004; 34: 728–35

96. Lindsay R, Hart DM, MacLean A, et al. Bone response to termination of oestrogen treatment. *Lancet* 1978; 1: 1325–7

97. Horsman A, Nordin BE, Crilly RG. Effect on bone of withdrawal of oestrogen therapy. *Lancet* 1979; 2: 33

98. Christiansen C, Christensen MS, Transbol I. Bone mass after withdrawal of oestrogen replacement. *Lancet* 1981; 11: 1053–4

99. Sulak PJ. Endometrial cancer and hormone replacement therapy. Appropriate use of progestins to oppose endogenous and exogenous estrogen. *Endocrinol Metab Clin North Am* 1997; 26: 399–412

100. Meier DE, Orwoll ES, Keenan EJ, Fagerstrom RM. Marked decline in trabecular bone mineral content in healthy men with age: lack of association with sex steroid levels. *J Am Geriatr Soc* 1987; 35: 189–97

101. Harman SM, Tsitouras PD. Reproductive hormones in aging men. I. Measurement of sex steroids, basal luteinizing hormone, and Leydig cell response to human chorionic gonadotropin. *J Clin Endocrinol Metab* 1980; 51: 35–40

102. Riggs BL, Wahner HW, Dunn WL, et al. Differential changes in bone mineral density of the appendicular and axial skeleton with aging: relationship to spinal osteoporosis. *J Clin Invest* 1981; 67: 328–35

103. Jones G, Nguyen T, Sambrook P, et al. Progressive loss of bone in the femoral neck in elderly people: longitudinal findings from the Dubbo osteoporosis epidemiology study. *Br Med J* 1994; 309: 691–5

104. Khosla S, Melton LJ III, Atkinson EJ, et al. Relationship of serum sex steroid levels and bone turnover markers with bone mineral density in

men and women: a key role for bioavailable estrogen. *J Clin Endocrinol Metab* 1998; 83: 2266–74

105. Khosla S, Melton LJ III, Atkinson EJ, O'Fallon WM. Relationship of serum sex steroid levels to longitudinal changes in bone density in young versus elderly men. *J Clin Endocrinol Metab* 2001; 86: 3555–61

106. Murphy S, Khaw KT, Sneyd MJ, Compston JE. Endogenous sex hormones and bone mineral density among community-based postmenopausal women. *Postgrad Med J* 1992; 68: 908–13

107. Slemenda CW, Longcope C, Zhou L, et al. Sex steroids and bone mass in older men. Positive associations with serum estrogens and negative associations with androgens. *J Clin Invest* 1997; 100: 1755–9

108. Smith EP, Boyd J, Frank GR, et al. Estrogen resistance caused by a mutation in the estrogen-receptor gene in a man. *N Engl J Med* 1994; 331: 1056–61

109. Morishima A, Grumbach MM, Simpson ER, et al. Aromatase deficiency in male and female siblings caused by a novel mutation and the physiological role of estrogens. *J Clin Endocrinol Metab* 1995; 80: 3689–98

110. Carani C, Qin K, Simoni M, et al. Effect of testosterone and estradiol in a man with aromatase deficiency. *N Engl J Med* 1997; 337: 91–5

111. Szulc P, Hofbauer LC, Heufelder AE, et al. Osteoprotegerin serum levels in men: correlation with age, estrogen, and testosterone status. *J Clin Endocrinol Metab* 2001; 86: 3162–5

112. Falahati-Nini A, Riggs BL, Atkinson EJ, et al. Relative contributions of testosterone and estrogen in regulating bone resorption and formation in normal elderly men. *J Clin Invest* 2000; 106: 1553–60

Calcium and vitamin D: regulation of mineral homeostasis

6

D. Goltzman

HORMONAL CONTROL OF EXTRACELLULAR CALCIUM

Extracellular fluid (ECF) calcium is maintained under tight control within a relatively narrow range because of the importance of the calcium ion (Ca^{2+}) as a regulator of many homeostatic processes. Fluxes of calcium across the intestine, kidney and bone are the most important determinants of ECF Ca^{2+}. If 1000 mg of dietary Ca^{2+} are ingested, about 400 mg are absorbed in the intestine. Approximately 200 mg are excreted in the urine and about 200 mg are deposited in bone, to compensate for 200 mg which is resorbed from bone daily. The major hormonal regulators of Ca^{2+} transport across the gut, bone and kidney are the peptide hormone, parathyroid hormone (PTH) and the secosteroid 1,25-dihydroxyvitamin D ($1,25(OH)_2D$).

The major glandular form of PTH is 84 amino acids in length, but most of the bioactivity resides in the amino-terminal region. A genetic relative of PTH is PTH-related peptide (PTHrP), which was initially discovered as the mediator of hypercalcemia of malignancy, and which shares weak amino-acid sequence homology with PTH. Because of this limited but important homology within the amino-terminal domain, the amino-terminal region of each molecule can cross-react with a common type I PTH/PTHrP membrane receptor in target tissues and induce many of the same biological responses. Nevertheless, recent studies have also shown that these molecules may exert independent effects.

Another hormonal contributor to calcium homeostasis is ECF Ca^{2+} itself, which can bind to a specific membrane receptor, the calcium-sensing receptor (CaR)[1]. Thus elevations in ECF Ca^{2+} will act via the CaR in the parathyroid cell and induce cell signaling, which inhibits PTH production and secretion. The CaR is expressed in multiple tissues, and in addition to the parathyroid cell also plays an important function in the renal tubule cell. Here, elevations in ECF Ca^{2+} can signal via the CaR to inhibit NaCl transport and thereby decrease Ca^{2+} reabsorption. This results in an elevation in the renal tubular luminal Ca^{2+} and ultimately in urine Ca^{2+}. An analogous situation appears to exist in lactating breast-tubule epithelium, where an increase in Ca^{2+} can, via the CaR, result in an increase in Ca^{2+} in milk[2].

The metabolic activation of vitamin D to its hormonal form is a multistep process (Figure 1)[3]. Ultraviolet (UV) irradiation of the skin converts a skin precursor, 7-dehydrocholesterol, to a pre-vitamin D_3 which is then converted to vitamin D_3 (cholecalciferol). Vitamin D_3 then enters the bloodstream and can circulate bound to a vitamin D-binding protein (DBP). Vitamin D_3 can also be absorbed from the diet via the gut, as can a plant-derived sterol, ergocalciferol or vitamin D_2. Vitamin D is then transported to the liver where it undergoes a first hydroxylation via a hepatic 25-hydroxylase to produce 25-hydroxyvitamin D (25(OH)D). This metabolite is the most abundant circulating and stored form of vitamin D. The generated 25(OH)D is then transported to the kidney where it can undergo a second hydroxylation at one of two major sites on the molecule. In the presence of increased PTH or decreased serum phosphorus (P_i), the renal enzyme, 25-hydroxyvitamin D 1α-hydroxylase (1α(OH)ase) is stimulated and 25(OH)D is converted to the active form, $1,25(OH)_2D$, which

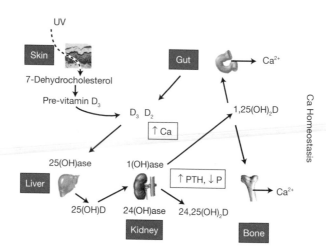

Figure 1 Metabolic activation of vitamin D. Ultraviolet (UV) light exposure of skin converts a precursor, 7-dehydrocholesterol, to pre-vitamin D_3, which is converted to vitamin D_3 (cholecalciferol), which then enters the bloodstream. Vitamin D_3 or vitamin D_2 (ergocalciferol) can also be absorbed from the diet via the gut. Vitamin D is then transported to the liver and 25(OH)D is formed via the action of a 25(OH)ase enzyme. The 25(OH)D can then be converted in the kidney either to bioactive 1,25(OH)$_2$D via the action of a 1α(OH)ase enzyme, or to bioinert 24,25(OH)$_2$D via the action of a 24(OH)ase. The 1α(OH)ase is stimulated by elevated parathyroid hormone (PTH) and low phosporus (P_i) and inhibited by elevated Ca^{2+} and by 1,25(OH)$_2$D. The bioactive 1,25(OH)$_2$D can then enhance Ca^{2+} absorption from the gut and resorb Ca^{2+} from bone

will then circulate and regulate Ca^{2+} homeostasis. Elevated Ca^{2+} and 1,25(OH)$_2$D can both inhibit the 1α(OH)ase. In the presence of high Ca^{2+}, low PTH, high P_i or high 1,25(OH)$_2$D, a renal 24-hydroxylase enzyme is stimulated and 25(OH)D is converted to 24,25(OH)$_2$D, which appears overall to be an inert metabolite.

Abundant evidence points to the prime importance of UV exposure as a source of vitamin D. Few unfortified foods other than fatty fish (such as salmon and herring) contain appreciable amounts of vitamin D. Even in countries where a variety of foods is fortified with vitamin D, circulating 25(OH)D concentrations will vary according to the month of the year, with peak values found at the end of the summer and lowest value during the winter[4]. This important role of UV exposure of the skin in generating vitamin D may be mitigated, even in sunny climates, by naturally occurring skin hyperpigmentation, use of sunscreen and sunblocks or clothing customs and traditions which shield the skin from UV exposure.

Metabolism of vitamin D may, however, be even more complex than previously appreciated. In recent years, extrarenal 1α(OH)ases have been described in many tissues, including immune cells, prostate, breast, colon, bone cells and muscle cells, which can apparently convert 25(OH)D to 1,25(OH)$_2$D locally. Locally produced 1,25(OH)$_2$D, acting as a paracrine/autocrine factor, may therefore have additional roles to play in such diverse functions as immunomodulation, cell growth, bone health and muscle health[3].

In target cells, the 1,25(OH)$_2$D sterol binds to its cognate receptor, the vitamin D receptor (VDR), which is found in multiple tissues. It heterodimerizes with the retinoid X receptor (RXR) and then mobilizes a variety of coregulatory molecules. The complex will bind to vitamin D response elements (VDREs) on target genes and then increase or decrease gene transcription.

The integrated control of ECF Ca^{2+} by PTH, Ca^{2+} and 1,25(OH)$_2$D appears to function as

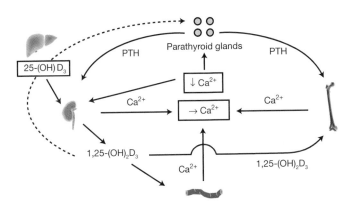

Figure 2 Hormonal regulation of extracellular fluid (ECF) Ca^{2+}. A reduction in ECF Ca^{2+} will stimulate parathyroid hormone (PTH) release. PTH then acts in the kidney to enhance Ca^{2+} reabsorption and increase $1,25(OH)_2D_3$ production. Low ECF Ca^{2+} will also enhance Ca^{2+} reabsorption. The $1,25(OH)_2D_3$ will increase intestinal Ca^{2+} absorption and, with PTH, resorb bone to release Ca^{2+}. The result is a normalization of ECF Ca^{2+} and a loss of the stimulus to increase PTH further

follows (Figure 2). A reduction in ECF Ca^{2+} acting via the CaR serves as a signal to increase PTH release from the parathyroid glands. PTH then acts on the kidney to enhance the renal reabsorption of Ca^{2+} and to stimulate the renal $1\alpha(OH)ase$, which then converts $25(OH)D$ to the active form, $1,25(OH)_2D$. Low ECF Ca^{2+}, acting via the CaR, may also contribute to increased renal calcium reabsorption. The $1,25(OH)_2D$ formed in the kidney will then increase intestinal calcium transport, and both PTH and $1,25(OH)_2D$ can increase bone resorption and liberate Ca^{2+} from bone. These combined effects on kidney, intestine and bone then lead to an increase in ECF Ca^{2+}, and turn off the signal for further PTH release. Phosphorus (P_i) will also be absorbed with Ca^{2+} from the intestine and will be resorbed from the bone with Ca^{2+}, but the phosphaturic effect of PTH prevents a net serum increase in P_i. This paradigm for the integrated control of ECF Ca^{2+} by hormones is somewhat idealized, however, and extensive modification of this scheme may occur at various stages during growth and development.

ACCRUAL AND LOSS OF SKELETAL MASS

Bone is by far the largest repository for calcium in the body, and calcium in turn provides bone with its unique tissue strength. Bone mass increases until it reaches a peak at approximately age 30–35 (Figure 3). Fracture predisposition in later life appears to be a function of both the quantity and quality of peak adult bone mass that is achieved, as well as the rate at which bone is subsequently lost. It is important, therefore, to understand how alterations in mineral homeostasis influence both the accrual of bone and its loss. Mineral homeostasis and its effect on bone will differ, however, through different stages of growth, development and aging. It is consequently of interest to examine the differing paradigms of mineral homeostasis during these stages.

Fetal mineral and skeletal homeostasis

Although fetal skeletal accrual provides a relatively minor quantitative component of total

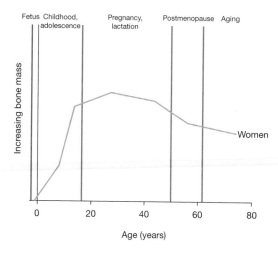

Figure 3 Stages of skeletal evolution. Bone mass begins to accrue in the fetus and accelerates markedly during adolescence. Further slower increases occur until about mid-life. In the postmenopausal period, the rate of bone loss accelerates. Bone loss continues at a lower rate during aging

skeletal mass, it is an important foundation which may markedly contribute to the subsequent quantity and quality of bone. Calcium is required by the fetus both for skeletal growth and to maintain an ECF level of Ca^{2+} that is higher than in the mother[4]. All fetal calcium is derived from maternal sources by transport across placental membranes. By the third trimester, this amounts to approximately 200 mg per day. Maintenance of ECF Ca^{2+} is also derived mainly from placental Ca^{2+} transport, but possibly also from fetal bone resorption and renal reabsorption from the kidney. Gut absorption seems to play a smaller role. From experiments in animals in which genetic ablation of genes encoding PTHrP[5], CaR[6] and PTH[7] have been performed, it appears that PTHrP and CaR play a critical role in the transport of Ca^{2+} across the placenta. PTHrP is also important for normal cartilaginous growth plate development[8], and PTH in the fetus is essential for normal trabecular bone formation[9], i.e. it is 'anabolic' for trabecular bone. Whether PTH or PTHrP helps to maintain the high fetal ECF Ca^{2+} by resorbing cortical bone or enhancing renal Ca^{2+} reabsorption in the fetal kidney is as yet unknown[10]. Studies of genetic ablation of

genes encoding the $1\alpha(OH)$ase and the VDR suggest that $1,25(OH)_2D_3$ may have little role to play in the physiologic modulation of ECF Ca^{2+} in the fetus.

Mineral and skeletal homeostasis during pregnancy

During pregnancy, total calcium may drop within the range of normal as a result of expansion of the ECF volume, but ionized Ca^{2+} remains normal[11]. PTH concentrations may decline to the lower limits of normal and then rise slightly within the normal range toward the end of pregnancy. A major increase in circulating $1,25(OH)_2D_3$, which originates from the maternal kidney, has been noted by a number of investigators. This increase appears to persist to the end of pregnancy. A few studies have also reported increases in PTHrP, particularly in the third trimester. The maternal increases in $1,25(OH)_2D_3$ that occur enhance Ca^{2+} absorption and may transiently increase ECF Ca^{2+}, decrease PTH and produce hypercalciuria. Maternal increases in PTHrP seem important for the transport of Ca^{2+} across the placenta to the fetus, but may also stimulate bone resorption. In the mother, the maternal urinary Ca^{2+} losses and losses of Ca^{2+} to the fetus may normalize the maternal ECF Ca^{2+}, by offsetting the transient increase in ECF Ca^{2+} caused by enhanced $1,25(OH)_2D_3$-induced Ca^{2+} transport and increased PTHrP-induced bone resorption. Overall, however, the main maternal source of Ca^{2+} for the fetus is derived from intestinal Ca^{2+} absorption, with some contribution of increased bone resorption. Urine Ca^{2+} losses represent an additional stress on maternal Ca^{2+} homeostasis. Consequently, it is important to ensure adequate vitamin D as a substrate for $1,25(OH)_2D_3$, and adequate dietary Ca^{2+} for the $1,25(OH)_2D_3$ to absorb. In many countries, the recommended intake of dietary calcium is 1 g per day, and the recommended consumption of vitamin D is 200–400 international units (IU) per day (5–10 µg per day). This recommended intake of vitamin D may be quite insufficient, according to some experts[12].

Mineral and skeletal homeostasis during lactation

During lactation, there is a stress on maternal calcium homeostasis caused by the need for providing Ca^{2+} in breast-milk. Total ECF calcium may increase in the mother within the normal range as the ECF volume returns to normal after pregnancy; ionized Ca^{2+} remains normal. PTH may decline within the normal range, but may transiently rise during and after weaning[4]. Circulating $1,25(OH)_2D_3$ concentrations fall into the normal range from their elevated levels during pregnancy, and may rise transiently after weaning. PTHrP concentrations appear to increase during lactation and then fall during weaning. The major source of calcium for milk in the lactating mother appears to be maternal bone. Reduced levels of estrogen caused by gonadotropin releasing hormone (GnRH) suppression by prolactin result in increased bone resorption, and the calcium liberated from bone can suppress PTH and $1,25(OH)_2D_3$ levels. Prolactin may also increase PTHrP from lactating breast tissue, which can contribute to the bone resorption[13,14]. Studies with targeted inactivation of the CaR gene in mice indicate that a fall in ECF Ca^{2+} can trigger, via CaR in breast tissue, increased PTHrP release from the lactating breast, which will resorb bone and restore ECF Ca^{2+} to normal. PTHrP action on enhancing bone resorption is supplemented by its effect on increasing urinary Ca^{2+} reabsorption. Therefore, to prevent excessive bone resorption during lactation, appropriate dietary intakes of calcium and vitamin D are required in order to provide the Ca^{2+} for breast milk. Whether the current recommendations of approximately 1000 mg of dietary calcium per day and 400 IU (10 µg) of vitamin D per day are appropriate is uncertain[12].

Mineral and skeletal homeostasis during childhood and adolescence

The largest increment in skeletal growth occurs during late childhood and adolescence. From age 9 to age 21, skeletal calcium deposition may increase from 900 to 2200 g, i.e. an increase of over 100 g per year[15]. At present, 200 IU per day

(5 µg per day) of vitamin D is generally recommended as sufficient vitamin D intake in children and adolescents. Approximately 500–1000 mg of calcium per day is generally recommended from ages 1 to 10, and approximately 1300 mg per day during adolescence. Whether this is sufficient is unclear[16]. What continues to be reported, however, is the persistence of vitamin D-deficient rickets in children[17–19]. Mild vitamin D deficiency may decrease calcium absorption and result in secondary hyperparathyroidism and increased bone resorption, and could lead to reduced bone mass in later life[20]. More severe vitamin D deficiency, however, may result in persistent hypocalcemia, more severe secondary hypoparathyroidism and rickets (i.e. a distorted cartilaginous growth plate with poor mineralization) and osteomalacia (i.e. excess osteoid or unmineralized trabecular and cortical bone). Because of the increased requirement for mineral during rapid skeletal growth, childhood and adolescence may present unique opportunities for development of these manifestations of severe vitamin D deficiency, even if calcium and vitamin D are only moderately limited.

Mineral and skeletal homeostasis in menopausal women

During the premenopausal era and especially during the postmenopausal era, reduction and loss of estrogen is the major determinant of increased bone resorption, leading to osteoporosis[15]. ECF Ca^{2+} generally does not rise because of the suppression of PTH and of $1,25(OH)_2D_3$ production and resulting increased losses of urinary Ca^{2+} and decreased Ca^{2+} absorption, respectively[15]. It is interesting to contrast this situation with the physiology prevailing during lactation. In lactation, estrogen deficiency is combined with PTHrP excess to resorb bone and direct Ca^{2+} into breast-milk. Losses of bone mineral can be more severe than after the menopause, but are reversible. In the menopausal situation, estrogen deficiency without the participation of PTHrP results in less severe bone loss but is more sustained and is irreversible. The estrogen withdrawal effect to increase bone resorption can therefore be viewed as a positive adaptive effect during lactation. The persistence of this effect in postreproductive menopausal women, however, represents a negative adaptation contributing to aging.

Mineral and skeletal homeostasis during aging

During the aging process, diminished vitamin D intake and synthesis along with reduced dietary calcium intake can contribute, via secondary hyperparathyroidism, to excessive bone resorption[21]. Studies have demonstrated reduced production of vitamin D after UV exposure in the elderly. Furthermore, lower 25(OH)D concentrations are more prevalent in the elderly, and decreasing mean 25(OH)D concentrations have been noted in elderly hip-fracture patients and institutionalized as compared with independent elderly.

Diminished bone formation may also play a role. Although the mediators of the decreased bone formation are unclear, recent work in animals suggests that PTHrP[9] and $1,25(OH)_2D_3$[22] have anabolic roles (as well as catabolic) in bone. This then is analogous to the biphasic effects of PTH on inducing both resorption and formation. Reduction in the levels or efficacy of these hormones with aging might contribute to the decreased bone formation seen in the elderly. In aging women, the role of reduced estrogen in enhanced bone resorption can continue to contribute to the development of osteoporosis (Figure 4)[15].

VITAMIN D DEFICIENCY IN ADULTS

Assessment of vitamin D deficiency

Current recommendations for adults in North America are generally for vitamin D intakes of 200–400 IU (5–10 µg) per day. Over 70 years of age, 600 IU (15 µg) may be recommended. In Europe, an intake of 400 IU per day is usually recommended for the elderly. How can we assess the vitamin D sufficiency of an individual and whether these levels of vitamin D intake are sufficient? Assays of both the active metabolite, $1,25(OH)_2D_3$, and of the most abundant circulating form, 25(OH)D, are both available.

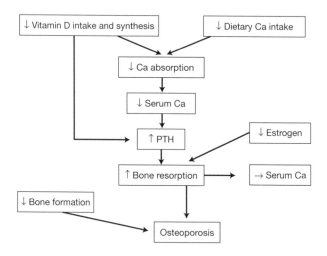

Figure 4 Postmenopausal and age-related bone loss. During aging, reduced vitamin D intake and synthesis and reduced dietary calcium intake occur, leading to decreased calcium absorption and secondary hyperparathyroidism. Decreased bone formation may also play a role. Estrogen withdrawal after the menopause also results in enhanced bone resorption. The increased bone resorption and decreased formation together contribute to progressive bone loss. PTH, parathyroid hormone

Assays of $1,25(OH)_2D_3$, a metabolite which circulates at considerably lower concentrations than $25(OH)D$, are still somewhat technically difficult. From a biological perspective, circulating $1,25(OH)_2D_3$ concentrations may be normal despite the presence of vitamin D deficiency, because of the compensatory stimulation of the renal $1\alpha(OH)$ase by hypocalcemia and secondary hyperparathyroidism. Furthermore, if local production of $1,25(OH)_2D_3$ is required for many of the actions of vitamin D, circulating levels may not reflect local levels inasmuch as the extrarenal $1\alpha(OH)$ase may be differently regulated compared with its renal enzyme. Consequently, $25(OH)D$ rather than $1,25(OH)_2D_3$ measurement has been accepted as a valid means to assess vitamin D deficiency. Measurement of $25(OH)D$ may also employ a variety of laboratory methods such that identical samples may be reported quite differently by different laboratories. Nevertheless, international cooperative groups such as the Vitamin D External Quality Assessment Scheme (DEQAS) have been developed to ensure quality control of these assays[23]. A more difficult caveat, however, is the issue of deciding what constitutes a normal, or abnormal, $25(OH)D$ concentration. A variety of indices have been suggested to define what a 'desirable' $25(OH)D$ concentration might be[24]. These include determining whether PTH concentrations are normal, whether bone marker concentrations are normal, whether bone mineral density is preserved, whether fractures are prevented and perhaps whether other health-related events such as cancer are prevented[25–27]. Others have suggested that the highest concentration that would avoid toxicity is what is required for a 'desirable' $25(OH)D$ concentration. Furthermore, it is not certain that 'desirable' concentrations are the same even for all adults, because of influences on mineral and skeletal homeostasis of variables such as age, sex, calcium intake and even exercise. Although the technical and biological variabilities which impinge on assay measurement make study comparisons difficult, in general, $25(OH)D$ concentrations of less than 12.5–25 nmol/l result in severe vitamin D deficiency and osteomalacia, concentrations less than 50 nmol/l are associated with secondary hyperparathyroidism and excessive bone resorption, which may lead to fractures, and concentrations less than 70–80 nmol/l may still provide suboptimal calcium absorption and perhaps mild secondary hyperparathyroidism (Figure 5). Toxicity, with hypercalciuria and hypercalcemia, generally occurs at concentrations of 250 nmol/l or higher[12].

Prevalence of vitamin D deficiency in adults

Low concentrations of $25(OH)D$ are prevalent worldwide in postmenopausal women, and have in fact been found to be more common in southern Europe and in Latin America than in northern Europe[24]. This may reflect the UV-protective effects of skin pigmentation and traditions of clothing in these countries, leading to hypovitaminosis D, versus the high intake of fatty fish in Scandinavian countries which may provide vitamin D sufficiency. Irrespective of the ubiquitous nature of vitamin D insufficiency, it is possible to raise circulating $25(OH)D$ concentrations even in the elderly by administering vitamin D. Nevertheless, the daily amounts required to achieve concentrations of 70–80 nmol/l may be considerably higher than the currently recommended doses of approximately 400 IU per day.

Effectiveness of vitamin D supplementation

Will increases in vitamin D consumption reduce the incidence of fractures in postmenopausal women? A number of studies have explored this issue; however, different study designs, including different study duration, use or non-use of calcium with vitamin D and the use or non-use of calcium for control groups, has made comparisons difficult. Nevertheless, meta-analyses of these studies suggest that either vitamin D or hydroxylated vitamin D supplements can reduce vertebral fractures by at least 30%. Although reductions are less clear for non-vertebral fractures, pooled estimates suggest that decreases of over 20% may occur. Consequently, relatively inexpensive therapy with vitamin D may provide

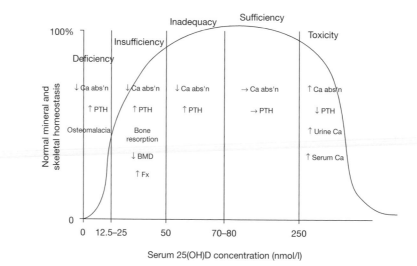

Figure 5 Concentrations of 25(OH)D required for mineral and skeletal homeostasis. Below 12.5–25 nmol/l, osteomalacia will generally occur. Hyperparathyroidism and bone resorption will occur below 50 nmol/l, and some residual reduced calcium absorption (abs'n) and secondary hyperparathyroidism may still be seen below 70–80 nmol/l. Concentrations of approximately 250 nmol/l or higher will produce evidence of vitamin D toxicity. PTH, parathyroid hormone; BMD, bone mineral density; Fx, fractures

considerable benefit even when introduced in the postmenopausal era.

CONCLUSIONS

Overall, understanding the physiology of mineral and skeletal homeostasis during sequential stages of growth, development and aging can provide insights into mineral and hormone requirements to achieve optimal peak bone mass and to reduce postmaturity bone loss. Nevertheless, more controlled, long-term prospective trials of vitamin D and calcium replacement are required, particularly to determine effects of supplementation of these nutrients on peak bone mass and subsequent fracture risk. This should lead to more effective measures to maximize skeletal development and to diminish the loss of bone that occurs during the aging process.

ACKNOWLEDGMENTS

This work was supported by grants from the Canadian Institutes for Health Research and the National Cancer Institute of Canada.

References

1. Brown EM, MacLeod RJ. Extracellular calcium sensing and extracellular calcium signaling. *Physiol Rev* 2001; 81: 239–97

2. VanHouten J, Dann P, McGeoch G, et al. The calcium-sensing receptor regulates mammary gland parathyroid hormone related protein production and calcium transport. *J Clin Invest* 2004; 113: 598–608

3. Holick MF. Vitamin D: a millennium perspective. *J Cell Biochem* 2003; 88: 296–307

4. Kovacs CS, Kronenberg HM. Maternal–fetal calcium and bone metabolism during pregnancy, puerperium lactation. *Endocr Rev* 1997; 18: 832–72

5. Kovacs CS, Lanske B, Hunzelman JL, et al. Parathyroid hormone-related peptide (PTHrP) regulates fetal–placental calcium transport through a receptor distinct from the PTH/PTHrP receptor. *Proc Natl Acad Sci* USA 1996; 93: 15233–8

6. Kovacs CS, Ho-Pao CL, Hunzelman JL, et al. Regulation of murine fetal–placental calcium metabolism by the calcium-sensing receptor. *J Clin Invest* 1998; 101: 2812–20

7. Kovacs CS, Manley NR, Moseley JM, et al. Fetal parathyroids are not required to maintain placental calcium transport. *J Clin Invest* 2001; 107: 1007–15

8. Amizuka N, Warshawksy H, Henderson JE, et al. Parathyroid hormone-related peptide-depleted mice show abnormal epiphysial cartilage development and altered endochondral bone formation. *J Cell Biol* 2001; 126: 1611–23

9. Miao D, Li J, Xue Y, Su H, et al. Parathyroid hormone-related peptide is required for increased trabecular bone volume in parathyroid hormone-null mice. *Endocrinology* 2004; 145: 3554–62

10. Kovacs CS, Chafe LL, Fudge NJ, et al. PTH regulates fetal blood calcium and skeletal mineralization independently of PTHrP. *Endocrinology* 2001; 142: 4983–93

11. Kovacs CS. Calcium and bone metabolism in pregnancy and lactation. *J Clin Endocrinol Metab* 2001; 86: 2344–8

12. Hollis BW, Wagner CL. Assessment of dietary vitamin D requirements during pregnancy and lactation. *Am J Clin Nutr* 2004; 79: 717–26

13. VanHouten JN, Wysolmerski JJ. Low estrogen and high parathyroid hormone-related peptide levels contribute to accelerated bone resorption and bone loss in lactating mice. *Endocrinology* 2003; 144: 5521–9

14. VanHouten JN, Dann P, Stewart AF, et al. Mammary-specific deletion of parathyroid hormone-related protein preserve bone mass during lactation. *J Clin Invest* 2003; 112: 1429–36

15. Marcus R. Post-menopausal osteoporosis. *Best Pract Res Clin Obstet Gynaecol* 2002; 16: 309–27

16. Gordon CM, Bachrach LK, Carpenter TO, et al. Bone health in children and adolescents: a symposium at the annual meeting of the Pediatric Academic Societies/Lawson Wilkins Pediatric Endocrine Society, May 2003. *Curr Probl Pediatr Adolesc Health Care* 2004; 34: 226–42

17. Krieter SR, Schwartz RP, Kirkman HN Jr, et al. Nutritional rickets in African American breast-fed infants. *J Pediatr* 2000; 137: 153–7

18. Pugliese MF, Blumberg DL, Hludzinski J, et al. Nutritional rickets in suburbia. *J Am Coll Nutr* 1998; 17: 637–41

19. Sills IN, Skuka KA, Horlick MN, et al. Vitamin D deficiency rickets. Reports of its demise are exaggerated. *Clin Pediatr* 1994; 33: 491–3

20. Zamora SA, Rizzoli R, Belli DC, et al. Vitamin D supplementation during infancy is associated with higher bone mineral mass in prepubertal girls. *J Clin Endocrinol Metab* 1999; 84: 4541–4

21. Peacock M. Nutritional aspects of hip fractures. *Chall Mod Med* 1995; 7: 213–22

22. Panda DK, Miao D, Bolivar I, et al. Inactivation of the 25-hydroxyvitamin D1 alpha-hydroxylase and vitamin D receptor demonstrates independent and interdependent effects of calcium and vitamin D on skeletal and mineral homeostasis. *J Biol Chem* 2004; 279: 16754–66

23. Hollis BW. Editorial: The determination of circulating 25-hydroxyvitamin D: no easy task. *J Clin Endocrinol Metab* 2004; 89: 3149–51

24. Lips P. Vitamin D deficiency and secondary hyperparathyroidism in the elderly: consequences for bone loss and fractures and therapeutic implications. *Endocr Rev* 2001; 22: 477–501

25. Lips P. Which circulating level of 25-hydroxyvitamin D is appropriate? *J Steroid Biochem Mol Biol* 2004; 89–90: 611–14

26. Vieth R. Why the optimal requirement for vitamin D3 is probably much higher than is officially recommended for adults. *J Steroid Biochem Mol Biol* 2004; 89–90:575–9

27. Papadimitropoulos E, Wells G, Shea B, et al. Meta-analyses of the efficacy of vitamin D treatment in preventing osteoporosis in post-menopausal women. *Endocr Rev* 2002; 23: 560–9

Genetic regulation of bone mass

7

S. H. Ralston

IMPORTANCE OF GENETICS IN OSTEOPOROSIS

Genetic factors play an important role in regulating several phenotypes revelant to the pathogenesis of osteoporosis. Data from twin and family studies have shown that between 50 and 85% of the variance in bone mass is genetically determined[1-4]. Other determinants of osteoporotic fracture risk such as quantitative ultrasound properties of bone[5], femoral neck geometry[5], muscle strength[6], bone turnover markers[7] and age at menopause[8] have also been shown to be genetically determined. Genetic factors play a less important role in the pathogenesis of fracture itself. Whilst family history of fracture has been shown to be an independent risk factor for fracture in several studies[9,10], twin studies have shown that environmental factors such as falls are a more important determinant of fracture than are genetic factors[11].

IDENTIFYING GENES WHICH PREDISPOSE TO OSTEOPOROSIS

Several approaches have been employed to identify the genes which contribute to the regulation of bone mass and the pathogenesis of fragility fractures. These include: linkage studies in families; linkage studies in experimental crosses of inbred strains of mice; and association studies of candidate genes in unrelated subjects.

Human linkage studies

Linkage studies are a tried and tested way of identifying genes responsible for monogenic diseases, and these have more recently been applied to the identification of chromosomal regions which contain genes that regulate quantitative traits such as bone mineral density. These regions are called quantitative trait loci (QTL). Linkage studies involve genotyping a large number of polymorphic markers, typically spread at 5–10 cM (million base pair) intervals throughout the genome and relating inheritance of these marker alleles to the inheritance of bone mass. An advantage of linkage studies is that they are statistically robust and unlikely to give false-positive results. A disadvantage is that they have limited power to detect genes of modest effect, such as those that have been implicated in the pathogenesis of osteoporosis.

Linkage studies have been used with greatest effect in the identification of genes responsible for monogenic bone diseases (Table 1). For example, mutations in the lipoprotein related receptor 5 (*LRP5*) gene have been shown to be responsible for two monogenic bone disease syndromes with opposing effects on bone mineral density (BMD): the high bone mass (HBM) syndrome, in which bone density is increased[18,19], and the osteoporosis pseudoglioma syndrome (OPPS), in which bone density is reduced[20]. It turns out that OPPS is caused by a variety of homozygous inactivating mutations in *LRP5*, whereas HMB is caused by heterozygous activating mutations in a specific region of the gene. Mutations in the latency-activating peptide domain of the transforming growth factor β1 (TGFβ1) gene have been shown to be responsible for Camaruti–Engelmann disease – a condition characterized by osteosclerosis mainly affecting the diaphysis of long bones[21], whereas inactivating mutations affecting the sclerostin (*SOST*) gene have been found to cause the syndromes of sclerosteosis and van Buchem disease[22], both of which are characterized by increased bone mass and generalized

Table 1 Monogenic bone disease genes

Gene	Disease	Function	Implicated in osteoporosis?
TCIRG1	recessive osteopetrosis	subunit of osteoclast proton pump	yes[12]
LRP5	high bone mass, osteoporosis, pseudoglioma syndrome	regulates osteoblast growth and bone formation	yes[13]
CLCN7	recessive osteopetrosis, dominant osteopetrosis	osteoclast chloride pump	yes[14]
CaII	recessive osteopetrosis with renal tubular acidosis	catalyzes formation of protons from CO_2 and H_2O in osteoclasts	not studied
CatK	pyknodysostosis	degrades bone matrix	no[15]
SOST	sclerosteosis, van Buchem disease	inhibitor of BMP action	yes[16]
COLIA1	osteogenesis imperfecta	major protein of bone matrix	yes[17]

BMP, bone morphogenetic protein

osteosclerosis. Osteopetrosis is a disease characterized by defects in osteoclast function[23], and positional cloning studies have identified mutations in several genes as the cause of this condition. These include the TCIRG1 gene which encodes a subunit of the osteoclast proton pump[24], the CLCN7 gene which encodes the osteoclast chloride channel[25] and the CATK gene which encodes a protease that is essential for the degradation of bone matrix[26].

Although the above-mentioned conditions are rare, it turns out that polymorphic variation in several of these genes contributes to regulation of bone mass in the normal population. For example, polymorphisms in the TGFβ1 gene have been found by several groups to be associated with BMD in the normal population[27], as have polymorphisms in the LRP5 gene[13], TCIRG1 gene[12]; SOST gene[16] and CLCN7 gene[14].

Linkage studies have also been performed in families with osteoporosis and in population-based cohorts of individuals to identify QTL for regulation of BMD in subjects who do not have monogenic bone diseases (reviewed by Liu and colleagues[28]). These studies have yielded mixed results, with little replication of QTL in different studies. At the present time, only one gene has been identified by this approach, and that is BMP2, which was shown to account (at least in part) for the osteoporosis susceptibility locus

identified on chromosome 20p12 in the Icelandic population[29].

Linkage studies in experimental animals

Linkage studies in experimental animals have long been used in the identification of genes responsible for complex traits[30], and, over recent years, many such studies have been performed to identify loci involved in the regulation of BMD and bone geometry in mice. These studies involve setting up crosses of inbred strains of mice with low and high bone density to create an F1 generation of mice that have intermediate levels of BMD due to inheritance of alleles with opposing effects on BMD from the parents. By interbreeding offspring from the F1 generation, a second generation of mice (F2) is established with varying levels of BMD, because of segregation of BMD-regulating alleles in the offspring. A genome-wide search can then be performed in the F2 generation and the inheritance of specific alleles related to the inheritance of BMD. Mice have several advantages as an experimental model: environment can be carefully controlled, thus minimizing the influence of confounding factors; large numbers of progeny can be generated, giving excellent statistical power; and fine mapping can be achieved by repeated back-crosses onto the parental strain.

There are some limitations of this approach. So far, it has proved difficult to move from identification of QTL to gene discovery, since the regions of linkage are typically large and can only be narrowed by the time-consuming process of repeated back-crossing. It is also uncertain whether the genes that are found to regulate BMD in mice will also be relevant to the regulation of BMD in humans.

Multiple QTL for peak bone mass have now been identified by linkage analysis in mice[31], and some of these QTL have also been shown to act as determinants of bone strength, structure and biomechanical responsiveness[32,33]. To date, however, only one gene has been identified as the result of positional cloning studies in mice, and that is *Alox15* which is situated within a BMD QTL identified by Klein and colleagues on mouse chromosome 11[34]. The *Alox15* gene was discovered by a microarray experiment which showed a 20-fold increase in *Alox15* mRNA levels in the low BMD-associated DBA2 mouse strain used to identify the QTL. Subsequent studies of *Alox15* knock-out mice and pharmacologic inhibitors of *Alox15* activity confirmed the importance of the *Alox15* gene as a regulator of bone metabolism and bone mass. Further studies are now in progress to determine whether genetic variation in the human homolog contributes to the regulation of bone mass in humans.

Candidate gene association studies

In the case of candidate gene studies, the investigator selects a gene that is thought to play a role in the regulation of bone turnover or bone mass and identifies polymorphisms in that gene, either by performing mutation screening or by analyzing online databases that hold information on polymorphic variations in genes throughout the genome. These polymorphisms (or groups of linked polymorphisms termed haplotypes) are then investigated for an association with BMD, fractures or other phenotypes of interest in population-based studies or in case–control studies. Candidate gene-association studies are relatively easy to perform, and can detect genetic variants which have modest effects on the phenotype of interest. Disadvantages of these studies include the possibility of false-positive (or false-negative) results due to confounding factors and population stratification. Moreover, demonstration of an association between a candidate gene polymorphism and a trait does not necessarily mean that the polymorphism is causally responsible for the effect observed. Another explanation is that the effect could be mediated by a linked polymorphism in the same gene or in a gene nearby. Mention should be made of the transmission disequilibrium test (TDT), which is a special type of association study that examines the frequency with which individuals inherit putative susceptibility alleles from a heterozygous parent[35]. The transmitted allele in the TDT acts as the 'case' and the non-transmitted allele acts as the 'control', thus circumventing the problem of population stratification. The TDT is statistically robust, but lacks power when the polymorphism of interest is uncommon. Another disadvantage is that it can only be used where parental samples are available, thus limiting its applicability to the study of late-onset diseases such as osteoporosis.

Individual candidate genes that have been implicated in the regulation of bone mass or osteoporotic fractures by association studies are discussed in more detail below.

Vitamin D receptor (VDR)

Vitamin D, by interacting with its receptor, plays an important role in calcium homeostasis by regulating bone cell growth and differentiation, intestinal calcium absorption and parathyroid hormone secretion. Morrison identified three common polymorphisms in the 3′ region of the *VDR* gene situated between exons 8 and 9, which are recognized by the restriction enzymes *Bsm*I, *Apa*I and *Taq*I. These were found to be associated with circulating levels of the osteoblast-specific protein osteocalcin and bone mass in twin studies and a population-based study[36]. Other studies of *VDR* in relation to bone mass have yielded conflicting results, but a recent meta-analysis concluded that the *VDR Bsm*I genotype is associated with modest effects on bone mass[37]. There is evidence to suggest that

VDR genotype could influence the skeletal response to both calcium intake and vitamin D intake, although many of the studies on this topic have been small with rather inconclusive results.

Another polymorphism affecting exon 2 of *VDR* has been described which creates an alternative translation start site, potentially resulting in the production of two isoforms of the VDR protein, which differ in length by three amino acids[38]. This has been associated with BMD in some, but not all, populations. A functional polymorphism has been identified in the promoter of *VDR* at a binding site for the transcription factor Cdx-2, which has been associated with BMD in Japanese subjects[39] and with fracture in Caucasians[40]. The mechanisms by which these polymorphisms modulate *VDR* function are incompletely understood. There is evidence to suggest that the 3′ polymorphisms may act as markers for RNA stability. Evidence has also been presented to suggest that the isoforms of *VDR* encoded by the different *Fok-1* alleles differ in terms of function, although other groups have failed to confirm these findings.

Type I collagen

The genes encoding type I collagen (*COLIA1* and *COLIA2*) are important candidates for the pathogenesis of osteoporosis. Grant and colleagues[41] described a common polymorphism affecting a binding site for the transcription factor Sp1 in the first intron of *COLIA1*, which was more prevalent in osteoporotic patients than in controls. Positive associations between the *COLIA1* Sp1 polymorphism and bone mass or osteoporotic fractures were subsequently reported in several populations, and a meta-analysis showed that the *COLIA1* genotype conferred differences in BMD of approximately 0.15 *Z* score units per copy of the 's' allele and an increase in fracture risk of approximately 62% per copy of the 's' allele[17]. Significant ethnic differences have been reported in population prevalence of *COLIA1* Sp1 alleles: the polymorphism is common in Caucasian populations, but is rare in Africans and Chinese[42]. The mechanism by which the Sp1 polymorphism predisposes to osteoporosis has

been investigated by Mann and colleagues[17], who found that the 's' allele had increased affinity for Sp1 protein binding and was associated with elevated allele-specific transcription in heterozygotes. These abnormalities were accompanied by increased production of the αI chain of collagen by osteoblasts cultured from 'Ss' heterozygotes, resulting in an increased ratio of α1/α2 chains, reflecting the presence of α1 homotrimer formation. Biomechanical testing of bone samples from 'Ss' heterozygotes showed reduced bone strength compared with 'SS' homozygotes and impairment in the mineralization of bone[43]. Overall, the data suggest that the *COLIA1* Sp1 polymorphism is a functional variant which has adverse effects on bone composition and mechanical strength.

Estrogen receptor α

The estrogen receptor α gene (*ESR1*) is a strong functional candidate for osteoporosis susceptibility. Most studies of *ESR1* have focused on a TA repeat polymorphism in the *ESR1* promoter[44], and two other polymorhisms within intron 1 of the *ESR1*, recognized by the restriction enzymes *Pvu*II and *Xba*I[45]. Most studies of *ESR1* alleles in osteoporosis have been small, but a meta-analysis of these studies has suggested that polymorphic variation at the *Xba*I site may act as a determinant of bone mass[46]. Recently, a large association study involving nearly 19 000 subjects showed that the *Xba*I polymorphism is associated with osteoporotic fracture independent of differences in BMD[47]. The TA repeat polymorphism in the *ESR1* promoter is in strong linkage disequilibrium with the *Xba*I and *Pvu*II polymorphisms[48], and it is currently uncertain which (if any) of these polymorphisms is functional. There is some evidence to suggest that the *Pvu*II polymorphism affects a Myb binding site, and that polymorphic variations at this site alter *ESR1* transcription *in vitro*[49]. This does not exclude the possibility that the *Xba*I and TA repeat polymorphisms also have functional consequences, or indeed the possibility that other linked polymorphisms at the *ESR1* locus may be responsible for the associations with osteoporosis phenotypes that have been observed.

Other genes

Polymorphisms of several other candidate genes have been associated with bone mass and/or osteoporotic fracture, and this subject has recently been reviewed[28,50]. Polymorphisms in the TGFβ1 gene have been associated with BMD, osteoporotic fracture and circulating TGFβ levels in various studies[27], although the mechanisms by which these influence TGFβ1 function are unclear. Polymorphisms in the 3' untranslated region of the *TNFRS1B* gene have been associated with femoral neck bone mass in women, and there is evidence to suggest that this might be mediated by an effect on RNA stability[51]. The *TNFRSF1B* gene is a functional candidate for regulation of BMD because it encodes the tumor necrosis factor (TNF) type 2 receptor, and is a positional candidate since it lies within a linkage region for BMD regulation on chromosome 1p36[52]. Another gene that lies close to *TNFRSF1B* on chromosome 1p36 is the methylene tetrahydrofolate reductase (MTHFR) gene, which plays a role in folate metabolism. A functional polymorphism affecting codon 667 of MTHFR has been associated with BMD and fracture in various studies[53,54], and it is thought that this effect may be mediated by altering homocysteine metabolism. Associations have been described between polymorphisms in the promoter of the interleukin-6 (IL-6) gene and BMD, and it appears that these polymorphisms affect transcriptional regulaton of IL-6 and influence bone turnover[55]. Other investigators have looked at possible associations between apolipoprotein E (apo E) alleles and osteoporosis. In Japanese women, the apo E4 allele was found to be associated with low bone mass, and, in another study of US women, the same allele was associated with osteoporotic fractures independent of bone mass. The mechanism by which apo E alleles influence susceptibility to osteoporosis are unclear, but may involve differences in hydroxylation of the osteoblast-specific protein osteocalcin. Other candidate genes which have been studied in relation to BMD include those for the calcitonin receptor, osteocalcin, parathyroid hormone, the parathyroid hormone receptor, the androgen receptor, aromatase, interleukin-1β and the interleukin-1 receptor antagonist (IL-1ra).

References

1. Pocock NA, Eisman JA, Hopper JL, et al. Genetic determinants of bone mass in adults: a twin study. *J Clin Invest* 1987; 80: 706–10

2. Smith DM, Nance WE, Kang KW, et al. Genetic factors in determining bone mass. *J Clin Invest* 1973; 52: 2800–8

3. Gueguen R, Jouanny P, Guillemin F, et al. Segregation analysis and variance components analysis of bone mineral density in healthy families. *J Bone Miner Res* 1995; 12: 2017–22

4. Krall EA, Dawson-Hughes B. Heritable and lifestyle determinants of bone mineral density. *J Bone Miner Res* 1993; 8: 1–9

5. Arden NK, Baker J, Hogg C, et al. The heritability of bone mineral density, ultrasound of the calcaneus and hip axis length: a study of postmenopausal twins. *J Bone Miner Res* 1996; 11: 530–4

6. Arden NK, Spector TD. Genetic influences on muscle strength, lean body mass, and bone mineral density: a twin study. *J Bone Miner Res* 1997; 12: 2076–81

7. Garnero P, Arden NK, Griffiths G, et al. Genetic influence on bone turnover in postmenopausal twins. *J Clin Endocrinol Metab* 1996; 81: 140–6

8. Snieder H, MacGregor AJ, Spector TD. Genes control the cessation of a woman's reproductive life: a twin study of hysterectomy and age at menopause. *J Clin Endocrinol Metab* 1998; 83: 1875–80

9. Torgerson DJ, Campbell MK, Thomas RE, Reid DM. Prediction of perimenopausal fractures by

bone mineral density and other risk factors. *J Bone Miner Res* 1996; 11: 293–7

10. Cummings SR, Nevitt MC, Browner WS, et al. Risk factors for hip fracture in white women. Study of Osteoporotic Fractures Research Group. *N Engl J Med* 1995; 332: 767–73

11. Kannus P, Palvanen M, Kaprio J, et al. Genetic factors and osteoporotic fractures in elderly people: prospective 25 year follow up of a nationwide cohort of elderly Finnish twins. *Br Med J* 1999; 319: 1334–7

12. Sobacchi C, Vezzoni P, Reid DM, et al. Association between a polymorphism affecting an AP1 binding site in the promoter of the TCIRG1 gene and bone mass in women. *Calcif Tissue Int* 2004; 74: 35–41

13. Ferrari SL, Deutsch S, Choudhury U, et al. Polymorphisms in the low-density lipoprotein receptor-related protein 5 (LRP5) gene are associated with variation in vertebral bone mass, vertebral bone size, and stature in whites. *Am J Hum Genet* 2004; 74: 866–75

14. Mirolo M, Taranta A, Albagha OME, et al. A missense polymorphism in exon 15 of the chloride channel 7 gene (CLCN7) is associated with hip bone density in women. *Calcif Tiss Int* 2003; 72: 421 (abst)

15. Giraudeau FS, McGinnis RE, Gray IC, et al. Characterization of common genetic variants in cathepsin K and testing for association with bone mineral density in a large cohort of perimenopausal women from Scotland. *J Bone Miner Res* 2004; 19: 31–41

16. Uitterlinden AG, Arp PP, Paeper BW, et al. Polymorphisms in the sclerosteosis/van Buchem disease gene (SOST) region are associated with bone-mineral density in elderly whites. *Am J Hum Genet* 2004; 75: 1032–45

17. Mann V, Hobson EE, Li B, et al. A COL1A1 Sp1 binding site polymorphism predisposes to osteoporotic fracture by affecting bone density and quality. *J Clin Invest* 2001; 107: 899–907

18. Little RD, Carulli JP, Del Mastro RG, et al. A mutation in the LDL receptor-related protein 5 gene results in the autosomal dominant high-bone-mass trait. *Am J Hum Genet* 2002; 70: 11–19

19. Van Wesenbeeck L, Cleiren E, Gram J, et al. Six novel missense mutations in the LDL receptor-related protein 5 (LRP5) gene in different conditions with an increased bone density. *Am J Hum Genet* 2003; 72: 763–71

20. Gong Y, Slee RB, Fukai N, et al. LDL receptor-related protein 5 (LRP5) affects bone accrual and eye development. *Cell* 2001; 107: 513–23

21. Janssens K, Gershoni-Baruch R, Guanabens N, et al. Mutations in the gene encoding the latency-associated peptide of TGF-beta1 cause Camurati–Engelmann disease. *Nat Genet* 2000; 26: 273–5

22. Balemans W, Patel N, Ebeling M, et al. Identification of a 52 kb deletion downstream of the SOST gene in patients with van Buchem disease. *J Med Genet* 2002; 39: 91–7

23. de Vernejoul MC, Benichou O. Human osteopetrosis and other sclerosing disorders: recent genetic developments. *Calcif Tissue Int* 2001; 69: 1–6

24. Frattini A, Orchard PJ, Sobacchi C, et al. Defects in TCIRG1 subunit of the vacuolar proton pump are responsible for a subset of human autosomal recessive osteopetrosis. *Nat Genet* 2000; 25: 343–6

25. Cleiren E, Benichou O, Van Hul E, et al. Albers–Schonberg disease (autosomal dominant osteopetrosis, type II) results from mutations in the ClCN7 chloride channel gene. *Hum Mol Genet* 2001; 10: 2861–7

26. Gelb BD, Shi GP, Chapman HA, Desnick RJ. Pycnodysostosis, a lysosomal disease caused by cathepsin K deficiency. *Science* 1996; 273: 1236–8

27. Hinke V, Seck T, Clanget C, et al. Association of transforming growth factor-beta1 (TGFbeta1) T29 → C gene polymorphism with bone mineral density (BMD), changes in BMD, and serum concentrations of TGF-beta1 in a population-based sample of postmenopausal german women. *Calcif Tissue Int* 2001; 69: 315–20

28. Liu YZ, Liu YJ, Recker RR, Deng HW. Molecular studies of identification of genes for osteoporosis: the 2002 update. *J Endocrinol* 2003; 177: 147–96

29. Styrkarsdottir U, Cazier J-B, Kong A, et al. Linkage of osteoporosis to chromosome 20p12 and association to BMP2. *PLoS Biol* 2003; 1: E69

30. Rogers J, Mahaney MC, Beamer WG, et al. Beyond one gene-one disease: alternative

strategies for deciphering genetic determinants of osteoporosis. *Calcif Tissue Int* 1997; 60: 225–8

31. Klein RF, Carlos AS, Vartanian KA, et al. Confirmation and fine mapping of chromosomal regions influencing peak bone mass in mice. *J Bone Miner Res* 2001; 16: 1953–61

32. Robling AG, Li J, Shultz KL, et al. Evidence for a skeletal mechanosensitivity gene on mouse chromosome 4. *FASEB J* 2003; 17: 324–6

33. Turner CH, Sun Q, Schriefer J, et al. Congenic mice reveal sex-specific genetic regulation of femoral structure and strength. *Calcif Tissue Int* 2003; 73: 297–303

34. Klein RF, Allard J, Avnur Z, et al. Regulation of bone mass in mice by the lipoxygenase gene Alox15. *Science* 2004; 303: 229–32

35. Spielman RS, McGinnis RE, Ewens WJ. Transmission test for linkage disequilibrium: the insulin gene region and insulin-dependent diabetes mellitus (IDDM). *Am J Hum Genet* 1993; 52: 506–16

36. Morrison NA, Qi JC, Tokita A, et al. Prediction of bone density from vitamin D receptor alleles. *Nature (London)* 1994; 367: 284–7

37. Thakkinstian A, D'Este C, Eisman J, et al. Meta-analysis of molecular association studies: vitamin D receptor gene polymorphisms and BMD as a case study. *J Bone Miner Res* 2004; 19: 419–28

38. Arai H, Miyamoto K-I, Taketani Y, et al. A vitamin D receptor gene polymorphism in the translation initiation codon: effect on protein activity and relation to bone mineral density in Japanese women. *J Bone Miner Res* 1997; 12: 915–21

39. Arai H, Miyamoto KI, Yoshida M, et al. The polymorphism in the caudal-related homeodomain protein Cdx-2 binding element in the human vitamin D receptor gene. *J Bone Miner Res* 2001; 16: 1256–64

40. Fang Y, van Meurs JB, Bergink AP, et al. Cdx-2 polymorphism in the promoter region of the human vitamin D receptor gene determines susceptibility to fracture in the elderly. *J Bone Miner Res* 2003; 18: 1632–41

41. Grant SFA, Reid DM, Blake G, et al. Reduced bone density and osteoporosis associated with a polymorphic Sp1 site in the collagen type I alpha 1 gene. *Nature Genet* 1996; 14: 203–5

42. Beavan S, Prentice A, Dibba B, et al. Polymorphism of the collagen type I alpha 1 gene and

ethnic differences in hip-fracture rates. *N Engl J Med* 1998; 339: 351–2

43. Stewart TL, Roschger P, Misof BM, et al. Association of COLIA1 Sp1 alleles with defective bone nodule formation *in vitro* and abnormal bone mineralisation *in vivo*. *Calcif Tiss Int* 2005; May 19 [Epub]

44. Sano M, Inoue S, Hosoi T, et al. Association of estrogen receptor dinucleotide repeat polymorphism with osteoporosis. *Biochem Biophys Res Commun* 1995; 217: 378–83

45. Kobayashi S, Inoue S, Hosoi T, et al. Association of bone mineral density with polymorphism of the estrogen receptor gene. *J Bone Miner Res* 1996; 11: 306–11

46. Ioannidis JP, Stavrou I, Trikalinos TA, et al. Association of polymorphisms of the estrogen receptor alpha gene with bone mineral density and fracture risk in women: a meta-analysis. *J Bone Miner Res* 2002; 17: 2048–60

47. Ioannidis JP, Ralston SH, Bennett ST, et al. Differential genetic effects of ESR1 gene polymorphisms on osteoporosis outcomes. *J Am Med Assoc* 2004; 292: 2105–14

48. Becherini L, Gennari L, Masi L, et al. Evidence of a linkage disequilibrium between polymorphisms in the human estrogen receptor alpha gene and their relationship to bone mass variation in postmenopausal Italian women. *Hum Mol Genet* 2000; 9: 2043–50

49. Herrington DM, Howard TD, Brosnihan KB, et al. Common estrogen receptor polymorphism augments effects of hormone replacement therapy on E-selectin but not C-reactive protein. *Circulation* 2002; 105: 1879–82

50. Ralston SH. The genetics of osteoporosis. *Bone* 1999; 25: 85–6

51. Albagha OME, Tasker PN, McGuigan FEA, et al. Linkage disequilibrium between polymorphisms in the human TNFRSF1B gene and their association with bone mass in perimenopausal women. *Hum Mol Genet* 2002; 11: 2289–95

52. Devoto M, Specchia C, Li HH, et al. Variance component linkage analysis indicates a QTL for femoral neck bone mineral density on chromosome 1p36. *Hum Mol Genet* 2001; 10: 2447–52

53. Jorgensen HL, Madsen JS, Madsen B, et al. Association of a common allelic polymorphism (C677T) in the methylene tetrahydrofolate

reductase gene with a reduced risk of osteoporotic fractures. A case control study in Danish postmenopausal women. *Calcif Tissue Int* 2002; 71: 386–92

54. Miyao M, Morita H, Hosoi T, et al. Association of methylenetetrahydrofolate reductase (MTHFR) polymorphism with bone mineral density in postmenopausal Japanese women. *Calcif Tissue Int* 2000; 66: 190–4

55. Ferrari SL, Garnero P, Emond S, et al. A functional polymorphic variant in the interleukin-6 gene promoter associated with low bone resorption in postmenopausal women. *Arthritis Rheum* 2001; 44: 196–201

Bone mineral acquisition during infancy and adolescence 8

G. Saggese and G. I. Baroncelli

THE CONCEPT OF PEAK BONE MASS

Peak bone mass (PBM) is defined as the highest level of bone mass achieved as a result of normal growth[1]. PBM represents a main determinant of osteoporotic fracture risk in adulthood, together with the maintenance of bone mass in adulthood, and the rate of bone loss in late adulthood[2].

In both sexes, the timing of PBM has been considered to occur from ages as early as 16–18 years[1,3,4]. Lumbar spine and femoral bone mineral density (BMD) show a rapid decline after the attainment of PBM[5,6], whereas radial, skull and total body BMD show a minimal increase until 50 years as a result of continuous periosteal expansion with age[1]. Matkovic and colleagues[1] showed that the timing of cessation of linear growth is 1–7 years earlier than cessation of the accumulation of bone mass at various skeletal sites, suggesting that a rapid consolidation of skeletal density occurs after the bulk of bone modeling has been completed. Nevertheless, mostly, PBM is reached in late adolescence within the second decade of life. Differences in examined skeletal sites and/or in densitometric techniques used to assess bone mineral status, as well as racial, genetic or environmental factors, may influence the pattern of bone mass accumulation and the value of PBM.

ACQUISITION OF BONE MASS DURING CHILDHOOD AND ADOLESCENCE

Before puberty, no consistent gender difference in bone mineral status assessed at the axial or appendicular skeleton has been reported. Moreover, there is no evidence for a gender difference in bone mass at birth. This lack of difference in bone mass between sexes is maintained up to the onset of puberty[7].

In both sexes, lumbar spine BMD, assessed by dual-energy X-ray absorptiometry (DXA), increases progressively during childhood and adolescence, and reaches a plateau around the ages of 15 and 17 years in girls and boys, respectively[3,4,8,9]. Subsequently, BMD values remain stable[1] or decline slightly[5]. BMD is higher in men than in women because the former have bigger bones, partly because prepubertal longitudinal growth continues for 2 years more in males than in females[9].

At the femoral neck, BMD values measured by DXA show a peak at the age of 14.5 years in females and 16.5 years in males; thereafter, BMD values remain stable[4,10] or decline slightly[6].

At the distal one-third of the radius, BMD values measured by single-photon absorptiometry increase progressively up to 18–19 years in males and 15–16 years in females[11].

At the proximal phalanges of the hand, studies using quantitative ultrasound have shown that PBM is reached at around 30 years[12–14].

The pattern of BMD values at the lumbar spine and femur during childhood and adolescence indicates that puberty has a crucial role in the acquisition of bone mass; indeed, a significant gain in skeletal mass occurs during the pubertal years, when approximately 40% of bone mass is accumulated[1,3,4]. In both sexes, maximal BMD accumulation at the lumbar spine and femoral neck occurs in the last stages of puberty, mainly in males[3,15].

It has been calculated that, at the time of peak height *velocity* (12–13 years in females and 14–15 years in males; pubertal stages 2 and 3), the percentage total height gain is greater than the percentage incremental areal BMD at the lumbar spine, femoral neck and femoral mid-shaft. In males, the greatest difference between height and BMD gains is more pronounced at the lumbar spine and femoral neck than at the femoral mid-shaft, whereas in females the difference appears to be of a lower magnitude than in males[10]. Moreover, Theintz and colleagues[4] demonstrated that the increment in bone mass at the lumbar spine as a function of height gain follows a loop pattern when pubertal stages are taken into consideration. The model suggests that there is a dissociation between the increment of bone mass and height gain; in the last stages of puberty, when height gain decreases abruptly, bone mass accumulation is sustained. Therefore, an accumulation of lumbar bone mass occurs after the attainment of peak height velocity in both sexes.

DETERMINANTS OF PEAK BONE MASS

Many factors, more or less independent, are known to influence the acquisition of bone mass during childhood and adolescence. These determinants include both endogenous and exogenous factors. Furthermore, some diseases may affect, *per se* or by their treatment, the acquisition of bone mass in children and adolescents[16].

Genetic factors

The main determinant of PBM appears to be genetic factors. Indeed, twin and family studies support a strong genetic component of BMD, accounting for approximately 70–80% of adult BMD[17–21]. Most studies have used methods that identify candidate genes which could be involved in the regulation of bone turnover, or polymorphisms for these genes. The involved genes are not clearly identified, but the most important are probably those related to body size[22]. It has been suggested that a polymorphism in the vitamin D

receptor gene (*VDR*) may be an important determinant of bone mass[23]. However, conflicting data have been reported in both adults[24,25] and children[26–30] regarding the association between *VDR* polymorphism and BMD values or predisposition to osteoporosis. Some genetic determinants of bone mass have been identified (Table 1), but their predictive role in children at risk of osteoporosis is not defined. The mechanism(s) by which the genetic factors determine BMD is unknown, but lean and fat mass, body weight, muscle strength, hormone secretion, timing of puberty and even physical and dietary tendencies may be influenced by hereditary factors.

However, it is important to consider that heredity and environment are not separable. Indeed, genetic factors could influence the efficiency with which an individual utilizes and conserves the nutrients needed for the acquisition of bone mass[22]. Moreover, some environmental factors may have different effects due to different expression of a genetic determinant.

Regarding racial factors, BMD values are higher in black than in white subjects, and lower in girls of Asian ethnicity than in Caucasian girls[7].

Hormones

Many hormones are involved in the acquisition of bone mass: sex steroids, the growth hormone (GH)–insulin-like growth factor-I (IGF-I) axis, 1,25-dihydroxyvitamin D (1,25(OH)$_2$D), thyroid hormones, insulin, glucocorticoids, parathy-

Table 1 Some genetic determinants of bone mass

Vitamin D receptor (*VDR*)
Estradiol receptor (*ER*)
Calcitonin receptor (*CTR*)
Calcium-sensing receptor (*CASR*)
Glucocorticoid receptor (*GR*)
Parathyroid hormone
Transforming growth factor β1 (*TGFβ1*)
Interleukin-6 (*IL-6*)
Insulin-like growth factor-I (*IGF-I*)
Collagen type I$_{a1}$ (*COL1A1*)
Osteocalcin (*BGP*)

roid hormone and calcitonin[9]. Some clinical evidence in patients with altered hormonal secretion suggested that sex steroids and the GH–IGF-I axis play a main role in the acquisition of bone mass[16,31,32]. Indeed, individuals with mutations of the estrogen receptor and aromatase genes have estrogen deficiency and osteoporosis[16,31,32]. The predominant effect of testosterone on bone mass accumulation occurs via its aromatization to estrogen, but it may cause indirect effects via its anabolic action on lean tissue mass and a weak direct effect via its action on osteoblasts[32]. Children with GH deficiency have reduced bone turnover and BMD, but long-term GH therapy is able to improve both[16]. The role of sex steroids and the GH–IGF-I axis in the acquisition of bone mass is mainly evident during puberty, when the gain of bone mass is maximal.

Balance studies showed that the percentage of intestinal calcium absorption is closely related to circulating $1,25(OH)_2D$ concentrations. Indeed, intestinal calcium absorption is approximately 40% when $1,25(OH)_2D$ levels are in the normal range, but it may be extremely low (< 10%) if $1,25(OH)_2D$ levels are reduced. Therefore, an optimal vitamin D status is a key factor in regulating intestinal calcium absorption[33].

Dietary calcium

Relationships between calcium intake and adult BMD have been reported from many cross-sectional and retrospective studies; however, other studies did not show this association[22,34–37]. Some meta-analyses have concluded that calcium intake is a significant determinant of BMD but the magnitude of the effect is probably small, at about 1% of the population variance[36]. At any rate, there is evidence that a reduced calcium intake may be associated with a low bone mass and fractures in children[38] and adolescents[39–41]. Moreover, it has been shown that women with a low calcium intake during childhood and adolescence have less bone mass in adulthood and a greater risk of fracture[42].

On the other hand, studies of calcium supplementation showed that a calcium intake above the recommended intakes was able to improve the accumulation of bone mass in prepubertal and pubertal healthy subjects[1–3]. The mechanism(s) by which calcium supplementation produces its effect is probably related to a reduced bone turnover, stimulating the acquisition of bone mass[43]. However, subsequent studies reported that the effect of calcium supplementation on BMD ceased after the discontinuation of supplementation[44,45], whereas others showed a persisting effect of calcium supplementation on BMD until 3–5 years after the end of intervention[46]. A longer period of calcium supplementation, up to the attainment of PBM, will give more information on the long-term effect of calcium intake on bone mass.

Exposure to risk factors such as excessive sodium, phosphate, animal protein, caffeine and alcohol intakes may affect the accumulation of bone mass[47].

Physical exercise

The role of physical exercise in the development and maintenance of skeletal mass is generally accepted, but the data are not univocal. This is due to the difficulty in quantifying the effect of physical exercise alone, independently of the other determinants of PBM. In adults, physical activity is associated with greater bone mass[48]. The dominant arm in tennis players has greater bone mass than the non-dominant arm[49]. In contrast, complete (e.g. prolonged bed-rest, space-flight, traumatic paraplegia, cerebral palsy) or partial immobilization (e.g. fractures) was shown to result in various degrees of bone loss[50,51], but bone formation dramatically increased when immobilized subjects resumed exercise[52].

Few studies of the effect of physical exercise on BMD have been performed in children or adolescents. It has been shown that weight-bearing exercises during, and to a lesser extent after, puberty may improve BMD, mainly at the hip[32]. Non-weight-bearing exercises, such as swimming, did not increase BMD[32]. Ruiz and colleagues[53] also demonstrated that physical activity was strongly correlated with lumbar BMD; the correlation was present both during the initial phase of puberty (Tanner stage 2) and during puberty (Tanner stages 4–5). Moreover, Nordstrom and associates[54] demonstrated that BMD (measured for total body, head, humerus, spine, femur and tibia/fibula) was significantly correlated with muscle strength measured at the quadriceps. These results confirm previous data showing a correlation of muscle strength in the back with BMD of the lumbar spine[55], and of grip strength with BMD at the mid-radius[56]. Furthermore, a study by Schonau[57] at the distal radius, using peripheral quantitative computed tomography, showed that parameters of bone geometry such as bone cross-sectional area and cortical area, and bone strength index (which derives from the section modulus and the volumetric density of the cortical area), were correlated with grip strength measured by hand dynamometer.

Regular weight-bearing activity probably has a greater influence on bone mass than dietary calcium[58]. In any case, physical activity and calcium intake may not act on bone independent of each other. Indeed, a positive effect of physical activity appeared only at calcium intakes greater than 1000 mg/day, and the beneficial effect of a high calcium intake appeared only when physical activity was carried out[59]. Regarding the interaction between genetic and environmental factors and the acquisition of bone mass, an interesting hypothesis has been suggested by Kelly and colleagues[60]: with low calcium intake or low physical activity there is little difference between subjects with high or low genetic potential. Therefore, in order to obtain maximal expression of the genetic potential to achieve PBM, association of a high dietary calcium intake and regular physical activity is necessary.

CONCLUSIONS AND RECOMMENDATIONS

(1) Peak bone mass (PBM) is attained during late adolescence, and puberty represents a critical period for bone mass accumulation.

(2) PBM is the result of the interaction of various factors: genetic, hormonal, racial, nutritional, life-style and physical exercise.

(3) Environmental factors modulate the expression of the genetic potential to achieve PBM.

(4) Calcium intake seems to be a main nutritional determinant in bone mass acquisition. In children and adolescents in whom calcium intake is deficient, calcium supplementation according to adequate intake for age is recommended.

(5) Vitamin D has a major role in stimulating intestinal calcium absorption. In children and adolescents having an insufficient vitamin D status, vitamin D supplementation according to adequate intake for age is recommended.

(6) Physical exercise (mainly regular weight-bearing activity) is a key factor for the acquisition and maintenance of bone mass.

References

1. Matkovic V, Jelic T, Wardlaw GM, et al. Timing of peak bone mass in Caucasian females and its implication for the prevention of osteoporosis. Inference from a cross-sectional model. *J Clin Invest* 1994; 93: 799–808

2. National Osteoporosis Foundation. Osteoporosis: review of the evidence for prevention, diagnosis, and treatment and cost-effectiveness analysis. *Osteoporos Int* 1998; 8 (Suppl 4): S1–88

3. Bonjour J, Theintz G, Buchs B, et al. Critical years and stages of puberty for spinal and femoral bone mass accumulation during adolescence. *J Clin Endocrinol Metab* 1991; 73: 555–63

4. Theintz G, Buchs B, Rizzoli R, et al. Longitudinal monitoring of bone mass accumulation in

healthy adolescents: evidence for a marked reduction after 16 years of age at the levels of lumbar spine and femoral neck in female subjects. *J Clin Endocrinol Metab* 1992; 75: 1060–5

5. Haapasalo H, Kannus P, Sievanen H, et al. Development of mass, density, and estimated mechanical characteristics of bones in Caucasian females. *J Bone Miner Res* 1996; 11: 1751–60

6. Lu PW, Cowell CT, Lloyd-Jones SA, et al. Volumetric bone mineral density in normal subjects, aged 5–27 years. *J Clin Endocrinol Metab* 1996; 81: 1586–90

7. Rizzoli R, Bonjour JP. Determinants of peak bone mass and mechanisms of bone loss. *Osteoporos Int* 1999; 9 (Suppl 2): S17–23

8. Del Rio L, Carrascosa A, Pons F, et al. Bone mineral density of the lumbar spine in white Mediterranean Spanish children and adolescents: changes related to age, sex, and puberty. *Pediatr Res* 1994; 35: 362–6

9. Bonjour J, Theintz G, Law F, et al. Peak bone mass. *Osteoporos Int* 1994; 8 (Suppl 1): S7–13

10. Fournier PE, Rizzoli R, Slosman DO, et al. Asynchrony between the rates of standing height gain and bone mass accumulation during puberty. *Osteoporos Int* 1997; 7: 525–32

11. Saggese G, Federico G, Ghirri P, et al. Densitometria ossea in età pediatrica. Valori normali tra 2 e 19 anni. Primi dati Italiani. *Minerva Pediatr* 1986; 38: 545–51

12. Wuster C, Albanese C, De Aloysio D, et al. Phalangeal osteosonogrammetry study: age-related changes, diagnostic sensitivity, and discrimination power. The Phalangeal Osteosonogrammetry Study Group. *J Bone Miner Res* 2000; 15: 1603–14

13. Montagnani A, Gonnelli S, Cepollaro C, et al. Quantitative ultrasound at the phalanges in healthy Italian men. *Osteoporos Int* 2000; 11: 499–504

14. Drozdzowska B, Pluskiewicz W. Skeletal status in males aged 7–80 years assessed by quantitative ultrasound at the hand phalanges. *Osteoporos Int* 2003; 14: 295–300

15. Boot AM, De Ridder MAJ, Pols HAP, et al. Bone mineral density in children and adolescents: relation to puberty, calcium intake, and physical activity. *J Clin Endocrinol Metab* 1997; 82: 57–62

16. Baroncelli GI, Bertelloni S, Sodini F, et al. Acquisition of bone mass in normal individuals and in patients with growth hormone deficiency. *J Pediatr Endocrinol Metab* 2003; 16(Suppl 2): 327–35

17. Smith DA, Nance WE, Won Kang K, et al. Genetic factors in determining bone mass. *J Clin Invest* 1973; 52: 2800–8

18. Dequeker J, Nijs J, Verstaeten A, et al. Genetic determinants of bone mineral content at the spine and the radius: a twin study. *Bone* 1987; 8: 207–9

19. Pokock NA, Eisman JA, Hopper JL, et al. Genetic determinants of bone mass in adults; a twin study. *J Clin Invest* 1987; 80: 706–10

20. Seeman E, Hopper JL, Bach LA, et al. Reduced bone mass in daughters of women with osteoporosis. *N Engl J Med* 1989; 320: 554–8

21. Krall EA, Dawson-Hughes B. Heritable and lifestyle determinants of bone mineral density. *J Bone Miner Res* 1993; 8: 1–8

22. Heaney RP, Abrams S, Dawson-Hughes B, et al. Peak bone mass. *Osteoporos Int* 2000; 11: 985–1009

23. Audì L, Garcia-Ramirez M, Carrascosa A. Genetic determinants of bone mass. *Horm Res* 1999; 51: 105–23

24. Eisman JA. Vitamin D receptor gene alleles and osteoporosis: an affirmative view. *J Bone Miner Res* 1995; 10: 1289–93

25. Peacock M. Vitamin D receptor gene alleles and osteoporosis: a contrasting view. *J Bone Miner Res* 1995; 10: 1294–7

26. Gunnes M, Berg JP, Halse J, et al. Lack of relationship between vitamin D receptor genotype and forearm bone gain in healthy children, adolescents, and young adults. *J Clin Endocrinol Metab* 1997; 82: 851–5.

27. Sainz J, Van Tornout JM, Loro ML, et al. Vitamin D-receptor gene polymorphisms and bone density in prepubertal American girls of Mexican descent. *N Engl J Med* 1997; 337: 77–82

28. Ferrari SL, Rizzoli R, Slosman DO, et al. Do dietary calcium and age explain the controversy surrounding the relationship between bone mineral density and vitamin D receptor gene polymorphisms? *J Bone Miner Res* 1998; 13: 363–70

29. Tao C, Yu T, Garnett S, et al. Vitamin D receptor alleles predict growth and bone density in girls. *Arch Dis Child* 1998; 79: 488–93

30. Baroncelli GI, Federico G, Bertelloni S, et al. Vitamin-D receptor genotype does not predict bone mineral density, bone turnover, and growth in prepubertal children. *Horm Res* 1999; 51: 150–6

31. Saggese G, Bertelloni S, Baroncelli GI. Sex steroids and acquisition of bone mass. *Horm Res* 1997; 48 (Suppl 5): 65–71

32. Cowell CT, Tao C. Nature or nurture: determinants of peak bone mass in females. *J Pediatr Endocrinol Metab* 2002; 15(Suppl 5): 1387–93

33. Wilz DR, Gray RW, Dominguez JH, et al. Plasma 1,25(OH)2-vitamin D concentrations and net intestinal calcium, phosphate and magnesium absorption in humans. *Am J Clin Nutr* 1979; 32: 2052–60

34. Nicklas TA. Calcium intake trends and health consequences from childhood through adulthood. *J Am Coll Nutr* 2003; 22: 340–56

35. Flynn A. The role of dietary calcium in bone health. *Proc Nutr Soc* 2003; 62: 851–8

36. Prentice A. Diet, nutrition and the prevention of osteoporosis. *Public Health Nutr* 2004; 7: 227–43

37. Kardinaal AF, Ando S, Charles P, et al. Dietary calcium and bone density in adolescent girls and young women in Europe. *J Bone Miner Res* 1999; 14: 583–92

38. Chan GM, Hess M, Hollis J, et al. Bone mineral status in childhood accidental fractures. *Am J Dis Child* 1984; 138: 569–70

39. Saggese G, Baroncelli GI. Nutritional aspects of calcium and vitamin D from infancy to adolescence. *Ann Ist Super Sanità* 1995; 31: 461–79

40. Goulding A, Cannan R, Williams SM, et al. Bone mineral density in girls with forearm fractures. *J Bone Miner Res* 1998; 13: 143–8

41. Goulding A, Jones IE, Taylor RW, et al. Bone mineral density and body composition in boys with distal forearm fractures: a dual-energy X-ray absorptiometry study. *J Pediatr* 2001; 139: 509–15

42. Tucker KL. Does milk intake in childhood protect against later osteoporosis? *Am J Clin Nutr* 2003; 77: 10–11

43. Johnston CC, Miller JZ, Slemenda CW, et al. Calcium supplementation and increases in bone mineral density in children. *N Engl J Med* 1992; 327: 82–7

44. Lee WT, Leung SS, Leung DM, et al. A follow-up study on the effects of calcium-supplement withdrawal and puberty on bone acquisition of children. *Am J Clin Nutr* 1996; 64: 71–7

45. Lee WT, Leung SS, Leung DM, et al. Bone mineral acquisition in low calcium intake children following the withdrawal of calcium supplement. *Acta Paediatr* 1997; 86: 570–6

46. Bonjour JP, Chevalley T, Ammann P, et al. Gain in bone mineral mass in prepubertal girls 3.5 years after discontinuation of calcium supplementation: a follow-up study. *Lancet* 2001; 358: 1208–12

47. Toss G. Effect of calcium intake vs. other life-style factors on bone mass. *J Intern Med* 1992; 231: 181–6

48. Nilsson BE, Westlin NE. Bone density in athletes. *Clin Orthop* 1971; 77: 177–82

49. Huddleston AL, Rockwell D, Kulund DN. Bone mass in lifetime tennis athletes. *J Am Med Assoc* 1980; 224: 1107–9

50. Leblanc AD, Schneider VS, Evans HJ, et al. Bone mineral loss and recovery after 17 weeks of bed rest. *J Bone Miner Res* 1990; 5: 843–50

51. Anderson SA, Cohn SH. Bone demineralization during space flight. *Physiologist* 1985; 28: 212–17

52. Marcus R. Mechanisms of exercise effects on bone. In *Principles of Bone Biology*, 1st edn. San Diego, CA: Academic Press, 1996; 1135–46

53. Ruiz JC, Mandel C, Garabedian M. Influence of spontaneous calcium intake and physical exercise on the vertebral and femoral bone mineral density of children and adolescents. *J Bone Miner Res* 1995; 10: 675–82

54. Nordstrom P, Thorsen K, Nordstrom G, et al. Bone mass, muscle strength, and different body constitutional parameters in adolescent boys with a low or moderate exercise level. *Bone* 1995; 17: 351–6

55. Sinaki M, McPhee M, Hodgson S, et al. Relationship between bone mineral density of spine and strength of back extensor in healthy postmenopausal women. *Mayo Clin Proc* 1986; 61: 116–22

56. Snow-Harter C, Bouxsein M, Lewis B, et al. Muscle strength as a predictor of bone mineral density in young women. *J Bone Miner Res* 1990; 5: 589–95

57. Schonau E. The development of the skeletal system in children and the influence of muscular strength. *Horm Res* 1998; 49: 27–31

58. Welten DC, Kemper HCG, Post GB, et al. Weight-bearing activity during youth is a more important factor for peak bone mass than calcium intake. *J Bone Miner Res* 1994; 9: 1089–96

59. Specker BL. Evidence for an interaction between calcium intake and physical activity on changes in bone mineral density. *J Bone Miner Res* 1996; 11: 1539–44

60. Kelly PJ, Eisman JA, Sambrook PN. Interaction of genetic and environmental influences on peak bone density. *Osteoporos Int* 1990; 1: 56–60

Osteoporosis: influence of life-style

9

R. Rizzoli

INTRODUCTION

Diagnosis of the disease relies on the quantitative assessment of bone mineral mass/density, which represents one major determinant of bone strength and, thereby, of fracture risk. However, indications for treatment are based on the evaluation of fracture risk, which also integrates other factors, clinical and biochemical, compared with osteoporosis diagnosis. The age-related increase in fracture risk depends on a progressive decrease in bone mass, and a rising risk of falling. However, a minority of falls in the elderly (less than 2%) result in hip fracture[1]. The incidence of osteoporotic fractures varies from region to region, and may be related to population age distribution, genetic background or life-style conditions. For instance, it appears that hip fracture incidence is higher in urban than in rural areas in a given population[2]. Up to 40% of hip fractures concern patients living in nursing-homes[3]. This is probably related to advanced age and to a high prevalence of comorbidities requiring long-term care.

EXTRASKELETAL DETERMINANTS OF OSTEOPOROTIC FRACTURES

Almost all fractures, even those qualifying as 'low trauma' fractures, occur as a result of some injury. Usually this is the result of a fall, or the application of a specific loading event in some cases of vertebral fracture, such as bending forward to lift a heavy object with the arms extended. The risk of falling increases with age. Most falls in the elderly are due to intrinsic and extrinsic or environmental factors (Table 1). Among the intrinsic factors, the risk of falling increases with the number of disabilities. Impair-

Table 1 Risk factors associated with falls. Adapted from reference 4

Impaired mobility, disability
Impaired gait and balance
Neuromuscular or musculoskeletal disorders
Age
Impaired vision
Neurological, heart disorders
History of falls
Medication
Cognitive impairment

ment of gait, mobility and balance are the most consistently identified risk factors for falls and fall-related injuries. The ability to maintain postural control and avoid environmental obstacles depends on proprioceptive, vestibular and visual input translated into appropriate motor responses. Thus, the risk of falling increases with reduced visual acuity or diminished sensory perception of the lower extremities. Chronic illnesses, such as various neurological disorders, heart diseases, stroke, urinary incontinence, depression and impaired cognitive functions, increase the risk of falling. Medications such as hypnotics, antidepressants or sedatives are associated with falls. Environmental factors include potential hazards that can be found in the home, such as slippery floors, unstable furniture or insufficient lighting. The orientation of falls influences the consequences of falling. Indeed, the points of impact of a fall determine the type and extent of injury. When falling, the elderly tend to land on the hip. In contrast, middle-aged adults tend to fall forward, with the main impact on the wrist. Several reflexes and postural responses are initiated during a fall which can prevent or reduce the injury. The effectiveness of reflex actions depends on the speed of execution and the strength of the muscles initiating the protective movement. The impact of falls can be absorbed by surrounding soft tissue. The apparent protective effect of higher body weight may be due, at least in part, to the local shock-absorbing capacity of muscle and fat.

RISK FACTORS

Risk factors for osteoporotic fractures are listed in Table 2. The onset of substantial bone loss occurs at the age of 50 and 65 years in women and men, respectively. In contrast with bone mineral accrual during adolescence, bone size varies little throughout life, beyond the continuous and slight expansion of bone outer dimensions, which is mainly found in men, and which affects both the axial and the peripheral skeleton. This periosteal expansion is less than the increase in bone marrow space, which results from continuous endosteal resorption. Under these conditions, bone cortex becomes thinner. This phenomenon, together with an increment in cortical porosity and the destruction of trabeculae through thinning and perforation, accounts for age-dependent bone loss. Thus, this modeling process could be interpreted as a response to bone loss, in an attempt to compensate for a reduction in mechanical resistance[6].

Nutritional causes of bone mass loss

Calcium intake, vitamin D and osteoporosis

Calcium contributes to preservation of the bony tissue during adulthood, particularly in the elderly. Without an appropriate supply of vitamin D, from cutaneous and/or exogenous sources, the bioavailability and metabolism of calcium are disturbed[7]. This results in accelerated bone loss.

In the elderly, several alterations contribute towards a negative calcium balance. Indeed, with aging there is a decrease in calcium intake because of a reduction in dairy products consumption, in intestinal absorption of calcium, in the absorptive capacity of the intestinal epithelium to adapt to a low calcium intake, in

Table 2 Risk factors for osteoporotic fractures. Adapted from reference 5

Female sex
Premature menopause
Age[*]
Primary or secondary amenorrhea
Primary and secondary hypogonadism in men
Asian or white ethnic origin
Previous fragility fracture[*]
Low bone mineral density
Glucocorticoid therapy[*]
High bone turnover[*]
Family history of hip fracture[*]
Poor visual acuity[*]
Low body weight[*]
Neuromuscular disorders[*]
Cigarette smoking[*]
Excessive alcohol consumption
Long-term immobilization
Low dietary calcium intake
Vitamin D deficiency

---

[*]Characteristics that capture aspects of fracture risk over and above that provided by bone mineral density

exposure to sunlight and the capacity of the skin to produce vitamin D, and in renal reabsorption of calcium; there is also a decrease in the tubular calcium reabsorptive capacity to respond to the stimulatory effect of parathyroid hormone (PTH). Furthermore, the mild renal insufficiency regularly observed in the elderly can contribute to a state of chronic hyperparathyroidism that favors negative bone mineral balance and thereby osteoporosis. Increasing the calcium intake is certainly an important strategy, which appears to be relatively easier to implement compared with other possible preventive measures.

Protein malnutrition

Nutritional deficiencies play a significant role in osteoporosis in the elderly. Indeed, undernutrition is often observed in the elderly, and appears to be more severe in patients with hip fracture than in the general aging population. A low protein intake could be particularly detrimental for the conservation of bone integrity with aging[8,9]. Protein undernutrition can favor the occurrence of hip fracture by increasing the propensity to fall as a result of muscle weakness and impairment in movement coordination; by affecting protective mechanisms, such as reaction time and muscle strength, and thus reducing the energy required to fracture an osteoporotic proximal femur; and/or by decreasing bone mass (Figure 1)[10]. Furthermore, a reduction in the protective layer of soft tissue padding decreases the force required to fracture an osteoporotic hip.

Protein and osteoporotic fracture

Either a deficient or an excessive protein supply could negatively affect the balance of calcium[10]. An indirect argument in favor of a deleterious effect of high protein intake on bone is that hip fracture appears to be more frequent in countries with a high protein intake of animal origin. However, as expected, countries with the highest incidence of hip fracture are those with the longest life expectancy. In a prospective study carried out in more than 40 000 women in Iowa, a higher protein intake was associated with a reduced risk of hip fracture. The association was particularly evident with protein of animal rather than vegetal origin[11]. Increasing protein intake

has a favorable effect on bone mineral density (BMD) in elderly subjects receiving calcium and vitamin D supplements[12].

Protein and bone mass

Regarding the relationship to bone mineral mass, there is a positive correlation with spontaneous protein intake in premenopausal women[9]. In a longitudinal follow-up in the frame of the Framingham Study, the rate of bone mineral loss was inversely correlated to dietary protein intake[13]. Taken together, these results indicate that a sufficient protein intake is mandatory for bone health, particularly in the elderly. Thus, whereas a gradual decline in calorie intake with age can be considered an adequate adjustment to the progressive reduction in energy expenditure, the parallel reduction in protein intake may be detrimental for maintaining the integrity and function of several organs or systems, including skeletal muscles and bone.

Protein replenishment and osteoporosis

A state of undernutrition on admission, which is consistently documented in elderly patients with hip fracture, followed by inadequate food intake

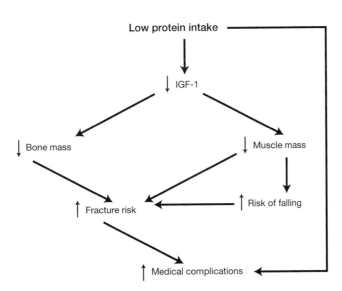

Figure 1 Protein undernutrition in the elderly. Possible role of insulin-like growth factor-I (IGF-I) in bone mass, muscle mass, risk of fracture and outcome after hip fracture

during the hospital stay, can adversely influence their clinical outcome[14]. An oral protein supplement that brought the intake from low to a level still below the recommended dietary allowance (RDA) (i.e. 0.8 g/kg body weight), thus avoiding the risk of an excess of dietary protein, improved the clinical course in the rehabilitation hospital, significantly lowering the rate of complications such as bed-sores, severe anemia or intercurrent lung or renal infections. The total length of stay in the orthopedic ward and rehabilitation hospital was significantly shorter by 25% in supplemented patients than in controls[14–16]. Normalization of protein intake, independent of that of energy, calcium and vitamin D, was in fact responsible for this more favorable outcome[15,16].

Vitamin K and osteoporosis

A low level of vitamin K_1 and K_2 has been reported in patients sustaining hip fracture[17]. The degree of vitamin K deficiency in humans can be assessed by measuring the undercarboxylated fraction of osteocalcin. This fraction increases with age and, therefore, is negatively related to BMD in elderly women. Hence, undercarboxylated osteocalcin has been found to be a predictor of hip fracture. Energy–protein undernutrition is usually associated with various vitamin deficiencies. To what extent vitamin K deficiency *per se* contributes to bone loss in undernourished patients sustaining hip fracture is still not known.

Other nutrients

By interfering with both the production and the action of parathyroid hormone, magnesium may indirectly affect bone metabolism. However, a specific role in the maintenance of bone mass during adulthood has not yet been identified. Several trace elements are required for normal bone metabolism. Various animal and/or ecological human studies suggest that aluminum, zinc, manganese, copper, boron, silicon and fluoride, at doses lower than those used in the treatment of osteoporosis, and vitamins B_6, B_{12} and C, could play a positive role in the normal metabolism of bone tissue. Selective intervention studies are still required to delineate their respective roles in the maintenance of bone mass, particularly in the elderly.

Mechanical causes of bone mass loss

Immobilization is an important cause of bone loss. The effect of disuse on bone mass is far greater than that of adding walking to an already ambulatory subject. Enforced immobilization in healthy volunteers results in a decrease in bone mineral mass. Motor deficit due to neurological disorders such as hemiplegia or paraplegia is a cause of bone loss. At the tissue level, immobilization results in negative balance, the amount of bone resorbed being greater than that formed. At the cellular level, immobilization results in increased osteoclastic resorption associated with a decrease in osteoblastic formation. The nature of the molecular signal(s) perceiving the reduced mechanical strain has not yet been clearly identified.

Toxic causes of bone mass loss

Excessive alcohol consumption appears to be a significant risk factor for osteoporosis, particularly in men[18]. Reduced rates of bone formation have been associated with alcohol abuse. A high intake of alcohol is often associated with marked dietary disturbance such as low protein intake, other changes in life-style, liver disease and decrease in testosterone production. These alterations can contribute to the osteoporosis observed in heavy drinkers. The use of tobacco appears to be associated with an increased risk of both axial and appendicular osteoporotic fractures in women and men[19]. This risk emerges with age. Smoking reduces the protective effects of obesity and of estrogen exposure. A reduced rate of bone formation and increased bone resorption might be responsible for bone loss, through a reduction in the production of and an acceleration in the degradation of estrogens.

GENERAL MANAGEMENT

The general measures to apply to reverse the negative impact of life-style disorders (Table 3) are based on the following reasons.

Table 3 General management

Treat any disease causing bone loss
Ensure dietary calcium intake ≥ 1000 mg/day
Ensure adequate dietary protein intake (1 g/kg body weight)
Correct or prevent vitamin D insufficiency (800 IU/day)
Promote weight-bearing physical exercise
Reduce falling risk
Reduce fall consequences (hip protectors)

There is a high prevalence of calcium, protein and vitamin D insufficiency in the elderly[6,9]. Calcium and vitamin D supplements decrease secondary hyperparathyroidism and, particularly in elderly subjects living in nursing-homes, reduce the risk of proximal femur fracture[20]. Sufficient protein intakes are necessary for homeostasis of the musculoskeletal system, but also in decreasing the complications occurring after an osteoporotic fracture[8,10,15]. Under these conditions, intakes of at least 1000 mg/day of calcium, 800 IU of vitamin D and 1 g/kg body weight of protein can be recommended in the general management of patients with osteoporosis. Regular physical exercise helps to maintain bone health, not only by stimulating bone formation and by retarding bone resorption, but also through a favorable influence on muscle function[21,22]. These measures, together with correction of decreased visual acuity, a reduction of drug consumption altering awareness and balance, and an improvement of the home environment (slippery floor, obstacles, insufficient lighting), are important steps aimed at preventing falls[4,23]. However, they have not been verified in randomized controlled trials fulfilling the requirements of evidence-based medicine. The wearing of hip protectors can significantly and specifically reduce hip fracture risk[24]. This has been shown in randomized controlled trials, and seems to be particularly efficient in the elderly living in nursing-homes. This population is at very high risk, since close to 40% of hip fractures occur in this kind of setting[3].

ACKNOWLEDGMENTS

Studies by our group cited in this chapter were supported by the Swiss National Science Foundation (grant nos. 32-49757.96, 32-58880.99 and 3200B0-100714). We would like to thank Marianne Perez for secretarial assistance.

References

1. Cummings SR, Melton LJ. Epidemiology and outcomes of osteoporotic fractures. *Lancet* 2002; 359: 1761–7

2. Chevalley T, Hermann FR, Delmi M, et al. Evaluation of the age-adjusted incidence of hip fractures between urban and rural areas: the difference is not related to the prevalence of institutions for the elderly. *Osteoporos Int* 2002; 13: 113–18

3. Schurch MA, Rizzoli R, Mermillod B, et al. A prospective study on socioeconomic aspects of fracture of the proximal femur. *J Bone Miner Res* 1996; 11: 1935–42

4. Myers AH, Young Y, Langlois JA. Prevention of falls in the elderly. *Bone* 1996; 18: 87S–101S

5. Kanis JA. Diagnosis of osteoporosis and assessment of fracture risk. *Lancet* 2002; 359: 1929–36

6. Seeman E. Pathogenesis of bone fragility in women and men. *Lancet* 2002; 359: 1841–50

7. Heaney RP. Calcium, dairy products and osteoporosis. *J Am Coll Nutr* 2000; 19: 83–99S

8. Rizzoli R, Bonjour JP. Nutritional approaches to healing fractures in the elderly. In Rosen CJ, Glowacki J, Bilezikian JP, eds. *The Aging Skeleton*. San Diego, CA: Academic Press, 1999: 399–409

9. Rizzoli R, Ammann P, Chevalley T, et al. Protein intake and bone disorders in the elderly. *Joint Bone Spine* 2001; 68: 383–92

10. Rizzoli R, Ammann P, Chevalley T, et al. Dietary protein intakes and bone strength. In Burckhardt P, Dawson-Hughes B, Heaney RP, eds. *Nutritional Aspects of Osteoporosis*. San Diego, CA: Elsevier Academic Press, 2004; 379–97

11. Munger RG, Cerhan JR, Chiu BC. Prospective study of dietary protein intake and risk of hip fracture in postmenopausal women. *Am J Clin Nutr* 1999; 69: 147–52

12. Dawson-Hughes B, Harris SS. Calcium intake influences the association of protein intake with rates of bone loss in elderly men and women. *Am J Clin Nutr* 2002; 75: 773–9

13. Hannan MT, Tucker KL, Dawson-Hughes B, et al. Effect of dietary protein on bone loss in elderly men and women: the Framingham Osteoporosis Study. *J Bone Miner Res* 2000; 15: 2504–12

14. Delmi M, Rapin CH, Bengoa JM, et al. Dietary supplementation in elderly patients with fractured neck of the femur. *Lancet* 1990; 335: 1013–16

15. Schurch MA, Rizzoli R, Slosman D, et al. Protein supplements increase serum insulin-like growth factor-I levels and attenuate proximal femur bone loss in patients with recent hip fracture. A randomized, double-blind, placebo-controlled trial. *Ann Intern Med* 1998; 128: 801–9

16. Tkatch L, Rapin CH, Rizzoli R, et al. Benefits of oral protein supplementation in elderly patients with fracture of the proximal femur. *J Am Coll Nutr* 1992; 11: 519–25

17. Booth SL, Broe KE, Gagnon DR, et al. Vitamin K intake and bone mineral density in women and men. *Am J Clin Nutr* 2003; 77: 512–16

18. Kanis JA, Borgstrom F, De Laet C, et al. Assessment of fracture risk. *Osteoporos Int* 2005; 16: 581–9

19. Kanis JA, Johnell O, Oden A, et al. Smoking and fracture risk: a meta-analysis. *Osteoporos Int* 2005; 16: 155–62

20. Chapuy MC, Arlot ME, Duboeuf F, et al. Vitamin D3 and calcium to prevent hip fractures in elderly women. *N Engl J Med* 1992; 327: 1637–42

21. Kelley GA, Kelley KS, Tran ZV. Exercise and bone mineral density in men: a meta-analysis. *J Appl Physiol* 2000; 88: 1730–6

22. Wolff I, van Croonenborg JJ, Kemper HC, et al. The effect of exercise training programs on bone mass: a meta-analysis of published controlled trials in pre- and postmenopausal women. *Osteoporos Int* 1999; 9: 1–12

23. Tinetti ME. Clinical practice. Preventing falls in elderly persons. *N Engl J Med* 2003; 348: 42–9

24. Kannus P, Parkkari J, Niemi S, et al. Prevention of hip fracture in elderly people with use of a hip protector. *N Engl J Med* 2000; 343: 1506–13

Postmenopausal osteoporosis and dental health

10

J. Wactawski-Wende

INTRODUCTION

Osteoporosis and periodontitis are diseases that affect a large number of men and women in the United States and worldwide, with increasing incidence with advancing age. Osteoporosis is a skeletal disorder characterized by compromised bone strength predisposing to increased risk of fracture, with bone strength determined by both bone density and bone quality[1]. Periodontitis has historically been described as an infection-mediated process characterized by resorption of the alveolar bone as well as loss of the soft tissue attachment to the tooth, and is a major cause of tooth loss in adults. It is assessed by oral examination, and typically characterized by determining the amount of loss of clinical attachment of the soft tissue adjacent to the teeth and the depth of pocket between the tooth and gum, or by measuring loss of alveolar crestal bone height (ACH) surrounding the teeth.

Periodontal disease is a major cause of tooth loss and edentulousness in adults[2], and has been associated with a number of chronic diseases[3-5] including osteoporosis. The association between osteoporosis and both periodontal disease and tooth loss in postmenopausal women has been addressed in a growing number of studies.

OVERVIEW OF PERIODONTAL DISEASES

Periodontal diseases include both gingivitis and periodontitis, which are infection-mediated inflammatory processes in the oral cavity. Both gingivitis and periodontitis are common in adults. Gingivitis usually affects only the gums and can result in inflammation, whereas periodontitis is usually more extensive, involving more of the soft tissue and the alveolar bone surrounding the teeth. Although milder forms of periodontitis are more common, the percentage of individuals with moderate to severe periodontitis increases with age. The more severe forms of periodontitis lead to the destruction of supporting tissue and resorption of the alveolar bone surrounding the teeth, and can, in the most severe cases, lead to tooth loss.

Although gingivitis may never proceed to periodontitis, it is usually the precursor to this more severe form of disease. Gingival inflammation is chararacterized by swelling, bleeding and reddening of the gums, which can be tender. Bacteria accumulate in the biofilm (plaque) at the gingival margins and result in a local immune response. Dental hygiene including brushing, flossing and cleaning, which reduce plaque formation, can reverse this process. However, gingivitis can lead to chronic infection and periodontitis in those instances where the amount of plaque and infection are left unchecked. The infectious agents that lead to destructive periodontal disease are typically gram-negative anaerobes. Factors that can influence gingival inflammation include sex steroid hormone levels, certain medications, cigarette smoking and certain diseases (human immunodeficiency virus, HIV). Most forms of adult periodontitis are moderately progressive and responsive to treatment.

In a healthy mouth, teeth are well supported by surrounding soft tissue and bone. The periodontal membrane or ligament attaches the surrounding soft tissue to the cementum of the tooth. Bony structure surrounds the tooth and

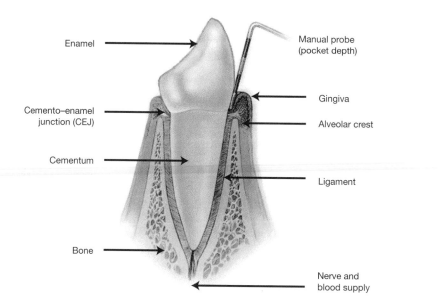

Enamel

Cemento–enamel
junction (CEJ)

Cementum

Bone

Manual probe
(pocket depth)

Gingiva

Alveolar crest

Ligament

Nerve and
blood supply

Figure 1 Tooth structures with major landmarks defined. Courtesy of the Florida Probe Corp.

provides support (Figure 1). In general, a chronic oral infection results in an immune response and gradual loss of attachment of the periodontal ligament to the gingiva. In addition, there is a loss of bone supporting the teeth. In the case of periodontitis, there is an accumulation of subgingival plaque. If the plaque is untreated, it becomes hardened, and this substance is known as calculus or tartar. As the condition progresses, the infectious agents in the biofilm continue to produce toxins that eventually destroy the periodontal ligament and bone, which over time results in the formation of a pocket between the tooth and adjacent tissues. This pocket harbors subgingival plaque and calculus and continues to cause damage to the surrounding tissues. If not treated, the disease progresses further until so much soft tissue and bone are lost that the tooth becomes unstable and can in some instances be lost. The progression of periodontal disease is illustrated in Figure 2.

The extent and severity of periodontal disease are determined through a series of measurements, including assessing the extent of gingival inflammation and bleeding, the probing depth of the pocket to the point of resistance, the clinical attachment loss of the periodontal ligament

measured from a fixed point on the tooth (usually the cemento–enamel junction) and the loss of adjacent alveolar bone as measured by X-ray[3]. Tooth loss due to periodontal disease can also be used to describe the extent and severity of disease. Severity is determined by both the extent of disease at any point in time and also the rate of disease progression over time and response of the tissues to treatment.

Gram-negative bacterial agents that have been implicated in the occurrence of periodontal disease include *Porphyromonas gingivalis*, *Prevotella intermedia*, *Tannerella forsythensis* (*Bacteroides forsythus*), *Treponema denticola* and *Actinobacillus actinomycetemcomitans*[3,6–9]. In reaction to the infection, neutrophils and antibodies respond to the site of the attack. In addition, cytokines and prostaglandin E_2 (PGE_2) are secreted by immune cells in response, and are known to affect bone, epithelial and connective tissues. Several of the cytokines that have been associated with periodontal diseases and local bone and tissue destruction are interleukin-1 (IL-1), tumor necrosis factor α (TNFα), and interferon γ (IFNγ), among others[10]. These cytokines mediate the processes of bone resorption and connective tissue destruction.

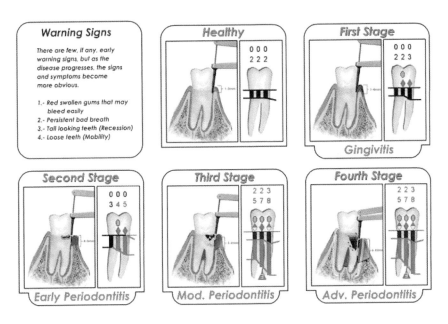

Figure 2 Stages of periodontal disease. Courtesy of the Florida Probe Corp.

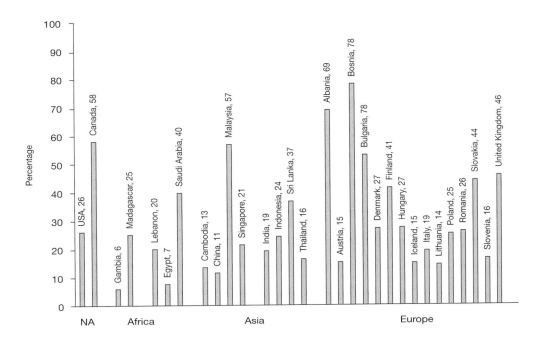

Figure 3 Edentulousness by selected countries. NA, North America. Source: reference 11

EPIDEMIOLOGY OF PERIODONTAL DISEASE AND TOOTH LOSS

Periodontal disease and tooth loss are quite prevalent, but vary by region. Figure 3 presents the prevalence of edentulousness for selected regions of the world for subjects aged 65 years and older. The rates range from less than 10% to over 60%. Although, in adults, tooth loss is primarily due to periodontal disease, extraction practices in various regions and trauma also have an impact on prevalence. In the United States, by the sixth decade of life, an average person has lost 12.1 teeth, including the third molars. Men and women are nearly equally likely to be edentulous. The rate of edentulousness increases with age, so that about a third (33.1%) of those aged 65 and older are edentulous, although this rate has declined over the past two decades in the USA[11,12].

The prevalence of clinical attachment loss increases with age, and varies to some degree by gender. In the United States, the prevalence of severe periodontal attachment loss increases dramatically with age, with nearly one-third of subjects having one or more teeth with 6 mm or more of attachment loss (Figure 4). Men are more likely to have at least one site with 6 mm or more loss. In addition, people with lower socioeconomic status are proportionately more likely to have severe attachment loss.

Age is one important factor that has been found to be associated with periodontal disease. In addition to increasing age, factors that have been associated with prevalence and severity of periodontitis include tobacco use[13], suboptimal dental care, low education level, low income, race, gender, genetics and certain medical conditions such as diabetes[3,13]. The risk factors and risk indicators for periodontal disease have been reviewed by Albandar[5]. Understanding the independent role of each of these factors is complicated by the fact that tobacco use, oral hygiene, professional prophylaxis and routine dental care are highly correlated with socioeconomic status, as are race and ethnicity.

CHARACTERIZATION OF PERIODONTAL DISEASE

Periodontal disease is assessed by oral examination, and typically characterized by determining the degree of loss of clinical attachment of the soft tissue adjacent to the teeth (CAL) and the depth of the pocket between the tooth and gum (PD), or by measuring the loss of alveolar crestal bone height surrounding the teeth (ACH). A thorough discussion of the classification of periodontal disease can be found elsewhere[14].

Pocket depth measurement

The sulcus or pocket depth is one measure of periodontal disease. It is usually determined by a probe inserted between the tooth and the gum. It is the distance in millimeters (mm) from the gingival margin (GM) to the base of the sulcus/pocket (see Figure 1). In research settings it is typically measured on six surfaces per tooth (distobuccal, mid-buccal, mesiobuccal, distolingual, mid-lingual and mesiolingual) of all the teeth present, except the third molars. Both manual probes and electronic probes can be used to assess PD. In general, pocket depth is considered a measure of recent infection, and is influenced by both depth of the pocket *per se* and hyperplasia or recession of the gum.

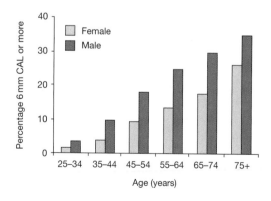

Figure 4 Percentage of US population with at least one tooth 6 mm or more clinical attachment loss (CAL) by age and gender. Adapted from reference 12 and National Center for Health Statistics data

Clinical attachment level

Clinical attachment level assesses the loss of attachment of the soft tissue from the surrounding teeth, and is defined as the distance in millimeters from a fixed point on the tooth, the cemento–enamel junction (CEJ), to the base of the pocket. The clinical attachment level is thought to be representative of the historical loss of attachment; however, this loss can be influenced by factors other than periodontal destruction, such as aggressive brushing. Periodontal severity increases as the amount of attachment loss and number of tooth sites affected increase. More severe disease can be defined as having 4 mm or more loss of attachment in at least one site. Attachment loss of 6 mm or more is considered very severe disease, and likely associated with later tooth loss.

Alveolar crestal height

Alveolar crestal height is typically assessed using oral radiographs. The ACH is a measure of the distance from the CEJ to the bone crest adjacent to the tooth, both mesially and distally. Although studies vary, typically a set of oral radiographs is taken including all teeth present in the mouth, with the exception of the third molars[15]. Standardization of the radiographs is critical, especially if the intent is to use the radiographs in studies of longitudinal change. Techniques employed in research to standardize these radiographs include the use of positioning devices such as ear-rods, as first described by Jeffcoat and colleagues[16], or a lateral cephalostat head-holder. In addition, positioning aids such as lasers are used in standardization. Other important considerations include beam length and angular position to the X-ray film, as well as processing technique. The technique for collection of standardized radiographs has been described by Hausmann and co-workers[15,17].

To measure interproximal alveolar crestal height (ACH), the radiographs are digitized. Measurements of cross-sectional radiographs includes computerized assessment of the ACH distance in millimeters. Typically, the values obtained are averaged across the entire mouth to obtain a mean ACH level, or in some instances

thresholds are described with distances over a predefined level being considered diseased. A value of 2 mm or less in distance from the CEJ to the crest of the tooth is considered healthy.

For longitudinal assessment of change, the technique usually includes a side-by-side comparison. Standardization of technique is critical for proper quantification of change. In longitudinal studies, the baseline radiograph and the follow-up radiograph are digitized and displayed side-by-side on a computer screen. The images are first aligned. Then the CEJs and alveolar crests are indicated on each image and a computer algorithm measures the distances and the difference. This routine requires the reader to determine whether the two images are aligned and comparable. Although there is considerable user interface, the error of the method has been demonstrated to be low with experienced examiners and standardized collection techniques[16,18–21]. Figure 5 includes two images from one individual taken 4 years apart. The loss in ACH is apparent.

Residual ridge resorption

The bone of the jaw where teeth are missing is called the residual ridge. Several studies have associated residual ridge resorption (RRR) with osteoporosis. Researchers have correlated the severity of osteoporosis with the degree of RRR. After a tooth is lost, there is resorption or recession of the oral bone in that region: this phenomenon is RRR. Most often, the extent of RRR is described in edentulous subjects, but RRR can be described in dentate subjects who have lost one or more teeth in the region of tooth loss. RRR can be described in cross-sectional studies, but more meaningful information can be obtained in prospective studies where the rate of RRR after tooth loss or extraction is described.

Clinical assessment for bleeding, plaque and calculus

Assessing plaque and calculus is typically done by examination, with a qualitative assessment given by the examiner. Plaque is usually assessed on three surfaces per tooth (buccal, mesiobuccal

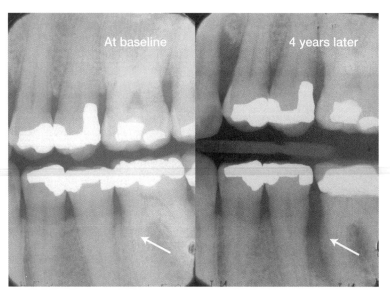

Figure 5 Alveolar crestal height change from baseline to 4 years later

and lingual) and scored as absent or present[22]. A calculus index is typically scored as absent, supragingival only or subgingival. Gingival bleeding is typically assessed in all teeth present, except for the third molars, by scoring bleeding (present or absent) upon gentle manipulation.

Tooth loss

Tooth loss is best assessed by an experienced examiner. Self-reported tooth loss is thought to be less reliable, and the location of lost teeth is usually unavailable. The reason for loss (caries, periodontal disease, trauma, other) is more difficult to obtain and often relies on recall of the subject, especially in large-scale studies. Also, the reason for tooth loss varies greatly across countries and regions, and may be the result of local practices and dentist preference, and may not reliably represent oral bone loss.

Radiographic assessment of oral bone density

The assessment of oral bone density is one of the most challenging of all in dental research. Measurement of oral bone density has been performed using a variety of techniques that include measurement of absolute density (dual energy X-ray absorptiometry (DXA); dual photon absorptiometry (DPA); quantitative computerized tomography (QCT); radiographic absorptiometry (RA)) of oral bones, and studies that approximate change in oral density over time, such as computer-assisted densitometric image analysis (CADIA). All techniques used to assess oral bone density are limited to some extent by either cost or precision. QCT provides perhaps the best assessment of oral density, since it allows assessment of the density in various regions of the oral bones without obstruction by teeth. However, this technique is relatively expensive and includes relatively high exposure to radiation. Both DPA and DXA have been used to assess oral bone density. However, positioning and reproducibility of oral density are difficult, and may require adaptations to the instrumentation[23]. RA has been used in several studies, employing bitewing radiographs taken with a calibrated step-wedge of known density in the field of X-ray. Reproducibility of this method is fairly good when positioning aids are used.

The region of the oral bone measured varies according to the technique used to assess oral density. Density assessments in human cadavers have shown variation across regions of the mandible, by edentulation and by age and gender[24,25]. QCT can measure virtually any region. RA is restricted to regions that can be accessed by bitewing radiographs. DXA and DPA can measure the mandible; however, obstruction by teeth in dentate subjects makes measurement of the basal bone easier to access and reproduce than regions surrounding the teeth. Most measurements are made in the mandible due to easier access. Within the mandible, subregions that may be measured include molar, premolar or incisor regions. Each region has the potential to be of different cortical thickness, which may affect density, especially using techniques that are two-dimensional and sensitive to thickness differences. Most (DXA, RA) but not all (QCT) measures of oral density are two-dimensional. The ability to measure oral bone density is restricted at least in part by whether or not teeth are present, with edentulous subjects being easier to assess without potential for tooth obstruction. However, edentulous subjects may have marked resorption of the residual ridge, which in turn affects the area of comparison and ultimately the density. Attempts to use radiomorphometric indices in panoramic radiographs to predict skeletal density have been largely disappointing[26].

For mandibular density using a step-wedge technique, an aluminum ramp of known distance is included in the periapical radiographs. The ramp generates a density gradient within the radiograph that is used after digitization to compare regions of bone surrounding the teeth. Here too, as in ACH determination, positioning is critical for both reliable assessment of the wedge (known density) and comparison with bone regions to determine bone density (g/cm²). The ramp needs to be properly aligned with respect to the X-ray beam. Various positioning aids assist in this, including use of ear-rods. These positioning aids are needed to ensure that the beam and ramp are perpendicularly aligned.

In addition to cross-sectional analysis of density, longitudinal assessment of change can be obtained by digitization of two radiographs after alignment, contrast correction and subtraction. The purpose of the digital subtraction is to iden-

tify the degree of change. An aluminum ramp included in the radiograph is used as an internal reference to measure mandibular bone density[20] in mg/mm². Newer techniques to optimize methods of subtraction and correction are currently under way.

STUDIES OF THE RELATIONSHIP OF OSTEOPOROSIS AND ORAL HEALTH

There is increasing evidence that osteoporosis, and the underlying loss of bone mass characteristic of this disease, is associated with oral bone loss, periodontal disease and tooth loss. Periodontitis has historically been defined as an infection-mediated destruction of the alveolar bone and soft tissue attachment to the tooth, responsible for most tooth loss seen in adult populations. Recent studies have shown low bone mass to be independently associated with measures of periodontal disease and tooth loss. Growing evidence supports the role of osteoporosis in the onset and progression of periodontal disease in humans, including several prospective studies.

Studies of osteoporosis and loss of soft tissue attachment

Studies of the relationship between measures of soft tissue attachment (CAL, PD) and osteoporosis have been mixed (Table 1). Phillips and Ashley[28] found that bone density assessed by the metacarpal index (MI) was associated with mesial pocket depth (Russell's periodontal index), and was significantly associated when limiting the assessment to posterior teeth, in 113 females aged 30–40 years. Ward and Manson[29] were able to find an association between periodontal disease index and loss of alveolar bone, but no relationship between metacarpal index and periodontal index. Elders and others[34] performed oral examinations and assessed spinal bone mineral density (BMD) and metacarpal cortical thickness (MCT) in 286 women aged 46–55 years. Sixty (21%) of the cohort were edentulous. In the dentate subjects, no significant correlation was observed between the clinical parameters of

Table 1 Studies of the relationship of osteoporosis and clinical attachment level (CAL)

Authors (year)	Oral measure	Osteoporosis assessment	Study design	Association
Groen et al.[27] (1968)	CAL	osteoporosis on X-ray	CS	+
Phillips and Ashley[28] (1973)	PD, Russell's index	metacarpal index	CS	+
Ward and Manson[29] (1973)	PD	metacarpal index	CS	−
Kribbs et al.[30] (1983)	PD	BMD forearm	CS	−
Kribbs et al.[31] (1989)	PD	BMD	CS	+
Kribbs et al.[32] (1990)	PD	BMD normal women	CS	−
Kribbs[33] (1990)	PD, CAL	osteoporosis – yes/no	CS	−
Elders et al.[34] (1992)	PD, bleeding	BMD spine	CS	−
von Wowern et al.[35] (1992)	CAL	BMC	P	−
von Wowern et al.[36] (1994)	CAL	fracture – yes/no	CS	+
von Wowern et al.[37] (1996)	CAL, bleeding	parenteral nutrition	CS	−
Hildebolt et al.[38] (1997)	CAL	BMD spine, hip	CS	−
Mohammed et al.[39] (1996)	CAL, GR	BMD spine	CS	+
Mohammed et al.[40] (1997)	CAL	BMD spine	CS	+
Weyant et al.[41] (1999)	CAL	BMD hip, spine, wrist	CS	+/−
Payne et al.[42] (2000)	bleeding, plaque	osteoporosis – yes/no	P	+
Tezal et al.[43] (2000)	CAL	BMD spine, hip, wrist	CS	+/−
Ronderos et al.[44] (2000)	CAL	BMD hip	CS	+
Inagaki et al.[45] (2001)	CPITN	metacarpal BMD	CS	+
Pilgram et al.[46] (2002)	CAL	BMD spine, hip	CS, P	+/−
Yoshihara et al.[47] (2004)	CAL	heel ultrasound	P	+

PD, pocket depth; GR, gingival recession; CPITN, Community Periodontal Index of Treatment Need; BMD, bone mineral density; BMC, bone mineral content; CS, cross-sectional; P, prospective; +, positive association; −, no association

periodontitis (mean probing depth, bleeding after probing and number of missing teeth) and BMD/MCT, nor between bone mass and alveolar bone height[34].

In two studies that had a primary intent to focus on the association between mandibular and skeletal density, Kribbs[31,32] showed that mandibular bone mass was significantly correlated with skeletal bone mass. However, periodontal pocket depth and bleeding showed no difference between women with osteoporosis and those with normal bone density. Plaque, calculus, smoking habits, reason for tooth extraction and other confounding factors were not assessed in this population. In another study comparing 112 normal and osteoporotic women aged 50–85, no differences were found in periodontal measures including mean pocket depth, distance from the CEJ to the pocket and bleeding on probing[33]. However, a previous study in osteoporotic

women found that periodontal pockets and bleeding on probing were significantly associated with mandibular bone mass[31].

In an earlier study in 30 postmenopausal women, Kribbs and others[30] found that neither forearm nor mandibular density was associated with periodontal measures (pocket depth, bleeding, root remaining); however, inflammation and pocket depth were significantly correlated. Although measures of periodontal disease were not found to be associated with density in this study, a significant correlation was found to exist between forearm density and oral bone density[30].

von Wowern and colleagues conducted a series of studies of periodontal disease and osteoporosis. In a recent case–control study that looked at oral and skeletal bone density in 26 female subjects, 12 with a history of osteoporotic fractures and 14 'normal' women, the authors found significantly more loss of periodontal attachment in osteoporotic women than in 'normal' women[36]. No difference was found for plaque or gingival bleeding between the two groups. Although the groups were similar with respect to age, menopausal age and smoking status, no control for confounding was done in the analysis.

A prior study that included 17 men and women being treated with glucocorticoid steroids found no significant associations between loss of bone mineral content and plaque, gingival bleeding or periodontal attachment loss[35]. In a study of men and women with short bowel syndrome on home parenteral nutrition, mean periodontal attachment loss was 2.51 mm in young females and 2.67 mm in the male subjects. All older women in this study were edentulous. No comparison group was available to assist with interpretation of these findings; however, additional periodontal variables (visible plaque, gingival bleeding) were similar to those expected from the published literature[37]. In another study, von Wowern and colleagues showed that periodontal attachment loss was significantly greater in women who had an osteoporotic fracture, compared with those with no previous fracture[36].

One of the earliest reports of the relationship between periodontal attachment loss and osteoporosis was a non-controlled study of the effects of osteoporosis on periodontal disease[27]. Groen and others[27] found toothlessness and severe periodontal disease among 38 patients, aged 43–73, who exhibited clinical and radiographic signs of advanced osteoporosis.

Hildebolt and others found no cross-sectional association between spine or femur BMD and periodontal attachment loss among 135 orally healthy subjects, although enrollment criteria may have limited the study's ability to detect an association if one existed[38]. In two longitudinal reports[42,48] designed to determine the association between skeletal and oral bone density, bleeding, plaque and periodontal attachment loss were also assessed. One study assessed the role of smoking in this relationship and found no difference in any periodontal variables between smokers and non-smokers, although the sample was small, consisting of 59 postmenopausal females. A second study of 38 postmenopausal women focused on the difference in bleeding and plaque between osteoporotic and non-osteoporotic females. Bleeding but not plaque was found to be worse in osteoporotic subjects. Pilgram and others[46], however, did not find a strong association between BMD of the spine and hip and attachment loss in 135 women participating in a clinical trial of hormone therapy. The association of BMD with CAL at baseline was insignificant; however, there was a suggestion that longitudinal changes in BMD were correlated with changes in CAL.

Several more recent studies have found an association. Mohammad and others[39] examined a subgroup of 42 postmenopausal Caucasian women participating in a larger study of 565 females. This small study found that those with low BMD had more gingival recession and a worse periodontal attachment level. In a 1997 study of 44 postmenopausal Caucasian females, Mohammad found that periodontal attachment loss varied according to spinal BMD, with greater loss of attachment seen in the group with the worst bone density.

Weyant and others[41] studied 292 white dentate women (mean age 75.5 years) randomly selected from participants of the Study of Osteoporotic Fractures, an ongoing study of risk factors for fracture in women over age 65. This study found an association between trochanteric region BMD and mean periodontal attachment level; however, the association did not reach statistical significance ($p = 0.09$) after adjustment for potential confounding variables. Although insignificant, 90% of the associations examined suggested worse periodontal disease with worse bone density measures.

In a study of 70 postmenopausal women from Buffalo[43], a relationship was found between spinal osteopenia and probing attachment loss. The relationship between CAL and BMD did not reach statistical significance after controlling for various confounding factors; however, the associations were consistent and may have been limited by the small sample size.

Yoshihara and colleagues[47] conducted a longitudinal study of periodontal attachment loss and bone density in a group of elderly Japanese men and women. There were differences in the mean number of progressive sites in the osteoporotic group (4.65 ± 5.51) compared with those without osteoporosis (3.26 ± 3.01) in females. Differences were also observed in males $(6.88 \pm 9.41$ vs. $3.41 \pm 2.79)$[47]. A small cross-sectional study of 30 Asian-American women found significant negative correlations for BMD and tooth loss and BMD and clinical attachment loss $(p < 0.01)$. Those with normal BMD had lost, on average, 6.8 teeth, compared with 10.5 teeth in the osteopenic group, and 16.5 teeth in the osteoporotic group $(p < 0.001)$[49]. Periodontal status was determined by the Community Periodontal Index of Treatment Need (CPITN). Periodontal severity was found to be increased in another study of Japanese subjects with lower metacarpal BMD, in both pre- and post-menopausal women. Among postmenopausal women, those with very low BMD had fewer teeth present than women with normal BMD[45].

Ronderos and colleagues[44] found that females with high calculus scores and low BMD had significantly more CAL than females with normal BMD and similar calculus scores $(p < 0.0001)$. No association was observed among women with low and intermediate levels of calculus. After adjustment for possible confounders, post-menopausal women who used hormone therapy had significantly less mean CAL than those who never used hormones.

Although the results of studies of the association of soft tissue attachment and bone density are mixed, several recent studies including one large population-based study have found an association. The relationship between osteoporosis and measures of soft tissue is not particularly strong, and likely requires larger, well-characterized studies in people at high risk.

Studies of osteoporosis and alveolar crestal height loss and residual ridge resorption

Most, but not all, studies of the relationship between osteoporosis or low skeletal BMD and ACH have shown an association (Table 2). However, the studies published to date are limited in number, and are largely cross-sectional in nature. The data from several prospective studies, however, support this association. Loss of ACH and RRR is more predominant in females than in males, and most predominant in older subjects. Presumably, the stronger consistent association found in older female subjects is due to lower bone density in these groups.

Residual ridge resorption has been shown to be affected by age; however, age was an important factor in loss of height in the residual ridge in edentulous adult mandibles only in females, but not in males[50]. Ortman and colleagues[51] assessed a random sample of 459 radiographs

Table 2 Studies of the relationship of osteoporosis and alveolar crestal height (ACH)

Authors (year)	*Oral measure*	*Osteoporosis assessment*	*Study design*	*Association*
Ward and Manson[29] (1973)	ABL/rapidity	metacarpal index	CS	+/–
Elders et al.[34] (1992)	ABH	BMD spine, MCT	CS	–
Humphries et al.[50] (1989)	RRR	gender, age	CS	+
Ortman et al.[51] (1989)	RRR	gender, age	CS	+
Hirai et al.[52] (1993)	RRR	osteoporosis – yes/no	CS	+
Wactawski-Wende et al.[53] (1996)	ACH	BMD spine, hip	CS	+
Payne et al.[42] (2000)	ACH	BMD spine, ABD	P	+
Tezal et al.[43] (2000)	ACH	BMD spine, hip	CS	+
Wactawski-Wende et al.[54] (2004)	ACH	*T*-score worst site	CS	+

ABL, alveolar bone loss; ABH, alveolar bone height; RRR, residual ridge resorption; BMD, bone mineral density; MCT, metacarpal cortical thickness; ABD, alveolar bone density; CS, cross-sectional; P, prospective; +, positive association; -, no association from edentulous patients, and found a significantly higher percentage of women with severe RRR than of men. Older female subjects (> 55 years) were more likely to be edentulous than older males and both male and female younger subjects. Hirai and others[52] found that skeletal osteoporosis strongly affected RRR in edentulous patients ($r = -0.42, p < 0.01$), as did female gender and increasing age.

A small study assessing the relationship between ACH and systemic BMD was conducted in 70 postmenopausal women[43,53]. Lower BMD of the femur was significantly correlated with worse mean ACH. The significant association between mean ACH and femur BMD persisted after adjustment for age, years since menopause, estrogen use, body mass index and smoking. More recently, a large cohort study of women was completed that examined the relationship between osteoporosis and severity of alveolar crestal bone loss. This well-controlled, large, cross-sectional study of over 1300 postmenopausal women showed a strong association between *T*-score category and ACH. This association was most evident in women 70 years of age or older, who were over three times more likely to have moderate to severe ACH if they were osteoporotic (Figure 6)[54].

Subject selection can influence the ability of a study to find an association. Studies that have included younger subjects have not found a consistent association between skeletal BMD and ACH. Elders and others assessed the association between alveolar bone height, spinal BMD and metacarpal cortical thickness (MCT) in 286 women aged 46–55 years, 21% of whom were edentulous[34]. The MCT and spinal BMD of dentate and edentulous subjects were not found to be different. In the dentate subjects, mean ACH was not correlated with spinal BMD, MCT, age or years since menopause. The lack of an association may have been limited by the selection of relatively young subjects (46–55 years), when the prevalence of osteoporosis may be low. Similarly, Ward and Manson were unable to show a significant relationship between ACH and metacarpal bone density in a younger group (mean age 41 years)[29]. However, 'rapidity' (alveolar bone loss divided by age) was associated with the metacarpal bone index in females, but not in males[29].

Prospective studies of the association of ACH and skeletal BMD are limited. However, one well-designed 2-year longitudinal study in 59 postmenopausal women determined that smokers ($n = 21$) had a higher frequency of ACH loss and worse oral density in the crestal and subcrestal regions than did non-smokers ($n = 38$). A significant interaction between spinal BMD and smoking on change in alveolar bone

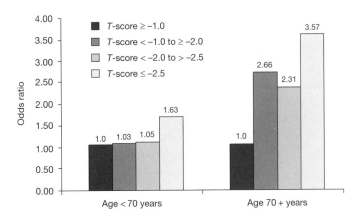

Figure 6 Odds ratios (adjusted for age, weight, school, current hormone therapy use, current calcium use, current vitamin D use, smoking status (ever/never)) for moderate to severe alveolar crestal height (ACH) by *T*-score group, age stratified

Table 3 Studies of the relationship of osteoporosis and tooth loss

Authors (year)	Oral measure	Osteoporosis assessment	Study design	Association
Daniell[55] (1983)	edentulousness	metacarpal index	CS	+
Kribbs et al.[32] (1990)	tooth number	osteoporosis – yes/no	CS	+
Kribbs et al.[33] (1990)	edentulousness	osteoporosis – yes/no	CS	+
Aström et al.[56] (1990)	tooth loss	hip fracture	P	+
Krall et al.[57] (1994)	tooth number	BMD spine, forearm	CS	+
Taguchi et al.[58] (1995)	tooth number	mandibular cortical width	CS	+
Taguchi et al.[59] (1995)	tooth number	fracture spine	CS	+
Krall et al.[60] (1996)	tooth loss	BMD loss	P	+
Krall et al.[61] (1997)	tooth number	estrogen use – yes/no	CS	+
Bando et al.[62] (1998)	edentulousness	BMD spine	CS	+
Taguchi et al.[63] (1999)	tooth number (posterior/anterior)	BMD spine	CS	+/–
Xie and Ainamo[64] (1999)	edentulousness	fracture history	CS	+
Wactawski-Wende et al.[53] (1996)	tooth number	BMD spine, hip	CS	+/–
May et al.[65] (1995)	tooth loss	BMD (men/women)	CS	+/–
Klemetti and Vainio[66] (1993)	tooth loss	BMD	CS	–
Klemetti et al.[67] (1994)	tooth loss	BMD	CS	–
Hildebolt et al.[38] (1997)	tooth number	BMD spine, hip	P	–
Mohammed et al.[40] (1997)	tooth loss	BMD spine	CS	–
Earnshaw et al.[68] (1998)	tooth number	BMD	CS	–
Inagaki et al.[45] (2001)	tooth number	metacarpal BMD	CS	+/–

BMD, bone mineral density; CS, cross-sectional; P, prospective; +, positive association; -, no association

density was found, with the non-smoking subjects with normal spine BMD gaining oral density over time, and subjects with low BMD who smoked losing oral BMD over time[42].

Osteoporosis and tooth loss

Numerous studies have looked at the relationship between osteoporosis and tooth loss, and most have found a positive association (Table 3). A cross-sectional study of mandibular BMD in osteoporotic women found that tooth loss and edentulousness were significantly more common in the osteoporotic group[32,33]. On average, the osteoporotic women had lost 6.9 mandibular teeth, compared with 4.5 teeth in women with normal BMD ($p < 0.05$). In a second study, osteoporotic subjects were reported to be edentulous more often than normal subjects (20% vs. 7%), although the differences were statistically insignificant[32,33]. In a previously reported study

of osteoporotic women, 20% of all women studied were edentulous[31]. The contributions of both osteoporosis severity and cigarette smoking to tooth loss were evaluated in 208 postmenopausal Caucasian women, aged 60–69, enrolled at a private dental office setting[55]. A strong association between smoking and edentulousness was found, and the pattern of denture need by age was worse for the women with osteoporosis.

Taguchi and co-workers studied the relationship between tooth loss and oral bone density. The first study included 269 subjects, 99 men and 170 women, aged 3–88 years. In males, no relationship was seen between mandibular cortical width and tooth loss; however, in female subjects, a decrease in mandibular cortical bone width was positively correlated with tooth loss. In women past their seventh decade of life, the association was most apparent[58,59]. In a cross-sectional study of 64 women aged 50–70 years, tooth loss was found to be highly correlated with the prevalence of spinal fracture[58,59]. A positive relationship between loss of the posterior teeth and alveolar and spinal bone density has been reported; however, no association was found between anterior teeth and density of the spine or oral cavity[63]. Bando and others[62] conducted a small study of 26 Asian postmenopausal subjects, 12 edentulous and 14 periodontally healthy dentate subjects. Spinal BMD was significantly lower in the edentulous subjects. One study of risk factors for edentulousness found self-reported fracture, as well as smoking and asthma, to be associated with edentulousness in 293 randomly selected elderly subjects from Helsinki[64]. Wactawski-Wende and others[53] reported a cross-sectional association between tooth loss and bone density in several regions of the hip, but not the spine, in a small study of 70 postmenopausal women. Significant correlations were found between fewer number of remaining teeth and bone density of several regions of the femur, including the total femur ($r = 0.21$, $p = 0.09$), Ward's triangle ($r = 0.31$, $p = 0.01$) and intertrochanter ($r = 0.23$, $p = 0.07$). A recent study found that periodontal status was related to low metacarpal bone density in both pre- and postmenopausal Japanese women. The number of teeth present was found to be associated with metacarpal bone density, but only in postmenopausal subjects[45].

A large cross-sectional study of the association of tooth loss with BMD of the spine and hip in 608 men and 874 women found that skeletal BMD in male subjects correlated with self-reported tooth loss, after controlling for age, BMI and smoking. However, the association of tooth loss with BMD was insignificant in the females studied, after controlling for the effects of age, BMI and smoking. Overall, 24% of the men and 27% of the women were edentulous, less than expected from previous estimates from this region. No information was available on the use of hormone replacement therapy in females[65].

Krall and co-workers[57] found a significant positive relationship between number of teeth and BMD of the spine ($p < 0.05$) and radius ($p < 0.01$) in a cross-sectional study of 329 postmenopausal women. The association persisted after controlling for pack-years of smoking, years since menopause, education and body mass. A subsequent analysis of participants in one of three prospective clinical trials of calcium and vitamin D assessed the relationship between bone loss in the hip, spine and total body and tooth loss in healthy, white, dentate, postmenopausal women[60]. In 189 women followed, 45 had lost at least one tooth during the next 7 years. Those who had lost teeth were significantly more likely than those who retained their teeth to lose BMD in the whole body, femur and spine (relative risk = 4.83, 1.50, 1.45, respectively), after controlling for years since menopause, body mass index (BMI), number of teeth at baseline, smoking and intervention assignment. Interestingly, all women enrolled had relatively normal spinal BMD values at baseline (i.e. no osteoporosis), and therefore the relationship of systemic bone loss to tooth loss would be predicted to be low over the 7-year study period. Of note was that half the women recruited reported ≤ 400 mg daily calcium dietary intake at baseline.

A related study of estrogen replacement use after the menopause and tooth retention in 488 women found that estrogen users had more teeth than non-users (12.5 vs. 10.7, $p = 0.046$), and duration of estrogen use independently predicted the number of remaining teeth ($p = 0.05$). Long-term users of estrogen had more teeth than never-users (14.3 vs. 10.7, $p < 0.02$). Estrogen use was shown to be protective for tooth loss, regardless of type of tooth or location in the mouth. Users of estrogen (1–4 years) had 1.1 more teeth than non-users[61].

A 3-year prospective Swedish study of 14 375 older men and women found that women with the fewest teeth at baseline (lowest tertile) had a risk of hip fracture that was twice that of women in the highest two tertiles. The association between tooth loss and hip fracture was stronger in the men studied, with the risk of fracture three-fold higher in men with the fewest teeth at baseline, although the absolute number of hip fractures was greatest in women[56].

Not all studies have found an association between bone density and tooth loss. Klemetti and Vainio[66] did not find an association between tooth loss and BMD in a group of 355 Finnish women; however, dental practice in Finland may have led to extractions for preventive purposes rather than as a result of underlying disease. Half of all the women studied had all their maxillary teeth and 25% of women had all their mandibular teeth extracted before the age of 30, suggesting that the reason for tooth loss was likely not periodontal in nature[66]. In a second report, Klemetti and colleagues[67] noted that tooth loss was greatest in those postmenopausal women in the lowest BMD category, although results were insignificant. The study included women between the ages of 48 and 56, who may not be at an age when the effects of osteoporosis on oral bone are yet detectable. Women with higher BMD retained their teeth in the presence of deep periodontal pockets better than those subjects with underlying osteoporosis. Mohammad and colleagues[40] conducted a study to assess the relationship between spinal bone density and tooth loss in a group of 44 white women. Tooth loss did not vary between groups with high and low spinal BMD overall, or after adjusting for age and periodontal status.

Several studies of younger women have not shown an association between bone density and periodontal disease. Hildebolt and others[38] found no association between spine or femur BMD and number of remaining teeth among 135 subjects enrolled in a hormone replacement study trial. Subjects were relatively young postmenopausal women who had ten or more teeth present and no periodontal pockets deeper than 5 mm at enrollment, limiting the ability to detect an association between BMD and tooth loss. Earnshaw and others[68] found no relationship between BMD and tooth number in 1365 white women aged between 45 and 59, who were within 12 years of the menopause. Analysis included adjustment for age, years since menopause, hormone replacement and center. This was a fairly large, well-controlled study; however, the underlying risk of tooth loss in this relatively young population may have been too small to observe in this study. Additional studies are needed to define this relationship further in larger cohorts of women, especially prospective cohorts where temporality can be established.

Osteoporosis and oral bone density

Oral bone density has been found to be associated with osteoporosis. Mandibular BMD was assessed by DPA and was found in a series of studies to be associated with total skeletal mass in osteoporotic women[35–37,69,70]. Mandibular density assessed by DPA was demonstrated to be highly accurate and precise[23]. Using this technique, von Wowern found that women had significantly lower bone mineral content (BMC) of the forearm and mandible, compared with men, and that, in older subjects mandibular density varied by sex and age, and rates of BMC loss were greater over time in older women than in men[69].

A 2-year prospective study of oral density in premenopausal and postmenopausal women before and following vestibulolingual sulcoplasty found baseline mandibular BMC to be related to the rate and percentage of mandibular BMC loss and RRR, particularly in older women[70]. BMC in the mandible and forearm was also found to decrease at a similar rate (5.6% per year) following glucocorticoid therapy in men and women[35].

In a case–control study of 12 women with a history of osteoporotic fractures and 14 normal controls, the osteoporotic women were found to have significantly lower mandibular and forearm BMC values compared with controls[36]. Mandibular BMC values in osteoporotic women were two standard deviations below those for young 'normal' women in 92% of the osteoporotic group and in 64% of the controls, suggesting that a large proportion of the controls also had mandibular osteopenia.

Kribbs and others[71] conducted a series of studies on the relationship between osteoporosis and oral bone density and other indicators of oral health in postmenopausal women, using a reproducible microdensitometry technique to determine mandibular density. In 30 postmenopausal women aged 55–71 years with a history of vertebral fracture, taking part in a larger randomized clinical trial, significant associations were found between RRR and bone height and radius density. Height of the mandible was correlated with tooth loss but not with density of the forearm regions or the mandible ($r = 0.21$). Mandibular density was correlated with total body calcium

($r = 0.89$) and forearm density ($r = 0.60$) in edentulous women ($n = 7$); however, only the correlation with total body calcium was statistically significant. A significant correlation was found to exist between forearm density and oral bone density[33]. Mandibular bone mass and cortical thickness at the gonion was found to be significantly correlated with BMD of the spine ($r = 0.39$) and radius ($r = 0.33$) in 50 women, aged 20–90, without vertebral fractures noted at enrollment. Associations were most apparent in the older (> 50) women. However, when spinal trabecular density was measured using QCT, only the association with cortical thickness at the gonion persisted[33]. In 112 women aged 50–85 years with or without prevalent vertebral fracture, women with vertebral fracture had significantly lower mandibular bone mass and density. Cortical thickness at the gonion was significantly higher in the normal subjects[33]. Kribbs and others[31] showed further that mandibular mass was correlated with all skeletal measures in osteoporotic women. The height of the edentulous ridge correlated with total body calcium and mandibular BMD.

Postmortem studies in edentulous female ($n = 24$) and male subjects ($n = 26$) found that specific gravity of the mandible and radius decreased with increasing age. Females had lower densities than males, and mandibular and radius measures were highly correlated ($r = 0.634$, $p < 0.01$)[72]. BMC in 25 edentulous mandibles taken from cadavers, measured by DPA, was found to increase in male subjects with advancing age, while mandibular BMC of female subjects tended to decrease with advancing age[73]. Mandibular density measured by QCT differed between partially and totally edentulous postmenopausal women who had been edentulous for more than 12 years, suggesting that years edentulous may be important when assessing the relationship between skeletal and mandibular density[74].

A prospective study of 69 women to determine the role of hormone therapy in the relationship between spinal density (DPA) and mandibular density (RA) found a significant, moderate correlation at baseline and at an average 5-year follow-up in 28 subjects. Density changes in the jaw and spine were also significantly correlated[75]. Oral density assessed by periapical radiographs in osteoporotic and normal women were associated ($p = 0.0534$) with skeletal density[76]. In a small study ($n = 24$) of estrogen levels (17β-estradiol (E_2)) among postmenopausal women, alveolar bone density was assessed using CADIA to measure the relative change in density in crestal and subcrestal regions of posterior interproximal alveolar bone. A net gain in alveolar density was found in E_2-sufficient women compared with those who were E_2-deficient ($p < 0.001$); however, the number of sites gaining/losing density were similar. CADIA does not allow calculation of absolute density changes[77]. In a 2-year study of oral bone density and bone height changes in 38 non-smoking postmenopausal women with periodontal disease, women with low BMD had higher rates of density loss and ACH loss than those with higher BMD. Estrogen deficiency was also found to be associated with greater loss of both oral BMD and ACH in women overall, and of crestal region density in osteopenic women[48]. These findings were supported by the results of a 3-year double-blind randomized clinical trial of hormone therapy that revealed that both oral and postcranial bone density were increased in postmenopausal women taking oral estrogen therapy, compared with placebo. In addition to the positive change in bone density, a significant increase in ACH was observed[78].

A 28-month prospective study of mandibular BMD (DXA) and hip BMD (DXA) and ultrasound assessment of the calcaneus and hand in 18 postmenopausal edentulous women found the largest change in density to occur in the mandible, with other significant loss seen in the femoral neck and Ward's triangle. Insignificant changes were seen in the trochanteric region and in all regions assessed by ultrasound. The change in mandibular density in this study was 7.54% per year. Although small, this study provided evidence of differential loss of BMD according to region[79].

Although there is evidence to support a correlation between systemic and oral bone density, several important issues remain, including: determination of normal ranges of mandibular density by age and sex, further comparison of mandibular density in normal and osteoporotic women, assessment of longitudinal progression of mandibular bone loss, comparison of rates of bone loss in the mandible and other skeletal regions, and the effects of different therapies on mandibular density compared with other skeletal sites[80]. Further study of measurement error in various techniques to assess oral density is also needed.

SUMMARY

Periodontitis results from bacteria that produce factors which cause loss of collagenous support of the tooth, as well as loss of alveolar bone. Osteoporosis is a skeletal disorder that results in loss of bone mineral throughout the body, including loss in the oral cavity. Reduction of bone in the oral cavity may result in more rapid alveolar crestal height loss after a challenge by bacteria. Systemic factors affecting bone remodeling may also modify the local tissue response to periodontal infection. Persons with systemic bone loss are known to have increased systemic production of cytokines (i.e. IL-1, IL-6) that may have effects on bone throughout the body, including the bones of the oral cavity. Periodontal infection has been shown to increase local cytokine production that, in turn, increases local osteoclast activity, resulting in increased bone resorption. Genetic factors that predispose a person to systemic bone loss also influence or predispose an individual to periodontal destruction. Last, certain life-style factors such as cigarette smoking and suboptimal calcium intake, among others, may put individuals at risk for development of both systemic osteopenia and oral bone loss.

A growing body of literature has accumulated regarding the role of osteoporosis in the onset and progression of periodontal disease and tooth loss, but further study is needed to understand this association. There is a need for additional studies, especially longitudinal studies to evaluate the temporal sequence of osteopenia and periodontal disease in large cohorts, where adequate assessment and control of confounding variables can be carried out.

Both osteoporosis and periodontal disease are major health concerns in older populations. Studies are needed to improve our understanding of the potential mechanisms by which osteoporosis is associated with periodontal disease and oral bone loss. Importantly, as further understanding of these common disorders is acquired, the consequences of osteoporosis on dental health can be better addressed. In addition, screening and treatment of the disease may be expanded to include dental-health professionals. This information will be increasingly important in the prevention of morbidity and mortality related to these very prevalent disorders in older Americans.

ACKNOWLEDGMENTS

The author would like to acknowledge Chris Gibbs and the Florida Probe Corp. for the use of illustrative diagrams in this manuscript.

References

1. National Institutes of Health. *Osteoporosis Prevention, Diagnosis, and Therapy*. NIH Consensus Statement. Washington, DC: NIH, March 2000; 17(1): 1–36

2. American Academy of Periodontology. *Glossary of Periodontal Terms*. 3rd edn. Chicago: American Academy of Periodontology, 1992

3. Genco R. Current view of risk factors for periodontal disease. *J Periodontol* 1996; 67S: 1041–9

4. Genco RJ, Löe H. The role of systemic conditions and disorders in periodontal disease. *Periodontology 2000* 1993; 2: 98–116

5. Albandar JM. Global risk factors and risk indicators for periodontal diseases. *Periodontology 2000* 2002; 29: 177–206

6. Socransky SS, Haffajee AD. The bacterial etiology of destructive periodontal disease: current concepts. *J Periodontol* 1992; 63: 322–31

7. Socransky SS, Haffajee AD. Microbial mechinisms in the pathogenesis of destructive periodontal diseases: a critical assesment. *J Periodontol Res* 1991; 26: 195–212

8. Li J, Helmerhorst EJ, Leone CW, et al. Identification of early microbial colonizers in human dental biofilm. *J App Microbiol* 2004; 97: 1311

9. Socransky SS, Haffajee AD. The nature of periodontal diseases. *Ann Periodontol* 1997; 2: 3–10

10. Genco RJ. Host responses in periodontal diseases: current concepts. *J Periodontol* 1992; 63: 338–55

11. Petersen PE. World Health Organization. *BULL WHO* 2005; 80(1)

12. US Surgeon General. Report on Oral Health, 2002. http://www.surgeongeneral.gov/library/oralhealth/

13. Grossi SG, Genco RJ, Machtei EE, et al. Assessment of risk for periodontal disease. II. Risk indicators for alveolar bone loss. *J Periodontol* 1995; 66: 23–9

14. Armitage GC. Classifying periodontal diseases – a long-standing dilemma. *Periodontology 2000* 2002; 30: 9–23

15. Hausmann E, Allen K, Dunford R, Christersson L. A reliable computerized method to determine the level of the radiographic alveolar crest. *J Periodont Res* 1989; 24: 368–9

16. Jeffcoat MK, Reddy MS, Webber RL, et al. Extra-oral control of geometry for digital subtraction radiography. *J Periodont Res* 1987; 22: 396–402

17. Hausmann E, Allen K, Clerehugh V. What alveolar crest level on a bite-wing radiograph represents bone loss? *J Periodontol* 1991; 62: 570–2

18. Hausmann E, Allen K, Carpio L, et al. Computerized methodology for detection of alveolar crestal bone loss from serial intraoral radiographs. *J Periodontol* 1992; 63: 657–62

19. Hausmann E, Allen K, Nordyerd J, et al. Studies on the relationship between changes in radiographic bone height and probing attachment. *J Clin Periodontol* 1994; 21: 128–32

20. Hausmann E, Allen K, Loza J, et al. Validation of quantitative digital subtraction radiography using electronically guided alignment device/impression technique. *J Periodontol* 1996; 67: 895–9

21. Hausmann E, Allen K. Reliability of bone height measurements made on serial radiographs. *J Periodontol* 1997; 68: 839–41

22. Machtei EE, Norderyd J, Koch G, et al. Rate of periodontal attachment loss in subjects with established periodontitis. *J Periodontol* 1993; 64: 713–18

23. von Wowern N. Dual-photon absorptiometry of mandibles: in vitro test of a new method. *Scand J Dent Res* 1985; 93: 169–77

24. Schwartz-Dabney CL, Dechow PC. Edentulation alters material properties of cortical bone in the human mandible. *J Dent Res* 2002; 81: 613–17

25. D'Amelio P, Panattoni GL, DiStefano M, et al. Densitometric study of dry human mandible. *J Clin Densitometry* 2002; 5: 363–7

26. Devlin, H, Horner K. Mandibular radiomorphometric indices in the diagnosis of reduced skeletal bone mineral density. *Osteoporos Int* 2002; 13: 373–8

27. Groen JJ, Menczel J, Shapiro S. Chronic destructive periodontal disease in patients with presenile osteoporosis. *J Periodontol* 1968; 39: 19–23

28. Phillips HB, Ashley FP. The relationship between periodontal disease and a metacarpal bone index. *Br Dent J* 1973; 134: 237–9

29. Ward VJ, Manson JD. Alveolar bone loss in periodontal disease and the metacarpal index. *J Periodontol* 1973; 44: 763–9

30. Kribbs PJ, Smith DE, Chesnut CH. Oral findings in osteoporosis. Part I: Measurement of mandibular bone density. *J Prosthet Dent* 1983; 50: 576–9

31. Kribbs PJ, Chesnut CH, Ott SM, Kilcoyne RF. Relationships between mandibular and skeletal bone in an osteoporotic population. *J Prosthet Dent* 1989; 62: 703–7

32. Kribbs PJ, Chesnut CH, Ott SM, Kilcoyne RF. Relationships between mandibular and skeletal bone in a population of normal women. *J Prosthet Dent* 1990; 63: 86–9

33. Kribbs PJ. Comparison of mandibular bone in normal and osteoporotic women. *J Prosthet Dent* 1990; 63: 218–22

34. Elders PJM, Habets LLMH, Netelenbos JC, et al. The relation between periodontitis and systemic bone mass in women between 46 and 55 years of age. *J Clin Periodontol* 1992; 19: 492–6

35. von Wowern N, Klausen B, Olgaard K. Steroid-induced mandibular bone loss in relation to marginal periodontal changes. *J Clin Periodontol* 1992; 19: 182–6

36. von Wowern N, Klausen B, Kollerup G. Osteoporosis: a risk factor in periodontal disease. *J Periodontol* 1994; 65: 1134–8

37. von Wowern N, Klausen B, Hylander E. Bone loss and oral state in patients on home parenteral nutrition. *J Parenteral Enteral Nutr* 1996; 20: 105–9

38. Hildebolt CF, Pilgram TK, Dotson M, et al. Attachment loss with postmenopausal age and smoking. *J Periodont Res* 1997; 32: 619–25

39. Mohammad AR, Brunsvold M, Bauer R. The strength of association between systemic postmenopausal osteoporosis and periodontal disease. *Int J Prosthodont* 1996; 9: 479–83

40. Mohammad AR, Bauer RL, Yeh C-K. Spinal bone density and tooth loss in a cohort of postmenopausal women. *Int J Prosthodont* 1997; 10: 381–5

41. Weyant RJ, Pearlstein ME, Churak AP, et al. The association between osteopenia and periodontal attachment loss in older women. *J Periodontol* 1999; 70: 982–91

42. Payne JB, Reinhardt RA, Nummikoski PV, et al. The association of cigarette smoking with alveolar bone loss in postmenopausal females. *J Clin Periodontol* 2000; 27: 658–64

43. Tezal M, Wactawski-Wende J, Grossi SG, et al. The relationship between bone mineral density and periodontitis in postmenopausal women. *J Periodontol* 2000; 71: 1492–8

44. Ronderos M, Jacobs DR, Himes JH, Pihlstrom BL. Associations of periodontal disease with femoral bone mineral density and estrogen replacement therapy: cross-sectional evaluation of US adults from NHANES III. *J Clin Periodontol* 2000; 27: 778–86

45. Inagaki K, Kurosu Y, Kamiya T, et al. Low metacarpal bone density, tooth loss, and peri-odontal disease in Japanese women. *J Dent Res* 2001; 80: 1818–22

46. Pilgram TK, Hildebolt CF, Dotson M, et al. Relationships between clinical attachment level and spine and hip bone mineral density: data from healthy postmenopausal women. *J Periodontol* 2002; 73: 298–301

47. Yoshihara A, Seida Y, Hanada N, Miyazaki H. A longitudinal study of the relationship between periodontal disease and bone mineral density in community-dwelling older adults. *J Clin Periodontol* 2004; 31: 680–4

48. Payne JB, Reinhardt RA, Nummikoski PV, Patil KD. Longitudinal alveolar bone loss in postmenopausal osteoporotic/osteopenic women. *Osteoporos Int* 1999; 10: 34–40

49. Mohammad AR, Hooper DA, Vermilyea SG, et al. An investigation of the relationship between systemic bone density and clinical periodontal status in post-menopausal Asian-American women. *Int Dent J* 2003; 53: 121–5

50. Humphries S, Devlin H, Worthington H. A radiographic investigation into bone resorption of mandibular alveolar bone in elderly edentulous adults. *J Dent* 1989; 17: 94–6

51. Ortman LF, Hausmann E, Dunford RG. Skeletal osteopenia and residual ridge resorption. *J Prosthet Dent* 1989; 61: 321–5

52. Hirai T, Ishijima T, Hashikawa Y, Yajima T. Osteoporosis and reduction of residual ridge in edentulous patients. *J Prosthet Dent* 1993; 69: 49–56

53. Wactawski-Wende J, Grossi S, Trevisan M, et al. The role of osteopenia in oral bone loss and periodontal disease. *J Periodontol* 1996; 67: 1076–84

54. Wactawski-Wende J, Hausmann E, Hovey KM, et al. The association between osteoporosis and oral bone loss in postmenopausal women. *J Periodontol* 2005; in press

55 Daniell HW. Postmenopausal tooth loss. Contributions to edentulism by osteoporosis and cigarette smoking. *Arch Intern Med* 1983; 143: 1678–82

56. Aström J, Bäckström C, Thidevall G. Tooth loss and hip fractures in the elderly. *J Bone Joint Surg (Br)* 1990; 72: 324–25

57. Krall EA, Dawson-Hughes B, Papas A, Garcia RI. Tooth loss and skeletal bone density in healthy postmenopausal women. *Osteoporos Int* 1994; 4: 104–9

58. Taguchi A, Tanimoto K, Suei Y, Wada T. Tooth loss and mandibular osteopenia. *Oral Surg Oral Med Oral Pathol Oral Radiol Endod* 1995; 79: 127–32

59. Taguchi A, Tanimoto K, Suei Y, et al. Oral signs as indicators of possible osteoporosis in older women. *Oral Surg Oral Med Oral Pathol Oral Radiol Endod* 1995; 80: 612–16

60. Krall EA, Garcia RI, Dawson-Hughes B. Increased risk of tooth loss is related to bone loss at the whole body, hip, and spine. *Calcif Tissue Int* 1996; 59: 433–7

61. Krall EA, Dawson-Hughes B, Garvey AJ, Garcia RI. Smoking, smoking cessation, and tooth loss. *J Dent Res* 1997; 76: 1653–9

62. Bando K, Nitta H, Matsubara M, et al. Bone mineral density in periodontally healthy and edentulous postmenopausal women. *Ann Periodontol* 1998; 3: 322–6

63. Taguchi A, Suei Y, Ohtsuka M, et al. Relationship between bone mineral density and tooth loss in elderly Japanese women. *Dentomaxillofac Radiol* 1999; 28: 219–23

64. Xie Q, Ainamo A. Association of edentulousness with systemic factors in elderly people living at home. *Community Dent Oral Epidemiol* 1999; 27: 202–9

65. May H, Reader R, Murphy S, Khaw K-T. Self-reported tooth loss and bone mineral density in older men and women. *Age Ageing* 1995; 24: 217–21

66. Klemetti E, Vainio P. Effect of bone mineral density in skeleton and mandible on extraction of teeth and clinical alveolar height. *J Prosthet Dent* 1993; 70: 21–5

67. Klemetti E, Vainio P, Lassila V. Mineral density in the mandibles of partially and totally edentate postmenopausal women. *Scand J Dent Res* 1994; 102: 64–7

68. Earnshaw SA, Keating N, Hosking DJ, et al. for the EPIC Study Group. Tooth counts do not predict bone mineral density in early postmenopausal Caucasian women. *Int J Epidemiol* 1998; 27: 479–83

69. von Wowern N. Bone mineral content of mandibles: normal reference values – rate of age related bone loss. *Calcif Tissue Int* 1988; 43: 193–8

70. von Wowern N, Hjorting-Hansen E. The mandibular bone mineral content in relation to vestibulolingual sulcoplasty. A 2-year follow-up. *J Prosthet Dent* 1991; 65: 804–8

71. Kribbs PJ, Smith DE, Chesnut CH. Oral findings in osteoporosis. Part II: Relationship between residual ridge and alveolar bone resorption in generalized skeletal osteopenia. *J Prosthet Dent* 1983; 50: 719–24

72. Henrikson P-A, Wallenius K. The mandible and osteoporosis (1). A qualitative comparison between the mandible and the radius. *J Oral Rehab* 1974; 1: 67–74

73. Solar P, Ulm CW, Thornton B, Matejka M. Sex-related differences in the bone density of atrophic mandibles. *J Prosthet Dent* 1994; 71: 345–9

74. Klemetti E, Collin H-L, Forss H, et al. Mineral status of the skeleton and advanced periodontal disease. *J Clin Periodontol* 1994; 21: 184–8

75. Jacobs R, Ghyselen J, Koninckx P, van Steenberghe D. Long-term bone mass evaluation of mandible and lumbar spine in a group of women receiving hormone replacement therapy. *Eur J Oral Sci* 1996; 104: 10–16

76. Mohajery M, Brooks SL. Oral radiographs in the detection of early signs of osteoporosis. *Oral Surg Oral Med Oral Pathol Oral Radiol Endod* 1992; 73: 112–17

77. Payne JB, Zachs NR, Reinhardt, RA et al. The association between estrogen status and alveolar bone density changes in postmenopausal women with a history of periodontitis. *J Periodontol* 1997; 68: 24–31

78. Civitelli R, Pilgram TK, Dotson M, et al. Alveolar and postcranial bone density in postmenopausal women receiving hormone/estrogen replacement therapy: a randomized, double-blind, placebo-controlled trial. *Arch Intern Med* 2002; 162: 1409–15

79. Drozdzowska B, Pluskiewicz W. Longitudinal changes in mandibular bone mineral density compared with hip bone mineral density and quantitative ultrasound at calcaneus and hand phalanges. *Br J Radiol* 2002; 75: 743–7

80. Kribbs PJ, Chesnut CH. Osteoporosis and dental osteopenia in the elderly. *Gerodontology* 1984; 3: 101–6

Bone quality

11

C. E. Bogado

THE CONCEPT OF BONE QUALITY

Osteoporosis has been characterized as a disease of decreased bone mass. Bones were considered to fracture due to a reduction in their mass. Accordingly, osteoporosis has been diagnosed based on a surrogate for bone mass, the areal bone mineral density (BMD). Treatments have been developed to prevent bone loss or restore bone lost, and their efficacy measured by how well these outcomes are achieved. However, several observations from large clinical trials have exposed the limitations of BMD measurement. Many fractures occur among patients with normal BMD[1], small changes in BMD result in greater than expected reductions in fracture risk[2], reductions in fracture risk are evident before maximal changes in BMD are achieved[3] and changes in BMD following antiresorptive treatment explain only a small proportion of the variance in fracture risk reduction[4]. The term *bone quality* has been used to explain these and other clinical findings that cannot be explained by BMD measurements. During the past decade, interest in bone quality has increased dramatically, but the use of the term has been inconsistent, mainly due to the lack of a consensus on an operational definition.

Four years ago, the term bone quality was introduced in an updated definition of osteoporosis proposed by a National Institutes of Health (NIH)-sponsored Consensus Conference on Osteoporosis as 'a skeletal disorder characterized by compromised *bone strength* predisposing to an increased risk of fractures'. This statement asserted that bone strength reflects the integration of bone quality and bone density[5]. However, a definition of bone quality and/or bone strength was not provided. An operational definition of bone quality has been proposed as the 'totality of

features and characteristics that influence a bone's ability to resist fractures'[6]. What are those features and characteristics of bone that influence resistance to fractures?

As structural engineers have long recognized, the strength of a structure is a function of:

(1) The mechanical properties of the material;

(2) The three-dimensional arrangement of that material in space;

(3) The amount of material.

The same is true for bone. If we accept that, in this context, bone strength is the ability to resist stress and strain, avoiding fracture, bone strength is a function of material properties, such as the degree of mineralization, the organic matrix and the accumulation of microdamage; structural properties, including geometry and microarchitecture; as well as the amount of mass. Bone remodeling optimizes bone mass and distribution in response to mechanical demand, and also repairs damaged bone.

The impact of bone remodeling and age on bone quality

After the menopause, there is an increase in the rate of bone turnover. It happens immediately after the menopause and is sustained over time. Recently, Recker and colleagues[7] measured bone remodeling rates in transilial biopsy specimens from 50 premenopausal women before and 1 year after the menopause, and 34 women who were 13 years past the menopause. Activation frequency was nearly doubled 1 year after the menopause, and was tripled 13 years after the menopause. This rise in the rate of bone remodeling has for a long time been considered to be responsible for the loss of bone mass and the subsequent increase in the risk of fracture in postmenopausal osteoporosis. However, bone remodeling is now widely recognized to be a fragility factor by itself, independent of BMD. In a reanalysis of data from clinical trials with estrogen therapy in postmenopausal osteoporotic women, Riggs and colleagues[8] showed that vertebral fracture risk was directly related to the rate of bone turnover, and increased about four-fold between low and high levels of turnover, even in the presence of normal BMD.

Age also contributes to fracture risk. Hui and associates[9] studied the relationship of fracture risk to both bone mass and subject age. While this article confirmed the inverse relationship between BMD and fracture risk, it showed that the risk for fracture increases with age at any level of bone mass. Older subjects had several-fold the fracture risk of young subjects at the same bone mass.

Age and bone remodeling imbalance impact on both the material and structural determinants of bone strength.

The structural properties of bone

In order to avoid fracture, bone needs to be both stiff and tough. In part, this is achieved by structural adaptation. Long bones are fashioned as a cortex of highly mineralized tissue placed distant from the central long axis, a design that confers maximum resistance to bending (stiffness). In contrast, vertebral bodies consist of a mineralized interconnecting honeycomb of plates, a structure that can absorb energy by deformation (toughness).

Aging is accompanied by changes in trabecular bone microarchitecture that affect bone strength. There is progressive trabecular thinning, conversion from a plate-like to a rod-like structure and loss of connectivity, with preferential loss of horizontal trabeculae[10]. The loss of horizontal trabeculae results in a dramatic reduction in compressive strength[11]. According to Euler's theorem, the strength of a vertical trabecula is inversely proportional to the square power of its effective length[12]. Therefore, the loss of a horizontal strut or cross-tie increases the effective length of a vertical trabecula by a factor of two, but will reduce its compressive strength by a factor of four.

The remodeling process is also a source of structural weakness. The resorption cavities act as stress raisers by concentration of the mechanical stress imposed on bones. A high turnover rate produces an increase in the number and depth of resorption cavities, resulting in microdamage accumulation, trabecular perforation and loss of connectivity.

Cortical bone also deteriorates with age. Long bones suffer a continuous process of bone resorption at the endosteal surface that is compensated by periosteal apposition, resulting in bone expansion with age. In women, after the menopause, there is an increase in endocortical remodeling. Since periosteal apposition is insufficient to compensate for the bone loss at the endosteal surface, there is a progressive thinning of the cortex. The increase in cross-sectional area maintains the bending stress until a point where the structure becomes unstable and susceptible to fracture. Furthermore, there is an increase in cortical porosity with age, which is more evident in women, and contributes to bone fragility[13].

The material properties of bone

The required levels of toughness and stiffness can also be achieved by adaptation of the relative amounts of the organic and mineral constituents of bone. The degree of mineralization is one of the most, if not the most, important material property of bone.

After bone resorption, bone formation is a multistep process. At each bone remodeling unit, after the organic matrix is deposited, there is a fast process of primary mineral apposition that yields a low-mineralized bone. This is followed by a slow and gradual secondary mineralization, including an increase in crystal number and crystal size. The duration of this process depends on the level of bone remodeling. Therefore, an imbalance in the rate of bone remodeling affects the bone tissue mineral content. If the remodeling rate is high, older, more mineralized bone is replaced by younger, less mineralized bone. In contrast, if remodeling decreases, more time is available for secondary mineralization. The degree of mineralization of bone shows a high correlation with bone strength when it is measured by compressive testing of bone biopsy samples[14]. However, there is a complex relationship between mineralization and bone strength. The greater is the tissue mineral content, the greater are the stiffness and the peak stress that the bone will tolerate. However, increasing mineral content is associated with declining toughness. Highly mineralized bone becomes brittle and will not be able to absorb energy without cracking upon impact loading. Animal studies have suggested that high mineralization following pharmaceutical suppression of remodeling is associated with microdamage accumulation[15]. Microdamage accumulation significantly reduces toughness and may decrease fracture resistance[16]. Moreover, it has been suggested that microfractures need less energy to propagate in homogeneous composite materials, as is the case in older, highly mineralized bone[17]. However, the extent of damage accumulation necessary to increase fracture risk significantly is unclear, and it has been suggested that, while the accumulation of microdamage is associated with reduced toughness, the ability of a material to undergo microcracking may increase its toughness. The role of damage accumulation in fracture risk remains unclear.

CAN BONE QUALITY BE MEASURED?

At present, there are no suitable techniques for the measurement of material properties of bone in the clinical setting. Similarly, the assessment of trabecular microarchitecture has been restricted to invasive techniques such as histomorphometry or micro-computed tomography (CT) of bone biopsy samples, because most available non-invasive imaging techniques lack the resolution required for such purposes. However, a new generation of high-resolution peripheral quantitative CT scanners with acceptable levels of radiation dose for clinical use have recently become

available. It allows the measurement of both densitometric and architectural parameters for cortical and trabecular bone separately. Even more important, three-dimensional (3-D) images can be obtained, opening the door to *in vivo* assessment of bone mechanical competence in the near future[18].

Another recent development is the combination of a specifically designed magnetic resonance (MR) detection coil and image processing software that provides a highly detailed 3-D model of bone architecture using a standard clinical magnetic resonance imaging (MRI) scanner. In addition to standard structural histomorphometry, topology parameters, such as plate-to-rod ratio, can be obtained. Structural parameters could be more sensitive to individual differences than bone density. A study using this micro-MRI technique showed that two groups of postmenopausal women – with and without vertebral fractures – with similar BMD values at both hip and lumbar spine could be discriminated based on the deterioration of topology parameters[19].

There is also some progress in the assessment of cortical bone geometry. It is mentioned above that at some point the aging cortical cortex can become unstable and susceptible to fracture. Engineers estimate the stability of thin-walled tubes under bending stress by calculation of the buckling ratio. The buckling ratio has been calculated from estimated geometric parameters obtained from standard dual-energy X-ray absorptiometry (DXA) scans of the hip, a technique known as hip structure analysis[20]. It has been suggested that estimation of the buckling ratio can predict the risk of fracture. Crans and colleagues[21] calculated the baseline buckling ratio in patients from the placebo arm of the Multiple Outcomes of Raloxifene Evaluation (MORE) study, using hip structure analysis. There was a significant relationship between baseline femoral neck buckling ratio and 3-year vertebral fracture risk, and a significant relationship between the baseline intertrochanter buckling ratio and vertebral, non-vertebral and hip fracture risk at 3 years. The estimation of buckling ratio could also be a sensitive tool for the assessment of treatment efficacy. A study in a subset of patients from a large clinical trial on the effects of daily injections of PTH (1–34) (teriparatide) in postmenopausal osteoporotic women showed a decrease in femoral neck buckling ratio after 18 months of treatment[22]. Hip structure analysis has severe limitations, and these results should be considered as preliminary. However, the buckling ratio could be calculated from imaging techniques other than DXA that allow more precise measurements of geometric properties of bone, such as quantitative computed tomography (QCT) or peripheral QCT (pQCT).

CONCLUSIONS

There are opportunities for improvement in the identification of those at greatest risk for fracture, and monitoring the response to treatment.

New techniques for non-invasive measurement of structural determinants of bone strength could very soon find their way from research to the clinic.

In contrast, the non-invasive measurement of bone material properties remains elusive, and worthy of additional research effort.

References

1. Wainwright S, Phipps K, Stone J, et al. A large proportion of fractures in postmenopausal women occur with baseline bone mineral density T-score > −2.5. *J Bone Miner Res* 2001; 16: S155

2. Cranney A, Tugwell P, Zytaruk N, et al. Meta-analysis of therapies for postmenopausal osteoporosis. IV. Meta-analysis of raloxifene for the prevention and treatment of postmenopausal osteoporosis. *Endocr Rev* 2002; 23: 524–8

3. Watts NB, Josse RG, Hamdy RC, et al. Risedronate prevents new vertebral fractures in postmenopausal women at high risk. *J Clin Endocrinol Metab* 2003; 88: 542–9

4. Cummings SR, Karpf DB, Harris F, et al. Improvement in spinal bone mineral density and reduction in risk of vertebral fractures during treatment with antiresorptive drugs. *Am J Med* 2002; 112: 281–9

5. NIH Consensus Development Panel. Osteoporosis prevention, diagnosis and therapy. *J Am Med Assoc* 2001; 285: 785–95

6. Bouxsein ML. Bone quality: where do we go from here? *Osteoporos Int* 2003; 14 (Suppl 5): S118–27

7. Recker R, Lappe J, Davies KM, et al. Bone remodeling increases substantially in the years after menopause and remains increased in older osteoporosis patients. *J Bone Miner Res* 2004; 19: 1628–33

8. Riggs BL, Melton LJ III, O'Fallon WM. Drug therapy for vertebral fractures in osteoporosis: evidence that decreases in bone turnover and increases in bone mass both determine antifracture efficacy. *Bone* 1996; 18: 197S–201S

9. Hui SL, Slemenda CW, Johnston CC Jr. Age and bone mass as predictors of fracture in a prospective study. *J Clin Invest* 1988; 81: 1804–9

10. Mosekilde L. Age-related changes in vertebral trabecular bone architecture assessed by a new method. *Bone* 1988; 9: 247–50

11. Thomsen JS, Ebbesen EN, Mosekilde L. Age-related differences between thinning of horizontal and vertical trabeculae in human lumbar spine as assessed by a new computerized method. *Bone* 2002; 31: 136–42

12. Bell GH, Dunbar O, Beck JS, et al. Variations in strength of vertebrae with age and their relation to osteoporosis. *Calcif Tissue Res* 1967; 1: 75–86

13. Bousson V, Meunier A, Bergot C, et al. Distribution of intracortical porosity in human mid-femoral cortex by age and gender. *J Bone Miner Res* 2001; 16: 1308–17

14. Follet H, Boivin G, Rumelhart C, et al. The degree of mineralization is a determinant of bone strength: a study on human calcanei. *Bone* 2004; 34: 783–9

15. Mashiba T, Hirano T, Turner CH, et al. Suppressed bone turnover by bisphosphonates

increases microdamage accumulation and reduces some biomechanical properties in dog rib. *J Bone Miner Res* 2000; 15: 613–20

16. Norman TL, Yeni YN, Brown CU, et al. Influence of microdamage on fracture toughness of the human femur and tibia. *Bone* 1998; 23: 303–6

17. Kendall K. Control of cracks by interfaces in composites. *Proc R Soc London* 1975; 341: 409–28

18. Müller R. Bone microarchitecture assessment: current and future trends. *Osteoporos Int* 2003; 14 (Suppl 5): S89–99

19. Wehrli FW, Gomberg BR, Saha PK, et al. Digital topological analysis of in-vivo magnetic resonance microimages of trabecular bone reveals

structural implications of osteoporosis. *J Bone Miner Res* 2001; 16: 1520–31

20. Beck TJ, Ruff CB, Warden KE, et al. Predicting femoral neck strength from bone mineral data. A structural approach. *Invest Radiol* 1990; 25: 6–18

21. Crans GG, Beck TJ, Semanik LM, et al. Baseline buckling ratio derived from hip structure analysis predicts the risk of nonvertebral fractures. *J Bone Miner Res* 2004; 19 (Suppl 1): S92

22. Uusi-Rasi K, Semanick LM, Zanchetta JR, et al. Effects of teriparatide [rhPTH (1–34)] treatment on structural geometry of the proximal femur in elderly osteoporotic women. *Bone* 2005; 36: 948–58

Diagnosis: clinical, hormonal and biochemical evaluation   12

D. M. Reid

INTRODUCTION

This paper examines the value of clinical risk factors for osteoporosis and their role in identifying, first, risk factors that are associated with fracture and, second, risk factors associated with low bone density that can be used to stimulate a measurement of bone mass to enable a clinical diagnosis. Hormonal assessments are generally required to identify secondary osteoporosis and the causes of secondary osteoporosis. The tests frequently carried out to exclude these disorders are described. Finally, the role of biochemical measurements of bone turnover for predicting fracture, identifying secondary osteoporosis, targeting successful treatment and monitoring treatment efficacy are discussed.

A good starting point is to examine the definition of osteoporosis as discussed in the National Institutes of Health Consensus 2001[1]. The consensus statement defines osteoporosis as 'a skeletal disorder characterized by reduced bone strength predisposing a person to an increased risk of fracture'. The consensus statement progresses to describe bone strength as primarily reflecting an integration of *bone density* and *bone quality*.

The consensus statement further defines the main predictors of *low* bone density in an individual as low body mass index, a family history of osteoporosis, smoking and prior fracture, late menarche, early menopause and low estrogen levels. Predictors of *high* bone density include grip strength and current exercise. The role of predictors of falls is not ignored and these include slow gait speed, decreased quadriceps strength, impaired cognition, impaired vision and presence of environmental hazards. There are also identified predictors of fracture occurring after a fall, and these include those of a tall disposition, those individuals who fall to the side and bone geometry, for example femoral neck length or shape.

PREDICTORS OF FRACTURES

It is useful to review which factors are associated with site-specific osteoporotic fractures and those that are associated with all fractures of bone sites considered to relate to osteoporosis. Multiple risk factors for fracture have been described as shown in Table 1. While low bone mineral density (BMD) is a major risk factor, it is important to realize that some known factors are independent, or partly independent, of BMD[2]. Prominent among these are age and previous fragility fracture, which may in part be due to the influence of falls, which increase in incidence with age and pre-date most, but not all, fractures.

Some of the relationship to fall risk and an interaction with low BMD can be seen in a recent analysis that has been published from the OFELY (Os des Femmes de Lyon) study, of a 5-year follow-up of 672 women who suffered 81 fractures (24 vertebral, 16 risk, nine hip, five humerus, 11 ankle, etc.)[3]. Significant predictors of fracture from the study are shown in Table 2. It will be seen that the most prominent factors amongst those identified are previous fracture, low total hip bone density, low physical activity score, low grip strength and increasing age, which, in this particular study, applied to those over the age of 65. A further paper has very recently been published from the United Kingdom examining a shorter follow-up of a larger

Table 1 Risk factors for fracture which are dependent or partially or completely independent of bone mineral density (BMD). Adapted from reference 2

BMD-related	Partly or completely BMD-independent
Female gender	age
BMD	Asian or Caucasian race
Premature menopause	vitamin D deficiency
Primary or secondary amenorrhea	cigarette smoking
Prolonged immobilization	excessive alcohol consumption
Low dietary calcium intake	neuromuscular disorders
	family history of hip fracture
	poor visual acuity
	previous fragility fracture
	glucocorticoid therapy
	low body weight
	high bone turnover

Table 2 Predictors for all fractures from the OFELY (Os des Femmes de Lyon) study[3]

Variable	OR	95% CI	p Value
Fracture after age 45	3.33	1.42–7.79	0.006
Total hip BMD $\leq 0.736\,g/cm^2$	3.15	1.75–5.66	0.001
Physical activity score ≤ 14	2.08	1.17–3.69	0.01
Grip strength ≤ 60 bar	2.05	1.15–3.64	0.01
Age ≥ 65	1.90	1.04–3.47	0.04
Maternal history of fragility fracture	1.77	1.01–3.09	0.04
Past falls	1.76	1.00–3.09	0.05

BMD, bone mineral density; OR, odds ratio; CI, confidence interval

cohort of 4292 women over the age of 70, who were followed for 2 years[4]. During that time, 330 fractures occurred, including 125 risk factors and 51 hip fractures. The only significant factors which showed an excess odds ratio (OR) were previous fracture (OR 2.67, 95% confidence interval (CI) 2.10–3.40), a fall in the previous 12 months (OR 2.06, 95% CI 1.63–2.59) and increased age (OR per year increase 1.03, 95% CI 1.01–1.05). The authors examined separately significant factors for hip fracture and wrist fracture, and the only factors that were consistent across both subgroups were previous fracture, with odds ratios of around 2.3, and falling in the previous 12 months, which showed ratios of between 1.6 and 2.92. Age was only a significant

risk factor for hip fracture, as was low body weight[4].

Colles' fractures

Larger studies have reported on the risk factors for specific fractures. The Study of Osteoporotic Fractures (SOF) database has been examined to determine specific factors for Colles' fracture, with 527 cases occurring during a follow-up of 9.8 years. Here the relative risk of wrist fracture was increased: by 80% in those who had *decreased forearm BMD* (per 0.1 g/cm²); in those who had *recurrent falls*, where the increased risk was 60% compared with subjects who had no falls; and in those with *previous fracture since the age of 50*,

Table 3 Risk factors for hip fractures from the Study of Osteoporotic Fractures[6]

Factor	Relative risk	95% CI
Relative deficit		
Age (per 5-year increase)	1.5	1.3–1.7
History of maternal hip fracture	2.0	1.4–2.9
Height at age 25 (per 6 cm)	1.2	1.1–1.4
Self-related health (per 1 point decrease)*	1.7	1.3–2.2
History of hyperthyroidism	1.8	1.2–2.6
Current use of long-acting benzodiazepines	1.6	1.1–2.4
Current use of anticonvulsants	2.8	1.2–6.3
Current caffeine intake (per 190 mg/day)	1.3	1.0–1.5
On feet less than 4 h/day	1.7	1.2–2.4
Inability to rise from chair	2.1	1.3–3.2
Lowest quartile for distance depth perception	1.5	1.1–2.0
Low frequency contrast sensitivity (1 SD decrease)	1.2	1.0–1.5
Resting pulse > 80 beats/min	1.8	1.3–2.5
Relative benefit		
Increase in weight since age 25 (per 20%) gain	0.6	0.5–0.7
Walking for exercise	0.7	0.5–0.9

*Health was rated as poor (1 point), fair (2 points), or good to excellent (3 points); CI, confidence interval

where there was a 30% increased risk[5]. Current oral estrogen reduced the chance of Colles' fracture by 40%[5].

Hip fractures

The often quoted work of Cummings from the Study of Osteoporotic Fractures (SOF) demonstrated comprehensively how multiple significant risk factors contribute to hip fracture risk (Table 3). Eleven separate factors increased risk, while two factors (weight gain and walking for exercise) reduced the risk[6]. In their article, Cummings and colleagues described almost for the first time how combinations of risk factors plus low calcaneal bone density could increase risk of fracture exponentially when considered together. For example, calcaneal BMD in the lowest third of the normal range associated with the presence of more than five risk factors increased the risk of hip fracture about 25-fold, when compared with those with calcaneal bone density in the highest third of the normative range and with 0–2 risk factors[6].

New risk factors for hip fracture have recently been described. It is recognized that patients with homocystinuria have increased skeletal deformities and osteoporosis[7]. In the Framingham study, in the female population where follow-up was 15 years, patients with a baseline homocysteine level in the highest quartile of the population range had a highly significant 90% increase in hip fracture, compared with those with the lowest quartile homocysteine levels[8]. In a study from The Netherlands, three separate cohorts were also shown to have significantly increased risk of hip fracture if their serum homocysteine level was in the highest quartile of the normative range, compared with the lowest quartile[9]. In the largest cohort from this study followed for 8.1 years, the highest quartile had a doubling of the fracture risk[10].

A further factor associated with fractures is increased levels of vitamin A or retinol, which are present in many foods including liver, kidney and milk. High levels of retinol stimulate osteoclast activity and increase bone resorption, and also increase periosteal bone formation[7]. In a recent

Table 4 Risk factors for osteoporosis approved as indications for bone mineral density measurement

Royal College of Physicians, UK[14]	*National Osteoporosis Foundation*[15]
Radiographic osteopenia	All women aged 65 and older regardless of risk factors
Vertebral deformity	Younger postmenopausal women with one or more risk factors
Previous fragility fracture	Postmenopausal women who present with fractures
Prolonged corticosteroids	
Premature menopause	
Prolonged amenorrhea	
Primary hypogonadism	
Other diseases associated with osteoporosis	
Maternal history of hip fracture	
Low body mass index ($<19\,kg/m^2$)	

study, those who had the highest quintile of vitamin A intake amounting to more than 3 mg per day had an increased relative risk of hip fracture, compared with those of the lowest quintile, of almost 50% (95% CI 1.05–2.07)[10], and at least in men higher serum retinol levels are associated with excess fracture risk[11].

Vertebral fractures

A recent study from van der Klift and colleagues[12] reported the risk factors for vertebral fracture in a 6.3-year follow-up of 1624 women aged more than or equal to 55, in whom 113 morphometric vertebral fractures were detected. The significant positive clinical risk factors leading to excess risk of morphometric fractures included body mass index, walking-aid use, age at menopause and current smoker; the most prominent clinical risk factor for vertebral fracture was a prevalent vertebral fracture, where relative risk rose by over 500% compared with no prevalent fracture. Bone density was also predictive of fracture, with a one-standard-deviation reduction in either lumbar spine or femoral neck BMD being associated with an almost doubling of risk[12]. The only significant clinical risk factors for incident vertebral fracture in the small number of only 34 cases as recently reported by Papaioannou and colleagues[13] were femoral neck BMD and the physical functioning domain of the Short Form 36-item (SF-36) questionnaire.

CLINICAL RISK FACTORS FOR OSTEOPOROSIS

The multiple risk factors associated with low BMD have been examined and described as part of guidelines preparation in both the UK[14] and the USA[15] as the indicators allowed for bone density assessment. The similarities and differences between these guidelines can be seen in Table 4. As will be appreciated, the conceptual approach between the UK and North American guidelines differs fundamentally, and this will give rise to differences in the populations that can be identified for assessment and, thus, treatment[16]. The validity of the Royal College of Physicians criteria for the diagnosis of osteoporosis has recently been described by Kayan and colleagues[17], and compared with population norms. The presence of an indication as approved by the Royal College of Physicians guidelines for bone density measurement is associated with approximately half a standard deviation difference in bone density. The strongest association with bone density is radiological osteopenia, followed by estrogen lack, presence of secondary disorders and previous fracture. The use of corticosteroids in referred patients did not increase the risk of osteoporosis, compared with the population norm, nor did kyphosis, although it was not clear whether the kyphotic patients also had vertebral fractures. Nevertheless, these criteria performed rather better than non-Royal College of Physicians criteria, such as perimenopausal women, those with back pain and those who were treated without densitometry, where the bone density was on average more than one standard deviation above the age-matched mean[17].

Diseases and medications associated with osteoporosis

There are multiple medications, including glucocorticoids, gonadotropin releasing hormone antagonists, methotrexate, heparin and warfarin, that have all been associated with low bone density. These drugs and their associated disorders are listed in Table 5. As will be noted, they include hereditary skeletal and connective tissue diseases, endocrine and metabolic disorders, marrow disease including multiple myeloma, systemic lupus erythematosus (SLE) and rheumatoid arthritis. There are also a number of miscellaneous conditions, which include renal insufficiency and chronic hepatic disease. Recently, further evidence has become available that disorders such as celiac disease[18], Crohn's disease[19], peptic ulcer disease[20] and breast cancer treated with the aromatase inhibitor[21] are all associated with low bone density, and some

disorders may also be associated with fracture. Even patients who have already had a fall and who have two or more risk factors have been found to have increased incidence of osteoporosis[22], although this may simply be due to frailty.

Risk factor scores

This bewildering complex list of risk factors for fracture or low bone density has led to the development of assessment tools that combine many of these risk factors in a single score, which could be used to identify those individuals either who should have bone density testing or, in some cases, who are considered to be at such risk as to indicate the need for treatment directly. One of the most prominent of these indexes, which has been widely used, is the fracture index, as described by Black and colleagues[23]. A high-risk score of between 5 and 9 using the index is associated with a 5-year hip fracture risk of 8.2% without BMD as a risk factor, and adding BMD only marginally increases the fracture risk prediction at the hip. Similar data were described by Black and colleagues for non-vertebral and ver-

---

Table 5 Medications and diseases associated with secondary osteoporosis

Medications
Glucocorticoids, gonadotropin releasing hormone agonists, loop diuretics, methotrexate, thyroid replacement, heparin, depo-medroxyprogesterone acetate, anti-neoplastic agents, cyclosporin

Hereditary skeletal/connective tissue diseases
Osteogenesis imperfecta, rickets, hypophosphatasia, Marfan's syndrome

Endocrine and metabolic
Hypogonadism, hyperparathyroidism, hyperthyroidism, Cushing syndrome, acidosis, Gaucher's disease, hemochromatosis, insulin-dependent diabetes, androgen insensitivity

Marrow diseases
Myeloma, mastocytosis, thalassemia, leukemia

Rheumatologic diseases
Systemic lupus, ankylosing spondylitis, rheumatoid arthritis

Miscellaneous
Renal insufficiency, hypercalciuria, chronic hepatic disease, chronic obstructive pulmonary disease, depression, spinal cord injury, anorexia nervosa, malabsorption or malnutrition, cystic fibrosis, organ transplantation, pregnancy

New causes
Coeliac disease, peptic ulcer, Crohns' disease, breast cancer treated with aromatase inhibitor

---

tebral fractures, where again fracture risk increased only slightly by the addition of BMD as a risk factor in the SOF study population[23].

A number of other instruments have been derived in an attempt to detect those who will have low bone mineral density with increased specificity and sensitivity, compared with the simple one-off risk factors as described in the Royal College of Physicians and the National Osteoporosis Foundation guidelines. The sensitivity and specificity of these composite risk factor scores have been compared and contrasted in a recent publication[24]. Overall, these scores have a high sensitivity of around 90% in detecting those who have low bone density, but somewhat conservative specificity of no more than 50% indicating that many people with low bone density will be missed by using composite risk scores.

BIOCHEMICAL AND HORMONAL TESTING

In subjects who have presented with osteoporosis or indeed fracture, biochemical and hormonal testing is mainly used to detect secondary osteoporosis. The indications for testing and the tests used are described in Table 6, and have been described previously in guidelines[14,25].

USE OF BONE TURNOVER MARKERS

Bone turnover markers have been derived to reflect both bone resorption and bone formation. Formation markers can arise from matrix proteins such as osteocalcin or the procollagen type I propeptide from the C-terminal (PICP) or the N-terminal (PINP), or can be enzymatic such as the bone isoform of alkaline phosphatase. Resorption markers are derived from either collagen type I degradation, specifically the pyridinium cross-links of collagen from the C- or N-telopeptide region (CTX, NTX), or the cross-link protein, deoxypyridinoline (DPD). An enzymatic-derived bone marker associated with bone resorption is tartrate-resistant acid phosphatase

Table 6 Biochemical and hormonal tests used in the assessment of osteoporosis

Hematological disease and malignancy
Full blood count, erythrocyte sedimentation rate (ESR) or C-reactive protein (CRP)
Serum protein electrophoresis ± urinary Bence-Jones proteins

Chronic liver disease
Liver function tests – albumin, aspartate aminotransferase (AST), gamma glutamyl transferase (γGT)

Metabolic bone diseases
Serum calcium, phosphate, alkaline phosphatase

Chronic renal disease and malabsorption
Serum creatinine
Antiendomysial antibody

Endocrine disease
Serum thyroid stimulating hormone (TSH), parathyroid hormone (PTH), 25OH vitamin D
Serum estradiol, follicle stimulating hormone (FSH), testosterone, sex hormone binding globulin (SHBG)

type 5. These markers can be used in a variety of situations.

They have been used to predict spine bone loss where, in the individual patient, they have only moderate correlations with change in bone mineral density explaining just over 40% of the variability, rather similar to that explained by years since the menopause[26]. Perhaps a more promising use of the markers, however, is to enhance the predictive capacity of bone density for risk of hip or other fractures. Garnero and colleagues demonstrated in the EPIDOS (Epidémiologie de l'Ostéoporose) study that the risk of hip fracture with low hip bone density was increased 2.9-fold, while, if subjects had baseline urinary CTX above the upper limit of the young normal range, they had an increased risk of just over 2, and if both factors were combined the increased risk rose to around 4[27]. Kanis and associates proposed that including measurement of markers in a 10-year risk factor assessment for hip fracture would lead to a substantial increase in the relative risk of those who had a combination of low BMD, high CTX and a prior fracture, increasing the 10-year probability to over 50% if all three markers were present[28].

Use of bone markers to diagnose osteoporosis

Bone turnover markers are increased in only about 25% of women with postmenopausal osteoporosis, and hence cannot be used for diagnosis. Nor have bone markers been proved to be useful in a selection of patients who would effectively receive antifracture treatment. Seibel and colleagues have recently shown that bisphosphonates are effective at all levels of bone turnover in preventing fractures[29]. However, a high level of bone turnover may indicate the presence of secondary osteoporosis, such as in Paget's disease, secondary hyperparathyroidism, primary hyperparathyroidism, thyrotoxicosis or even hypogonadism. It may also be high in patients with malignancy or in those who have suffered a recent fracture. On the other hand, Cushing's syndrome will be associated with low osteocalcin levels, and osteogenesis imperfecta with low PICP[30].

MONITORING OF TREATMENT

Bone turnover markers have an increasing role in this situation. It is important to identify non-responders to hormone replacement therapy (HRT), for example, as any errors in dosing instructions can then be considered. Further, the detection of non-response could lead the clinician to consider secondary osteoporosis or to change treatment. Also, bone turnover markers have been used to encourage adherence with therapy[31].

Changes in biochemical markers are usually large, and occur more rapidly than changes in bone mineral density. Further, an increase in bone density only explains 4% of the antifracture efficacy with raloxifene[32], 17% with alendronate[33] and up to 28% with risedronate[34]. In contrast, changes in urinary NTX or CTX may explain as much as two-thirds of vertebral fracture reduction[34].

CONCLUSIONS

Risk factors are multiple, but can be used in conjunction with bone mineral density measurements and possibly bone markers to assist in prediction of the risk of incident fractures. The most persistent risk factors for fracture at all sites are *age* and *previous fracture*, with risk of falls a significant risk factor for hip and wrist fractures. Biochemical and hormonal testing should be used to exclude secondary osteoporosis, while bone turnover markers may be used soon to monitor therapy. However, to date, the only risk factor that has been shown to be a suitable target for effective treatment is bone mineral density.

References

1. Consensus Development Panel on Osteoporosis Prevention, Diagnosis and Therapy. Osteoporosis prevention, diagnosis and therapy. *J Am Med Assoc* 2001; 285: 785–95

2. Kanis JA. Diagnosis of osteoporosis and assessment of fracture risk. *Lancet* 2002; 359: 1929–36

3. Albrand G, Munoz F, Sornay-Rendu E, et al. Independent predictors of all osteoporosis-related fractures in healthy postmenopausal women: the OFELY study. *Bone* 2003; 32: 78–85

4. Porthouse J, Birks YF, Torgerson DJ, et al. Risk factors for fracture in a UK population: a prospective cohort study. *Q J Med* 2004; 97: 569–74

5. Vogt MT, Cauley JA, Tomaino MM, et al. Distal radius fractures in older women: a 10-year follow-up study of descriptive characteristics and risk factors. The study of osteoporotic fractures. *J Am Geriatr Soc* 2002; 50: 97–103

6. Cummings SR, Nevitt MC, Browner WS, et al. Risk factors for hip fracture in white women.

Study of Osteoporotic Fractures Research Group. [see Comment]. *N Engl J Med* 1995; 332: 767–73

7. Lips P. Hypervitaminosis A and fractures. *N Engl J Med* 2003; 348: 347–9

8. McLean RR, Jacques PF, Selhub J, et al. Homocysteine as a predictive factor for hip fracture in older persons. *N Engl J Med* 2004; 350: 2042–9

9. van Meurs JB, Dhonukshe-Rutten RA, Pluijm SM, et al. Homocysteine levels and the risk of osteoporotic fracture. *N Engl J Med* 2004; 350: 2033–41

10. Feskanich D, Singh V, Willett WC, Colditz GA. Vitamin A intake and hip fractures among postmenopausal women. *J Am Med Assoc* 2002; 287: 47–54

11. Michaelsson K, Lithell H, Vessby B, Melhus H. Serum retinol levels and the risk of fracture. *N Engl J Med* 2003; 348: 287–94

12. van der Klift M, de Laet CE, McCloskey EV, et al. Risk factors for incident vertebral fractures in men and women: the Rotterdam Study. *J Bone Miner Res* 2004; 19: 1172–80

13. Papaioannou A, Joseph L, Ioannidis G, et al. Risk factors associated with incident clinical vertebral and nonvertebral fractures in postmenopausal women: the Canadian Multicentre Osteoporosis Study (CaMos). *Osteoporos Int* 2005; 16: 568–78

14. Royal College of Physicians. *Osteoporosis: Clinical Guidelines for Prevention and Treatment*. London: Royal College of Physicians, 1999

15. National Osteoporosis Foundation. *Physician's guide to prevention and treatment of osteoporosis*. 99. NOF, 2004. http://www.nof.org/physguide

16. Kanis JA, Torgerson D, Cooper C. Comparison of the European and USA practice guidelines for osteoporosis. *Trends Endocrinol Metab* 2000; 11: 28–32

17. Kayan K, de Takats D, Ashford R, et al. Performance of clinical referral criteria for bone densitometry in patients under 65 years of age assessed by spine bone mineral density. *Postgrad Med J* 2003; 79: 581–4

18. West J, Logan RF, Hill PG, et al. Seroprevalence, correlates, and characteristics of undetected coeliac disease in England. *Gut* 2003; 52: 960–5

19. Siffiledeen JS, Fedorak RN, Siminoski K, et al. Bones and Crohn's: risk factors associated with low bone mineral density in patients with Crohn's disease. *Inflamm Bowel Dis* 2004; 10: 220–8

20. Sawicki A, Regula A, Godwod K, Debinski A. Peptic ulcer disease and calcium intake as risk factors of osteoporosis in women. *Osteoporos Int* 2003; 14: 983–6

21. Ramaswamy B, Shapiro CL. Osteopenia and osteoporosis in women with breast cancer, [Review]. *Semin Oncol* 2003; 30: 763–75

22. Newton JL, Kenny RA, Frearson R, Francis, RM. A prospective evaluation of bone mineral density measurement in females who have fallen. *Age Ageing* 2003; 32: 497–502

23. Black DM, Steinbuch M, Palermo L, et al. An assessment tool for predicting fracture risk in postmenopausal women. *Osteoporos Int* 2001; 12: 519–28

24. Wehren LE, Siris ES. Beyond bone mineral density: can existing clinical risk assessment instruments identify women at increased risk of osteoporosis? *J Intern Med* 2004; 256: 375–80

25. Anonymous. *Glucocorticoid Induced Osteoporosis: Guidelines for Prevention and Treatment*. London: Royal College of Physicians, 2002

26. Rogers A, Hannon RA, Eastell R. Biochemical markers as predictors of rates of bone loss after menopause. *J Bone Miner Res* 2000; 15: 1398–404

27. Garnero P, Hausherr E, Chapuy MC, et al. Markers of bone resorption predict hip fracture in elderly women: the EPIDOS Prospective Study. *J Bone Miner Res* 1996; 11: 1531–8

28. Kanis JA, Johnell O, Oden A, et al. Ten-year risk of osteoporotic fracture and the effect of risk factors on screening strategies. *Bone* 2002; 30: 251–8

29. Seibel MJ, Naganathan V, Barton I, Grauer, A. Relationship between pretreatment bone resorption and vertebral fracture incidence in postmenopausal osteoporotic women treated with risedronate. *J Bone Miner Res* 2004; 19: 323–9

30. Clowes JA, Eastell R. The role of bone turnover markers and risk factors in the assessment of osteoporosis and fracture risk. *Baillière's Best Pract Res Clin Endocrinol Metab* 2000; 14: 213–32

31. Clowes JA, Peel NF, Eastell R. The impact of monitoring on adherence and persistence with antiresorptive treatment for postmenopausal osteoporosis: a randomized controlled trial. *J Clin Endocrinol Metab* 2004; 89: 1117–23

32. Johnell O, Kanis JA, Black DM, et al. Associations between baseline risk factors and vertebral fracture risk in the Multiple Outcomes of Raloxifene Evaluation (MORE) Study. *J Bone Miner Res* 2004; 19: 764–72

33. Cummings SR, Karpf DB, Harris F, et al. Improvement in spine bone density and reduction in risk of vertebral fractures during treatment with antiresorptive drugs. *Am J Med* 2002; 112: 281–9

34. Eastell R, Barton I, Hannon RA, et al. Relationship of early changes in bone resorption to the reduction in fracture risk with risedronate. *J Bone Miner Res* 2003; 18: 1051–6

Advanced imaging assessment of bone quality 13

H. K. Genant and Y. Jiang

INTRODUCTION

More than standard bone densitometry[1], non-invasive and/or non-destructive techniques are capable of providing macro- or microstructural information about bone[2]. While bone densitometry provides important information about osteoporotic fracture risk, numerous studies indicate that bone strength is only partially explained by bone mineral density (BMD). Quantitative assessment of macrostructural characteristics such as geometry, and microstructural features such as relative trabecular volume, trabecular spacing and connectivity, may improve our ability to estimate bone strength.

The methods available for quantitatively assessing macrostructure include computed tomography and, particularly, volumetric quantitative computed tomography (vQCT). Non-invasive and/or non-destructive methods for assessing the microstructure of trabecular bone include high-resolution computed tomography (hrCT), micro-computed tomography (μCT), high-resolution magnetic resonance (hrMR) and micro-magnetic resonance (μMR). Volumetric QCT, hrCT and hrMR are generally applicable *in vivo*, while μCT and μMR are principally applicable *in vitro*.

VOLUMETRIC COMPUTED TOMOGRAPHY

The use of standard QCT has centered on two-dimensional characterization of vertebral trabecular bone, but there is also interest in developing three-dimensional, or vQCT, techniques to improve spinal measurements and to extend QCT assessments to the proximal femur. These three-dimensional techniques encompass the entire object of interest with stacked slices or spiral CT scans, and can use anatomic landmarks to define coordinate systems automatically for reformatting CT data into anatomically relevant projections.

Volumetric CT (Figure 1) can determine bone mineral content (BMC) or BMD of the entire bone or subregion, such as a vertebral body or femoral neck, as well as provide separate analysis of the trabecular or cortical components. Since a true and highly accurate volumetric rendering is provided, important geometrical and biomechanically relevant assessments such as cross-sectional moment of inertia and finite element

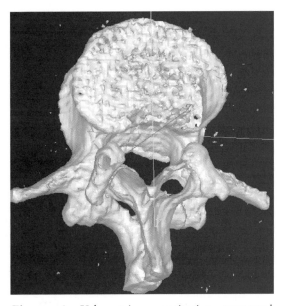

Figure 1 Volumetric quantitative computed tomography (QCT) of the spine may be used to analyze bone mineral density in bone compartments and to measure accurately vertebral geometry. Courtesy of Thomas Lang

analyses can be derived[2–8]. Highly accurate assessment of bone size and density, independent of the artifacts of projectional radiographic and densitometric techniques (such as absorptiometry), can also be derived for epidemiologic studies, and for studies of nutritional, racial and genetic influences on bone size and density[9].

Because of the complex anatomy of the proximal femur and its dramatic three-dimensional (3-D) variations in bone density, vQCT has particularly important ramifications for both research and clinical applications at this biologically relevant site (Figure 2). vQCT and finite element analysis modeling have been used by Lotz and colleagues[7] and by Keyak and associates[4] to improve estimations of proximal femoral strength over global projectional densitometry. *In vitro* studies by Lang and co-workers[5,6] have shown enhanced prediction of *in vitro* fracture load using subregional vQCT of the hip. QCT 3-D finite element modeling of the proximal femur shows moderate reproducibility in postmenopausal women[10]. QCT-based finite element models of the hip in 51 women aged 74 years showed different risk factors for hip fracture during single-limb stance and falls, which agree with epidemiologic findings of different risk factors for cervical and trochanteric fractures[11].

Finite element models derived from QCT scans may improve the prediction of vertebral strength, because they mechanically integrate all the geometrical and material property data within the scans. QCT BMD values of each bone voxel can be converted into elastic modulus values using predetermined correlation between the elastic modulus and QCT-derived BMD. Finite element models integrate mechanically all of the anisotropic, inhomogeneous and complex geometry of the bone structure examined. It has been demonstrated that voxel-based finite element model-derived estimates of strength are better predictors of *in vitro* vertebral compressive strength than are clinical measures of bone density derived from QCT with or without geometry[12]. Although imaging resolution is not critical in cross-sectional studies using clinical CT scanners, longitudinal studies that seek to track more subtle changes in stiffness over time should

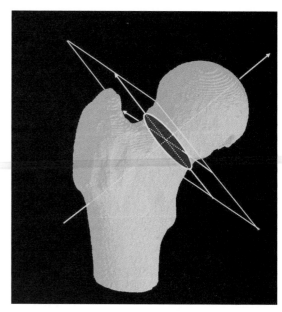

Figure 2 Volumetric quantitative computed tomography (QCT) of the hip may be used to analyze bone mineral density in bone compartments and to measure accurately proximal femoral geometry, as well as provide a basis for finite element analyses. Courtesy of Klaus Engelke

account for the small but highly significant effects of voxel size[13]. However, as these data were generated in the laboratory with excised bone specimen without soft tissue, they remain to be confirmed by clinical studies and epidemiological studies. In addition, the compressive loading experiments used in the laboratory differ from *in vivo* conditions.

HIGH-RESOLUTION COMPUTED TOMOGRAPHY

There is much research under way in the areas of high-resolution computed tomography (hrCT). The spatial resolution of clinical CT scanners (typically > 0.4 mm) is inadequate for highly accurate cortical measurements and for analysis of discrete trabecular morphological parameters, and new CT developments address this issue. There are two main approaches: the development of new image acquisition and analysis protocols using state-of-the-art clinical CT scanners;

and the development of new hrCT scanners for *in vivo* investigations of the peripheral skeleton, or of new μCT scanners for *in vitro* two- or three-dimensional structural analysis of very small bone samples (typically < 2 cm³).

State-of-the-art spiral CT scanners utilize a relatively high-resolution (~ 0.4 mm × 0.4 mm) thin slice (1–1.5 mm) to provide images of the spine and hip that clearly display structural information. However, this requires a higher radiation exposure than is employed for standard QCT. Also, extraction of the quantitative structural information is difficult, and the results vary substantially according to the threshold and image processing techniques used. This is due to substantial partial volume effects at this resolution, relative to the typical dimensions of trabeculae (100–400 μm) and trabecular spaces (200–2000 μm). hrCT has been employed to measure a feature called the trabecular fragmentation index (length of the trabecular network divided by the number of discontinuities) in an effort to separate osteoporotic subjects from normal subjects[14], and a similar trabecular textural analysis approach has been reported by Ito and colleagues[15]. Gordon and associates[16] reported a hrCT technique that extracts a texture parameter reflecting trabecular hole area, analogous to star volume, that appears to enhance vertebral fracture discrimination relative to BMD. One *in vitro* study showed that a combination of BMD and trabecular structural parameters of bone cubes examined by peripheral QCT improved prediction of bone biomechanical properties[17]. Recently, Link and colleagues have provided a comprehensive analysis of multislice hrCT with hrMR applied to the peripheral skeleton[18].

Higher-resolution CT scanners for peripheral skeletal measurements *in vivo* have been developed and evaluated by Rüegsegger, Durand and Müller and their group[19–21]. The images show trabecular structure in the radius, with a spatial resolution of 170 μm isotropic. The images can be used for quantitative trabecular structure analysis (Figure 3) and also for a separate assessment of cortical and trabecular BMD. Note, however, that these state-of-the-art scanners approach the limits of spatial resolution achievable *in vivo* with acceptable radiation exposure[22].

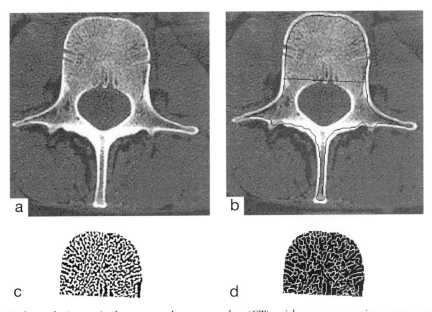

Figure 3 High-resolution spinal computed tomography (CT) with post-processing steps used to assess trabecular structure from CT image (a). The structure is segmented by defining the boundary between cortical and trabecular bone (b). The trabecular network is reduced to a binary image (c), which is then thinned to produce a representation of the trabecular form (d). Courtesy of Christopher Gordon

More recent studies of high-resolution and volumetric CT have further documented the unique capabilities of these techniques. They have shown that trabecular structural analysis from multidetector row CT images can better discriminate postmenopausal women with vertebral fracture than can dual-energy X-ray absorptiometry (DXA)[23]. High-resolution spiral CT assessment of the trabecular structure of the vertebral body in combination with BMD improves the prediction of biomechanical properties[24]. In elderly men, there is an independent association of sex steroid levels with cortical and trabecular area and their QCT volumetric BMD, but such an association is lacking in young men[25].

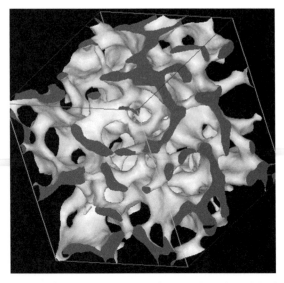

Figure 4 Three-dimensional (3-D) digital model of trabecular bone based on micro-computed tomography (μCT) image at approximately 60 mm^3 resolution. Courtesy of Klaus Engelke

MICRO-COMPUTED TOMOGRAPHY

To achieve very high spatial resolution images, Feldkamp and co-workers[26,27] constructed a unique μCT system for three-dimensional *in vitro* analyses of small bone samples (Figure 4). The system employed cone-beam geometry and a three-dimensional reconstruction algorithm. The spatial resolution of ~60 μm clearly visualized individual trabeculae, allowing three-dimensional analysis of the trabecular network. Goulet and colleagues[28] utilized images of bone cubes generated by this system to examine standard histomorphometric parameters, as well as additional parameters such as Euler number, an index of connectivity, and mean intercept length, a means of determining anisotropy. They also related these image-based parameters to Young's modulus, a measure of elasticity of bone. Based on data sets from Feldkamp's μCT, Engelke and colleagues[29,30] developed a 3-D digital model of trabecular bone for comparing two- and three-dimensional structural analysis methods, and to investigate the effects of spatial resolution and image processing techniques on the extraction of structural parameters. Three-dimensional data sets from these μCT systems can be used for calculating classical histomorphometric parameters such as trabecular thickness and separation[31–33], as well as for determining topological measurements such as Euler number and connectivity.

Another *in vitro* μCT scanner with a spatial resolution of 15–20 μm^3 was developed by Rüeggsegger and co-workers[34,35], and has been used extensively in laboratory investigations. Its high accuracy in relation to standard two-dimensional histomorphometry as well as to serial grindings and their derived three-dimensional parameters has been reported[16]. The relationship of these parameters to *in vitro* measures of strength and their application to microfinite element modeling have been shown[36,37]. More recently, additional special-purpose ultrahigh-resolution μCT systems have been developed for imaging bone microstructure at resolutions approaching 10 μm or better[38]. These various μCT systems have found wide application in both preclinical animal studies and clinical research settings[39]. Similarly, in animal studies, micro-CT has recently found application in the assessment of skeletal phenotype in gene knockout or knock-in mice[40–43], and in osteoporotic[44] or arthritic rodents[45].

In a human study by Jiang and colleagues, the rapid deterioration in trabecular microarchitecture in women experiencing the menopause was documented by paired iliac crest biopsies before and approximately 5 years after the menopause (Figure 5). Prominent thinning of trabeculae and conversion of plate-like to rod-like trabecular structure were observed[39].

Jiang and colleagues also used micro-CT with 3-D analyses, compared with standard 2-D histomorphometry, to study the longitudinal impact of teriparatide (PTH 1-34) treatment versus placebo on the skeleton of post-menopausal women (Figure 6). In this analysis, the changes of the more simple 2-D indices pertaining to cancellous bone structure, such as trabecular number, thickness and spacing, did not reach significance after PTH treatment. However, more stereologically correct indices, such as marrow star volume and μCT-based 3-D indices, revealed significant changes, further corroborating the superiority of these techniques for structural analysis of small samples, such as bone biopsies. The root mean square coefficient of variation (CV) as reproducibility of μCT examination after rescanning and reanalyzing 20 human biopsy specimens was 2–6% for trabecular structural parameters[46,47].

While the μCT scanners described above use an X-ray tube as radiation source, other investigators have explored the potential of high-intensity, tight-collimation synchrotron radiation, which allows either faster scanning or higher spatial resolution in imaging bone specimens. These systems have been referred to as X-ray tomographic microscopy (XTM), and can achieve spatial resolution of 10 μm or better. Bonse, Graeff and Engelke and their group[18,48–50] were among the first to apply this approach to the imaging of bone specimens. Kinney and Lane and co-workers[51,52] have applied the XTM approach to imaging the rat tibia at ultrahigh resolution, both *in vitro* and *in vivo*, and have documented the impact of oophorectomy and PTH treatment on two- and three-dimensionally derived trabecular bone indices. Ritman and Peyrin's group[53] have utilized synchrotron-based XTM to image trabecular bone ultrastructure at resolutions approaching 1–2 μm, thereby providing the capability to assess additional features such as resorption cavities. In recently reported studies using synchrotron radiation, micro-CT examination of sequential iliac biopsies showed that

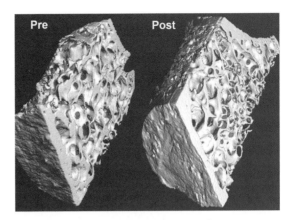

Figure 5 Micro-computed tomography (CT) image at ~ 20 μm³ resolution of trabecular structure of serial iliac crestng biopsies from a postmenopausal woman before and 2 years after estrogen replacement therapy. Courtesy of Yebin Jiang

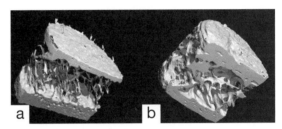

Figure 6 Paired biopsy samples were obtained from a 65-year-old woman treated with teriparatide (PTH). Compared to the baseline biopsy (a), PTH treatment (b) increased trabecular bone volume, trabecular connectivity and cortical thickness, and shifted trabecular morphology from a rod-like structure to a more plate-like pattern. Courtesy of Yebin Jiang

treatment with a bisphosphonate did not cause significant hypermineralization but did increase the mineralization at the tissue level[54]. Also, standard micro-CT and histomorphometric assessments of serial iliac crest bone biopsies from postmenopausal women treated with another bisphosphonate for 10 years showed normal microarchitecture[55].

At recent international congresses there have been many reports of additional studies using micro-CT, including technical developments and various applications. An *in vivo* human micro-CT scanner developed in Europe has been used to examine the distal radius or distal tibia with isotropic resolution of about $100 \mu m$[56]. Its application in the USA and other places remains to be seen. Advanced micro-finite analyses with models based on these 3-D peripheral micro-CT systems (isotropic voxel resolution of $165 \mu m$) have predicted the failure load of human radius Colles' fractures better than by DXA or bone morphology and geometry measurements[57]. Micro-CT (and micro-MRI, see below) replicate the complex trabecular architecture on a macroscopic scale for visual or biomechanical analysis. A complete set of 3-D image data provides a basis for finite element modeling using virtual biomechanics to predict mechanical properties[58].

MAGNETIC RESONANCE MICROSCOPY

High-resolution MR and micro-MR – referred to collectively as MR microscopy – have received considerable attention as research tools and as potential clinical tools for assessment of trabecular bone architecture. Magnetic resonance is a complex technology based on the application of high magnetic fields, transmission of radio-frequency (RF) waves and detection of RF signals from excited hydrogen protons. A non-invasive, non-ionizing radiation technique, MR can provide three-dimensional images in arbitrary orientations and can depict trabecular bone as a negative image by virtue of the strong signal generated by the abundant fat and water protons in the surrounding marrow tissue. The appearance of the MR image is affected by many factors beyond spatial resolution, including the field strength and specific pulse sequence used, the echo time and the signal-to-noise ratio achieved[59–61]. Analysis and interpretation of MR images are more complicated than for the X-ray-based images of CT. Nevertheless, MR microscopy holds much promise for improved quantitative assessment of trabecular structure both *in vivo* and *in vitro*.

Because of the relation of signal to field strength in MR, special-purpose, small-bore, high-field magnets have been employed to obtain very high-resolution or μMR images of

bone specimens *in vitro*. Wehrli and colleagues[62–65] obtained $78 \mu m$ isotopic resolution of human and bovine bone cubes using three-dimensional imaging at 9.4 T, and derived anisotropy ellipsoids from the analysis of mean intercept length. They also found good correlations between MR-derived parameters and standard histomorphometric measures. Antich and associates[66] have conducted similar experiments and found changes in accordance with histomorphometry measures. Kapadia and co-workers[67] extended the *in vitro* techniques to obtain images in an ovariectomized rat model, and were able to measure changes in trabecular structure following ovariectomy. Hipp and Simmons[68] examined bovine cubes in a small-bore microimaging spectrometer at $60 \mu m^3$ resolution, and found that three-dimensional results were heavily dependent upon the threshold and image processing algorithm. Majumdar and colleagues[69] examined human cadaver specimens using a standard clinical MR scanner at 1.5 T and a spatial resolution of $117 \times 117 \times 300 \mu m$, and compared these images with XTM images and with serial grindings to determine the impact of in-plane resolution and slice thickness on both two-dimensional and three-dimensional structural and textural parameters. Considerable resolution dependence was observed for traditional stereological parameters, some of which could be modulated by appropriate thresholds and image processing techniques.

Limitations of the signal-to-noise ratio, spatial resolution and total imaging time prevent resolution of smaller individual trabeculae *in vivo* at clinical field strengths, but images show the larger trabeculae and the texture of the trabecular network. The trabecular structure can still be quantified using standard techniques of stereology as well as textural parameters such as fractal analysis. In an early study by Majumdar and colleagues[60], establishing the feasibility of using such images to quantify trabecular structure, MR images of the distal radius were obtained using a modified gradient echo sequence, a 1.5-T imager and a spatial resolution of $156 \mu m^2$ and slice thickness of 0.7 mm. Representative axial sections from normal and osteoporotic subjects clearly depicted the loss of integrity of the trabecular network with the development of osteoporosis. Similar images of the calcaneus of normal subjects showed that the orientation of the trabeculae is significantly different in various anatomic regions. Ellipses, representing the mean intercept length, showed a preferred orientation and hence mapped the anisotropy of trabecular structure. In preliminary *in vivo* studies of the calcaneus, gray-scale reference values from fat, muscle and tendon were used to calculate reproducible threshold values[70]. This approach gave a mid-term, *in vivo* precision of ~ 3.5% CV for trabecular width and spacing.

Both Wehrli and colleagues[71] and Glüer and colleagues[72–74] have utilized clinical imagers at 1.5 T with special RF coil designs, and have measured trabecular and cortical bone in the phalanges, a convenient anatomic site particularly suitable for obtaining high signal-to-noise ratio and high spatial resolution images *in vivo*. Resolution of 78–150 μm and slice thickness of 300 μm have been achieved in the phalanges. Stampa and associates[74] used these phalangeal images to derive quantitative three-dimensional parameters based on an algorithm and model for defining trabecular rods and plates. Others, including Link[75], Majumdar[76] and Wehrli[77–79] and their groups have shown the ability to discriminate spine and/or hip fractures using trabecular structure or textural parameters from *in vivo* MR images of the radius or calcaneus. Recently, Engelke and colleagues have provided a comprehensive analysis of threshold effects in hrMR of the calcaneus when compared with ultrahigh-resolution anatomic sectioning *in vitro*[80]. Newitt and co-workers reported promising results for the application of micro-finite element analyses based on hrMR images of the distal radius *in vivo*[81] Structural parameters determined in high-resolution MR images of a proximal femur specimen correlated significantly with bone strength, with the highest correlations obtained combining DXA BMD and structural measures[82].

The resolution achievable *in vivo* by magnetic resonance imaging (MRI) is not sufficient to depict precisely individual trabeculae, and, thus, does not permit quantification of the 'true' trabecular bone morphology and topology.

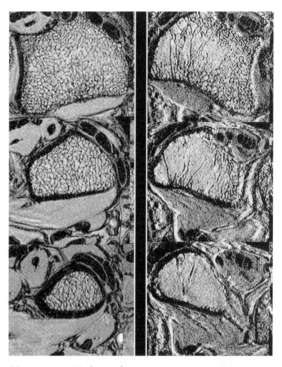

Figure 7 High-resolution (~ 150×150×500 μm) axial gradient echo magnetic resonance (MR) images of the distal radius of a young woman (left) and an elderly osteoporotic woman (right) clearly show the deterioration in trabecular and cortical structure. Courtesy of Sharmila Majumdar

Trabecular samples of the distal radius (Figure 7) imaged using MRI at 156×156×300 μm correlate well with micro-CT at 34×34×34 μm, with r^2 ranging from 0.57 to 0.64 for morphological measurements[83]. Trabecular bone structure parameters assessed in the distal radius on high-resolution MR and multislice CT images are significantly correlated with those determined on contact radiographs of the corresponding specimen sections. For MR imaging, the threshold algorithm used for binarizing the images substantially affected these correlations[84].

In an animal study by Jiang and colleagues, MRI microscopy showed that ovariectomy induces deterioration of trabecular microstructure and of the biomechanical properties in the femoral neck of ewes. Calcitonin treatment prevented ovariectomy-induced changes in a dose-dependent manner (Figure 8). The femoral neck

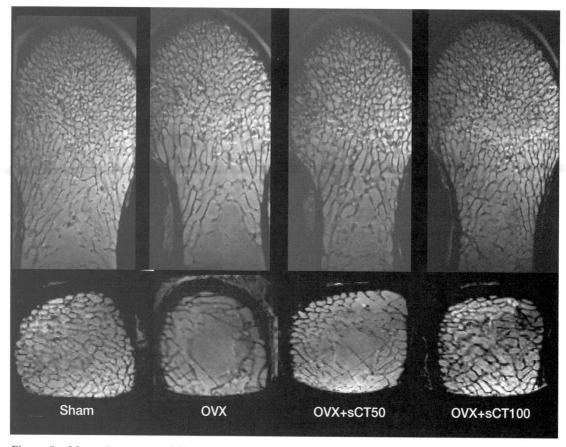

Figure 8 Magnetic resonance (MR) microscopic images of the proximal femur show that ovariectomy (OVX)-induced loss in trabecular microstructure in the femoral neck is prevented by treatment with salmon calcitonin (sCT) at 50 IU or 100 IU

trabecular microstructure correlated significantly with biomechanical properties, and its combination with BMD further improved the prediction of bone quality[85].

CHALLENGES FOR BONE IMAGING

Despite the considerable progress that has been made over the past decade in advanced bone imaging for osteoporosis assessment, a number of challenges remain. Technically, the challenges reflect the balances and trade-offs between spatial resolution, sample size, signal-to-noise ratio, radiation exposure and acquisition time, or between the complexity and expense of the imaging technologies versus their availability

and accessibility. Clinically, the challenges for bone imaging include balancing the advantages of standard BMD information versus the more complex architectural features of bone, or the deeper research requirements of the laboratory versus the broader needs of clinical practice. The biological differences between the peripheral appendicular skeleton and the central axial skeleton and their impact on the relevant bone imaging methods must be further clarified. Finally, the relative merits of these sophisticated imaging techniques must be weighed with respect to their applications as diagnostic procedures, requiring high accuracy or reliability, versus their applications as monitoring procedures, requiring high precision or reproducibility.

ACKNOWLEDGMENT

This chapter is adapted in part from Genant HK, Gordon C, Jiang Y, Lang TF, Link TM, Majumdar S. Advanced imaging of bone macro and micro structure. *Bone* 1999; 25: 149–52

References

1. Genant HK, Engelke K, Fuerst T, et al. Noninvasive assessment of bone mineral and structure: state of the art. *J Bone Miner Res* 1996; 11: 707–30

2. Faulkner KG, Cann CE, Hasegawa BH. CT-derived finite element model to determine vertebral cortex strength In Loew MH, ed. *Medical Imaging IC: Image Processing*. Newport Beach, CA: SPIE, 1990; 1233: 194–202

3. Lang TF, Guglielmi G, van Kuijk C, et al. Measurement of bone mineral density at the spine and proximal femur by volumetric quantitative computed tomography and dual-energy X-ray absorptiometry in elderly women with and without vertebral fractures. *Bone* 2002; 30: 247–50

4. Keyak JH, Rossi SA, Jones KA, Skinner HB. Prediction of femoral fracture load using automated finite element modeling. *J Biomech* 1998; 31: 125–33

5. Lang TF, Li J, Harris ST, Genant HK. Assessment of vertebral bone mineral density using volumetric quantitative computed tomography. *J Comput Assist Tomogr* 1999; 23: 130–7

6. Lang TF, Keyak JH, Heitz MW, et al. Volumetric quantitative computed tomography of the proximal femur: precision and relation to bone strength. *Bone* 1997; 21: 101–8

7. Lotz JC, Gerhart TN, Hayes WC. Mechanical properties of trabecular bone from the proximal femur: a quantitative CT study. *J Comput Assist Tomogr* 1990; 14: 107–14

8. McBroom RJ, Hayes WC, Edwards WT, et al. Prediction of vertebral body compressive fracture using quantitative computed tomography. *J Bone Joint Surg* 1985; 67: 1206–14

9. Jergas M, Breitenseher M, Glüer CC, et al. Estimates of volumetric bone density from projectional measurements improve the discriminatory capability of dual X-ray absorptiometry. *J Bone Miner Res* 1995; 10: 1101–10

10. Sode M, Keyak J, Bouxsein M, Lang T. Assessment of femoral neck torsional strength indices. *Bone Miner Res* 2004; 19: S238

11. Lang TF, Keyak JH, Yu A, et al. Determinants of proximal femoral strength in elderly women. *J Bone Miner Res* 2003; 18: S266

12. Crawford RP, Cann CE, Keaveny TM. Finite element models predict in vitro vertebral body compressive strength better than quantitative computed tomography. *Bone* 2003; 33: 744–50

13. Crawford RP, Rosenberg WS, Keaveny TM. Quantitative computed tomography-based finite element models of the human lumbar vertebral body: effect of element size on stiffness, damage, and fracture strength predictions. *J Biomech Eng* 2003; 125: 434–8

14. Chevalier F, Laval-Jeantet AM, Laval-Jeantet M, Bergot C. CT image analysis of the vertebral trabecular network in vivo. *Calcif Tissue Int* 1992; 51: 8–13

15. Ito M, Ohki M, Hayashi K, et al. Trabecular texture analysis of CT images in the relationship with spinal fracture. *Radiology* 1995; 194: 55–9

16. Gordon CL, Lang TF, Augat P, Genant HK. Image-based assessment of spinal trabecular bone structure from high-resolution CT images. *Osteoporos Int* 1998; 8: 317–25

17. Jiang Y, Zhao J, Augat P, et al. Trabecular bone mineral and calculated structure of human bone specimens scanned by peripheral quantitative computed tomography: relation to biomechanical properties. *J Bone Miner Res* 1998; 13: 1783–90

18. Link TM, Vieth V, Stehling C, et al. High-resolution MRI vs multislice spiral CT: which technique depicts the trabecular bone structure best? *Eur Radiol* 2003; 13: 663–71

19. Durand EP, Rüegsegger P. High-contrast resolution of CT images for bone structure analysis. *Med Phys* 1992; 19: 569–73

20. Muller R, Hahn M, Vogel M, et al. Morphometric analysis of noninvasively assessed bone biopsies: comparison of high-resolution computed tomography and histologic sections. *Bone* 1996; 18: 215–20

21. Muller R, Hildebrand T, Hauselmann HJ, Ruegsegger P. In vivo reproducibility of three-dimensional structural properties of noninvasive bone biopsies using 3D-pQCT. *J Bone Miner Res* 1996; 11: 1745–50

22. Engelke K, Graeff W, Meiss L, et al. High spatial resolution imaging of bone mineral using computed microtomography. Comparison with micro-radiography and undecalcified histologic sections. *Invest Radiol* 1993; 28: 341–9

23. Takada M, Kikuchi K, Unau S, Murata K. Three-dimensional analysis of trabecular bone structure of human vertebra in vivo using image data from multi-detector row computed tomography – correlation with bone mineral density and ability to discriminate women with vertebral fracture. *J Bone Miner Res* 2004; 19: S371

24. Bauer JS, Mueler D, Fischbeck M, et al. High resolution spiral-CT for the assessment of osteoporosis: which site of the spine and region of the vertebra is best suited to obtain trabecular bone structural parameters? *J Bone Miner Res* 2004; 19: S169

25. Khosla S, Melton LJ, Atkinson EJ, et al. Relationship of volumetric density, geometry and bone structure at different skeletal sites to sex steroid levels in men. *J Bone Miner Res* 2004; 19: S88

26. Feldkamp LA, Goldstein SA, Parfitt AM, et al. The direct examination of three-dimensional bone architecture in vitro by computed tomography. *J Bone Miner Res* 1989; 4: 3–11

27. Kuhn JL, Goldstein SA, Feldkamp LA, et al. Evaluation of a microcomputed tomography system to study trabecular bone structure. *J Orthop Res* 1990; 8: 833–42

28. Goulet RW, Goldstein SA, Ciarelli MJ, et al. The relationship between the structural and orthogonal compressive properties of trabecular bone. *J Biomech* 1994; 27: 375–89

29. Engelke K, Klifa C, Munch B, et al. Morphological analysis of the trabecular network: the influence of image processing technique on structural parameters. 10th International Bone Densitometry Workshop, Venice, Italy. *J Bone Miner Res* 1994; 25 (Suppl 2): S8

30. Engelke K, Song SM, Glüer CC, Genant HK. A digital model of trabecular bone. *J Bone Miner Res* 1996; 11: 480–9

31. Parfitt AM, Matthews C, Villanueva A. Relationships between surface, volume and thickness of iliac trabecular bone in aging and in osteoporosis. *J Clin Invest* 1983; 72: 1396–409

32. Parfitt AM. The stereologic basis of bone histomorphometry. Theory of quantitative microscopy and reconstruction of the third dimension. In Recker R, ed. *Bone Histomorphometry: Techniques and Interpretations*. Boca Raton: CRC Press, 1983: 53–87

33. Odgaard A, Gundersen HJG. Quantification of connectivity in cancellous bone, with special emphasis on 3-D reconstructions. *Bone* 1993; 14: 173–82

34. Ruegsegger P, Koller B, Muller R. A microtomographic system for the nondestructive evaluation of bone architecture. *Calcif Tissue Int* 1996; 58: 24–9

35. Müller R, Bauss F, Smith SY, Hannan MK. Mechano-structure relationships in normal, ovariectomized and ibandronate treated aged macaques as assessed by micro-tomographic imaging and biomechanical testing. *Trans Orthop Res Soc* 2001; 26: 66

36. Muller R, Ruegsegger P. Analysis of mechanical properties of cancellous bone under conditions of simulated bone atrophy. *J Biomech* 1996; 29: 1053–60

37. van Rietbergen B, Weinans H, Huiskes R, Odgaard A. A new method to determine trabecular bone elastic properties and loading using micromechanical finite-element models. *J Biomech* 1995; 28: 69–81

38. Engelke K, Karolczak M, Schaller S, et al. A cone beam micro-computed tomography (μCT) system for imaging of 3D trabecular bone structure. Presented at the 13th International bone Densitometry Workshop, October 1998, Wisconsin, USA

39. Jiang Y, Zhao, P, Liao EY, et al. Application of micro CT assessment of 3D bone microstructure in preclinical and clinical studies. *J Bone Miner Metab* 2005; 23S: 122–31

40. Sohaskey ML, Jiang Y, Zhao J, et al. Insertional mutagenesis of osteopotentia, a novel transmembrane protein essential for skeletal integrity. *J Bone Miner Res* 2004; 19: S21

41. Sorocéanu MA, Miao D, Jiang Y, et al. *Pthrp* haploinsufficiency impairs bone formation but potentiates the bone anabolic effects of PTH (1-34). *J Bone Miner Res* 2004; 19: S97

42. Takeshita S, Namba N, Zhao J, et al. SHIP-deficient mice are severely osteoporotic due to increased numbers of hyper-resorptive osteoclasts. *Nat Med* 2002; 8: 943–9

43. Bergo MO, Gavino B, Ross J, et al. Zmpste24 deficiency in mice causes spontaneous bone fractures, muscle weakness, and a prelamin A processing defect. *Proc Natl Acad Sci USA* 2002; 99: 13049–54

44. Lane NE, Balooch M, Zhao J, et al. Glucocorticoids induce changes around the osteocyte lacunae that reduces bone strength and bone mineral content independent of apoptosis: preliminary data from a glucocorticoid-induced bone loss model in male mice. *J Bone Miner Res* 2004; 19: S434–5

45. Jiang Y, Zhao JJ, Mangadu R, et al. Assessment of 3D cortical and trabecular bone microstructure and erosion on micro CT images of a murine model of arthritis. *J Bone Miner Res* 2004; 19: S474

46. Jiang Y, Zhao J, Mitlak BH, et al. Recombinant human parathyroid hormone (1-34) (teriparatide) improves both cortical and cancellous bone structure. *J Bone Miner Res* 2003; 18: 1932–41

47. Jiang Y, Zhao J, Eriksen EF, Genant HK. Reproducibility of micro CT quantification of 3D microarchitecture of the trabecular and cortical bone in the iliac crest of postmenopausal osteoporotic women and their treatment with teriparatide [rhPTH(1-34)]. Presented at RSNA'03, Chicago 2003: 571

48. Bonse U, Busch F, Gunnewig O, et al. 3D computed x-ray tomography of human cancellous bone at 8 μm spatial and 10-4 energy resolution. *Bone Miner* 1994; 25: 25–38

49. Engelke K, Dix W, Graeff W, et al. Quantitative microtomography and microradiography of bones using synchrotron radiation. Presented at the 8th International Workshop on Bone Densitometry, Bad Reichenhall, Germany, 1991, *Osteoporos Int*

50. Graeff W, Engelke K. Microradiography and microtomography. In Ebashi S, Koch M, Rubenstein E, ed. *Handbook on Synchrotron Radiation*. Amsterdam: North-Holland, 1991: 361–405

51. Kinney JH, Lane NE, Haupt DL. In vivo, three-dimensional microscopy of trabecular bone. *J Bone Miner Res* 1995; 10: 264–70

52. Lane NE, Thompson JM, Strewler GJ, Kinney JH. Intermittent treatment with human parathyroid hormone (hPTH[1-34]) increased trabecular bone volume but not connectivity in osteopenic rats. *J Bone Miner Res* 1995; 10: 1470–7

53. Peyrin F, Salome M, Cloetens P, et al. What do micro-CT examinations reveal at various resolutions: a study of the same trabecular bone samples at the 14, 7, and 2 micron level. Presented at a Symposium on Bone Architecture and the Competence of Bone, Ittingen, Switzerland, July 1998

54. Borah B, Ritman EL, Dufresne TE, et al. Five year risedronate therapy normalizes mineralization: synchrotron radiation micro-computed tomography study of sequential triple biopsies. *J Bone Miner Res* 2004; 19: S308

55. Recker R, Ensrud K, Diem S, et al. Normal bone histomorphometry and 3D microarchitecture after 10 years alendronate treatment of postmenopausal women. *J Bone Miner Res* 2004; 19: S45

56. Neff M, Dambacher M, Haemmerle S, et al. 3D evaluation of bone microarchitecture in humans using high resolution pQCT; a new in vivo, non invasive and time saving procedure. *J Bone Miner Res* 2004; 19: S236

57. Pistoia W, van Rietbergen B, Lochmuller EM, et al. Estimation of distal radius failure load with micro-finite element analysis models based on three-dimensional peripheral quantitative computed tomography images. *Bone* 2002; 30: 842–8

58. Borah B, Gross GJ, Dufresne TE, et al. Three-dimensional microimaging (MRmicroI and microCT), finite element modeling, and rapid prototyping provide unique insights into bone architecture in osteoporosis. *Anat Rec* 2001; 265: 101–10

59. Majumdar S, Genant H, Gies A, Guglielmi G. Regional variations in trabecular structure in the calcaneus assessed using high resolution magnetic resonance images and quantitative image analysis. *J Bone Miner Res* 1993; 8S: 351

60. Majumdar S, Genant H, Grampp S, et al. Analysis of trabecular bone structure in the distal radius using high resolution MRI. *Eur Radiol* 1994; 4: 517–24

61. Majumdar S, Newitt DC, Jergas M, et al. Evaluation of technical factors affecting the quantification of trabecular bone structure using magnetic resonance imaging. *Bone* 1995; 17: 417–30

62. Chung H, Wehrli FW, Williams JL, Kugelmass SD. Relationship between NMR transverse relaxation, trabecular bone architecture, and strength. *Proc Natl Acad Sci USA* 1993; 90: 10250–4

63. Chung HW, Wehrli FW, Williams JL, et al. Quantitative analysis of trabecular microstructure by 400 MHz nuclear magnetic resonance imaging. *J Bone Miner Res* 1995; 10: 803–11

64. Chung HW, Wehrli FW, Williams JL, Wehrli SL. Three-dimensional nuclear magnetic resonance microimaging of trabecular bone. *J Bone Miner Res* 1995; 10: 1452–61

65. Hwang SN, Wehrli FW, Williams JL. Probability-based structural parameters from three-dimensional nuclear magnetic resonance images as predictors of trabecular bone strength. *Med Phy* 1997; 24: 1255–61

66. Antich P, Mason R, McColl R, et al. Trabecular architecture studies by 3D MRI microscopy in bone biopsies. *J Bone Miner Res* 1994; 9S1: 327

67. Kapadia RD, High W, Bertolini D, Sarkar SK. MR microscopy: a novel diagnostic tool in osteoporosis research. In Christiansen C, ed. *4th International Symposium on Osteoporosis and Consensus Development Conference*, Hong Kong, 1993: 28

68. Simmons CA, Hipp JA. Method-based differences in the automated analysis of the three-dimensional morphology of trabecular bone. *J Bone Miner Res* 1997; 12: 942–7

69. Majumdar S, Newitt D, Mathur A, et al. Magnetic resonance imaging of trabecular bone structure in the distal radius: relationship with X-ray tomographic microscopy and biomechanics. *Osteoporos Int* 1996; 6: 376–85

70. Ouyang X, Selby K, Lang P, et al. High resolution magnetic resonance imaging of the calcaneus: age-related changes in trabecular structure and comparison with dual X-ray absorptiometry measurements. *Calcif Tissue Int* 1997; 60: 139–47

71. Jara H, Wehrli FW, Chung H, Ford JC. High-resolution variable flip angle 3D MR imaging of trabecular microstructure in vivo. *Magn Reson Med* 1993; 29: 528–39

72. Kühn B, Stampa B, Glüer C-C. Hochauflösende Darstellung und Quantifierung der trabekulären Knochenstruktur der Fingerphalangen mit der Magnetresonanztomographie. *Z Med Phys* 1997; 7: 162–8

73. Stampa B, Kühn B, Heller M, Glüer C-C. Rods or plates: a new algorithm to characterize bone structure using 3D magnetic resonance imaging. Presented at the 13th International Bone Densitometry Workshop, October 1998, Wisconsin, USA

74. Stampa B, Kuhn B, Liess C, et al. Characterization of the integrity of three-dimensional trabecular bone microstructure by connectivity and shape analysis using high-resolution magnetic resonance imaging in vivo. *Top Magn Reson Imaging* 2002; 13: 357–63

75. Link T, Majumdar S, Augat P, et al. In vivo high resolution MRI of the calcaneus: differences in trabecular structure in osteoporotic patients. *J Bone Miner Res* 1998; 13: 1175–82

76. Majumdar S, Genant HK, Grampp S, et al. Correlation of trabecular bone structure with age, bone mineral density and osteoporotic status: in vivo studies in the distal radius using high resolution magnetic resonance imaging. *J Bone Miner Res* 1997; 12: 111–18

77. Wehrli FW, Hwang SN, Ma J, et al. Cancellous bone volume and structure in the forearm: noninvasive assessment with MR microimaging and image processing. *Radiology* 1998; 206: 347–57

78. Wehrli FW, Gomberg BR, Saha PK, et al. Digital topological analysis of in vivo magnetic resonance microimages of trabecular bone reveals structural implications of osteoporosis. *J Bone Miner Res* 2001; 16: 1520–31

79. Wehrli FW, Saha PK, Gomberg BR, et al. Role of magnetic resonance for assessing structure and function of trabecular bone. *Top Magn Reson Imaging* 2002; 13: 335–55

80. Engelke K, Hahn M, Takada M, et al. Structural analysis of high resolution in vitro MR images

compared to stained grindings. *Calcif Tissue Int* 2001; 68: 163–71

81. Newitt DC, Majumdar S, van Rietbergen B, et al. In vivo assessment of architecture and micro-finite element analysis derived indices of mechanical properties of trabecular bone in the radius. *Osteoporos Int* 2002; 13: 6–17

82. Link TM, Vieth V, Langenberg R, et al. Structure analysis of high resolution magnetic resonance imaging of the proximal femur: in vitro correlation with biomechanical strength and BMD. *Calcif Tissue Int* 2003; 72: 156–65

83. Pothuaud L, Laib A, Levitz P, et al. Three-dimensional-line skeleton graph analysis of high-resolution magnetic resonance images: a validation study from 34-micron-resolution microcomputed tomography. *J Bone Miner Res* 2002; 17: 1883–95

84. Link TM, Vieth V, Stehling C, et al. High-resolution MRI vs multislice spiral CT: which technique depicts the trabecular bone structure best? *Eur Radiol* 2003; 13: 663–71

85. Jiang Y, Zhao J, Geusens P, et al. Femoral neck trabecular microstructure in ovariectomized ewes treated with calcitonin: MRI microscopic evaluation. *J Bone Miner Res* 2005; 20: 125–30

Quantitative ultrasonometry of bone in the management of postmenopausal women

14

P. Hadji

INTRODUCTION

The menopause represents a turning point in a woman's life at which a series of biological transformations take place, and each of these will individually, differently, affect general health as well as quality of life. In accordance with the increased life expectancy of women, physicians are confronted with an increasing number of diseases which occur during the postmenopausal period. From this point of view, management of the climacteric period is one of the major challenges for future gynecological routine.

Osteoporosis is a preventable disease that affects a large number of elderly women, and is responsible for increase of morbidity and mortality. Osteoporosis has perhaps the widest-ranging social, physical and economic impact associated with estrogen deficiency. Of those affected by osteoporosis, 80% are women, and there is a nearly 40% lifetime fracture risk among women who are aged 50. The most recent report by the World Health Organization (WHO) on osteoporosis[1], published in 1994, established that 23–30% of postmenopausal women are osteoporotic and that a further 25–40% present skeletal demineralization below normal values. Primary osteoporosis is a multifactorial state, and multiple mechanisms are involved in its pathogenesis. In women, the most frequent type is postmenopausal osteoporosis due to estrogen deprivation after the menopause[1–8]. The incidence of osteoporotic fracture in western societies is constantly increasing due to the increase of life expectancy.

Bone mass reaches its peak during the reproductive years, whereas a decrease of bone mineral content becomes relevant after the menopause. This sequence underlines the necessity of a central role of gynecologists in the assessment of female bone health at the time of the perimenopause, and consequently in establishing a 'biological zero'. The time after the menopause represents the scale on which to distinguish normal from increased bone changes. In fact, it is more appropriate to compare individual changes and characteristics of bone tissue on the basis of menopausal age than to compare subjects of the same age but with a different hormonal status.

The essential role of reproductive and endocrinological history has led many clinicians to use questionnaires to evaluate risk factors for osteoporosis, and also to perform instrumental examinations (dual-energy X-ray absorptiometry (DXA) and quantitative ultrasonometry (QUS)).

The diagnosis and clinical management of osteoporosis have been based on the measurement of bone mineral density (BMD) using DXA as the 'gold standard' method. Osteoporosis has been defined according to measurement of a BMD that is more than 2.5 standard deviations (SDs) below the young adult reference range (*T*-score). If the patient additionally has a history of fragility fracture, 'severe' osteoporosis is diagnosed. A *T*-score between -1 and -2 is categorized as 'low bone mass', or 'osteopenia'[1]. Bone densitometry has been selected as the standard used to establish the diagnosis, and it has also been considered the standard tool for clinical management of osteoporosis treatment and prevention. This corresponds to the measurement of blood pressure to assess the risk of stroke, or the measurement of blood glucose to assess the risk of diabetic complications.

The ideal technique for the measurement of bone mass should be reliable, fast and inexpensive, and give, if possible, no exposure to ionizing radiation. It should have a high level of accuracy in order to provide optimal evaluation of fracture risk in a given population. High precision is essential in the individual patient for monitoring the effects of treatment. Furthermore, the technique should give a validated prediction of risk of subsequent fracture.

Consequently, in recent years, the low cost and radiation-free method of quantitative ultrasonometry of bone (QUS) has emerged as an alternative to DXA in the assessment of bone structure, bone quality and fracture risk[9-36]. QUS is a method that is easy to use, and, although it is technologically very sophisticated, it is very versatile and suitable for out-patient use and has an excellent cost–benefit ratio. The most recent studies have demonstrated its advantages from a clinical point of view: its effectiveness in screening is greater than that of patient-history questionnaires[11,12,37-39], and it represents an independent risk factor for osteoporosis[40]. It is effective in longitudinal monitoring of the influence of menopause, exercise, hormone replacement therapy (HRT) and osteotropic therapies[34,36,41,42].

The aim of this chapter is to review the technical and biological aspects of bone tissue according to quantitative ultrasonometry and to evaluate its future role in clinical use in gynecological practice.

ABILITIES AND LIMITATIONS OF DXA MEASUREMENT

DXA has been considered the gold standard for measurement of bone mineral density in the diagnosis and follow-up of osteoporotic patients. However, recently, concerns about the clinical validity and utility of widespread use of the DXA technique have been raised. The attention of the medical community on BMD assessed by DXA has led to a kind of misconception of osteoporosis, which has somehow become synonymous with pathological BMD. Osteoporosis is a clinical diagnosis, and it is now evident that a low

BMD is not a disease *per se*, but a strong risk factor for fractures. DXA estimation cannot discriminate the entire population at risk for future fractures, and some 40–60% of fractures occur in women with a normal DXA measurement[43]. In addition, the results of fracture prevention trials clearly demonstrate that, with small increases of 3–8% of BMD, different antiresorptive agents can reduce the fracture incidence by 30–55%[44,45].

Therefore, fracture prevention following osteotropic treatment cannot be explained merely on the basis of an increase in BMD. It is necessary to take into consideration other properties and structural characteristics of bone tissue that cannot be measured by DXA, but can possibly be evaluated by QUS. Bone mineral density measured by DXA cannot discriminate the normal bone of a teenager with a BMD similar to that of an older woman[46]. This is relevant, since it shows the intrinsic limitation of a technique just measuring BMD. In fact, the mineral densities measured by DXA can be identical, although the structural characteristics of bone in young and elderly subjects are completely different. For similar reasons, DXA cannot discriminate subjects with osteomalacia from those with osteoporosis[47]. Conversely, QUS evaluates not only the density of bone, but also structural characteristics that allow differentiation between young and elderly bone, as well as osteoporotic from osteomalacic bone. Additionally, ultrasonometry measurements, which are correlated with the density and elasticity of bone tissue, represent a risk factor for fracture that is independent of densitometry values[11,12,38,39,48].

BONE ULTRASONOMETRY

Quantitative ultrasonometry (QUS) of bone uses ultrasound waves of frequencies ranging between 200 kHz and 1.5 MHz, considerably lower than the frequencies commonly used in echography. The first ultrasound parameters used to characterize bone tissue were speed of sound (SoS) and broadband ultrasound attenuation (BUA); other, more complex parameters were also developed from a combination of the former, including

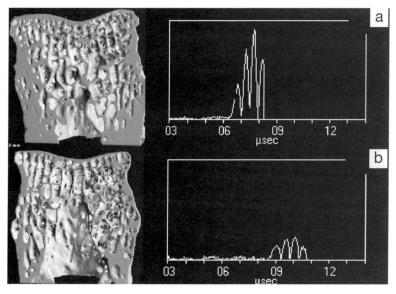

Figure 1 Image of phalanx (micro-quantitative computed tomography, μQCT) and relative ultrasound signal transmitted: normal bone (a) and osteoporotic bone (b)[54]

amplitude-dependent speed of sound (AD-SoS), stiffness index (SI) and quantitative ultrasound index (QUI). The latter have turned out to be more useful in identifying subjects with low bone mineral density or at high risk of fracture[36,49].

Experimental studies

The main interest for those studying the interaction of ultrasound and bone tissue has always been exact determination of the characteristics of the tissue measured. This can be evaluated by the shape of the ultrasound wave as it propagates though bone. Studies *in vitro* have clearly underlined that SoS is closely related to bone mineralization, leading to high correlation between SoS and BMD in the range of $r = 0.78–0.91$[50]. Hereby, SoS seems to be influenced more by mineral density than by the elastic characteristics of bone[51,52]. Broadband ultrasound attenuation (BUA), in contrast, seems to be influenced more by the structural characteristics of trabecular bone (porosity, etc.)[53]. Recent studies have also demonstrated that some morphological characteristics of the transmitted QUS wave are related to the structure and geometry of the bone segment analyzed[54,55] (Figure 1). Today it is possible

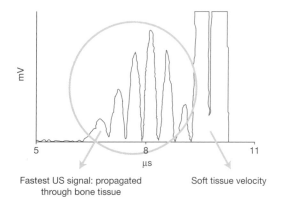

Figure 2 Ultrasound signal (US) transmitted through phalanx: fastest portion of the signal is circled. The right-hand part of soft tissue velocity (slow portion) is that corresponding to transmission through soft tissue

to perform more specific analysis, and to separate the part of the QUS signal relating to bone tissue alone: the fastest segment (Figure 2). Study of the fastest portion of the signal enables identification of a series of parameters able to describe the mechanical properties of the site analyzed, independent of the mineral density[47,51], whereas overall study of the signal (fastest and slow portions) appears unable to obtain the same results[56].

It has been demonstrated *in vitro* that bone architecture of the phalanx influences SoS, the shape of the QUS wave and the amplitude of the fastest part of the QUS signal differently[57]. In a study carried out on human phalanges of cadavers analyzed by QUS, DXA and micro-quantitative computed tomography (μQCT), Wüster and colleagues showed how the SoS and fast wave amplitude are more closely connected with the mineralized areas of the trabecular and cortical structure, while the frequency content of the signal, calculated by Fourier analysis, is linked with the areas occupied by the marrow and the organic matrix (Figure 3)[54].

In a clinical study of human phalanges analyzed also by nuclear magnetic resonance (NMR), it was shown that the duration (in microseconds) of the fastest QUS signal and the AD-SoS are able to reveal endosteal bone resorption, and are correlated with the dimensions of the cortical area and the moment of inertia of the bone itself[55].

Clinical studies

The clinical interest in QUS has stemmed mainly from its ability to assess fracture risk. A large number of studies have been conducted to assess

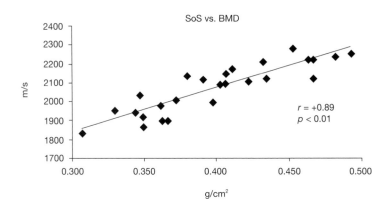

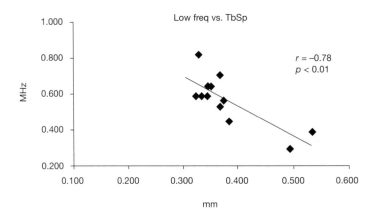

Figure 3 Associations between speed of sound (SoS) and bone mineral density (BMD) and between low frequency peak in the Fourier spectrum (low freq) and separation between trabeculae (TbSp)[54]

the efficacy of the measurement sites investigated as well as the performances of ultrasound devices in terms of stability, precision and capability to detect patients with osteoporotic fractures.

Measurement site

The measurement sites analyzed by QUS are all peripheral: phalanx, calcaneus, radius and tibia. The bone architecture (compact or trabecular bone), the type of bone (long or flat) and diaphyseal, epiphyseal or metaphyseal site are factors, based on the metabolic sensitivity of the bone tissue analyzed, that ultimately determine the performance of the device used.

Ultrasonographic measurements

The phalanx is measured with QUS at the metaphyseal level, where both trabecular (around 40%) and cortical bone are present.

The metaphysis of the phalanx is also characterized by high bone turnover, and turns out to be a site extremely sensitive to skeletal changes, whether physiological or due to the presence of metabolic diseases (hyperparathyroidism) or iatrogenc diseases (treatment with glucocorticoids)[58].

Measurement of the calcaneus (Figure 4) can be made, according to the device used, by immersing the foot in water or employing dry techniques. The calcaneus is composed almost entirely of trabecular bone, and has the advantage of having external surfaces that are flat, homogeneous, parallel and therefore suited to the geometry of propagation of the ultrasound beam.

The tibia and radius are studied by techniques of longitudinal transmission of the ultrasound wave. Propagation occurs mostly along the external surface of the bone, and therefore provides information mainly on the cortical bone tissue. Investigation of the tibia and radius is sensitive to phenomena of endosteal reabsorption[59].

Precision and stability of the measurements

The technology now allows fully reliable and reproducible measurements to be obtained. The extensive European multicenter Phalangeal Osteosonogrammetry Study (PhOS)[46] has clearly confirmed the precision and stability of the QUS method at the phalanx, showing a coefficient of variation of less than 1% in short- and long-term series. There are also large studies of QUS applied to the calcaneus that have shown a coefficient of variation of 1% for SoS, less than 4% for BUA and 1% for combination parameters such as the stiffness index[11,12,36,50].

Clinical performance

QUS was introduced in clinical practice as a technique for the investigation of bone tissue with regard to postmenopausal osteoporosis. Therefore, research has focused on its performance in terms of detecting osteoporotic subjects with and without fracture, and the assessment of fracture risk in postmenopausal women. The validity of peripheral densitometry has been investigated in the recent National Osteoporosis Risk Assessment (NORA) study[43]. Hereby, a population of more than 200 000 women have been investigated, showing a high degree of the ability to predict risk for future fracture with QUS at the phalanx, forearm or calcaneus. Table 1 reports the odds ratio values obtained (relative fracture risk by diminution of a standard deviation from the normal value). This study further confirms the ability of QUS to discriminate between normal and pathological conditions and to predict fracture risk, already underlined in

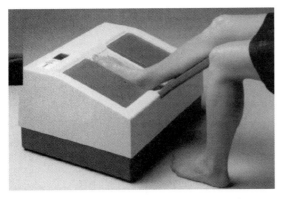

Figure 4 Ultrasound measurement at the calcaneus

Table 1 Relative risk calculated for each of the peripheral sites investigated in the National Osteoporosis Risk Assessment (NORA) study[43]

Site	Relative risk (odds ratio)
Phalanx	4.86
Forearm	2.86
Calcaneus	1.00

Table 2 Area below the receiver operating characteristics (ROC) curve (AUC) for detection of vertebral fractures

Technique	AUC
AD-SoS	0.823[*]
UBPI	0.867[*]
BMD L2 : L4	0.798[*]
BMD hip	0.779[*]
SoS	0.746[†]
BUA	0.760[†]
BMD L2 : L4	0.702[†]
BMD hip	0.723[†]

[*]Values reported for amplitude-dependent speed of sound (AD-SoS), ultrasound bone profile index (UBPI) at phalanx, bone mineral density (BMD) L2 : L4 and BMD hip, in total population, Phalangeal Osteosonogrammetry Study (PhOS)[46]. [†]Values reported for SoS and broadband ultrasound attenuation (BUA) at calcaneus, BMD L2 : L4 and BMD hip in the Basel Osteoporosis Study (BOS)[61]

cross-sectional[10,30,31,35,36,46,47,50] and several prospective, longitudinal studies[11,12,37,39].

The EPIDOS (Epidémiologie de l'Ostéoporose) study and the Study of Osteoporotic Fractures (SOF), two large-scale prospective, longitudinal studies, were the first to investigate the effectiveness of bone ultrasonometry at the calcaneus in comparison with DXA with regard to fracture risk prediction. The odds ratios (ORs) obtained for BUA and SoS were, respectively, 2.0 and 1.7[11,12]. Mele and colleagues. found values of OR of 1.5 (95% confidence interval (CI) 1.1–1.7) for AD-SoS measured at the phalanx in evaluating low-energy peripheral fractures[37]. The PhOS study, performed in 10 000 women, clearly demonstrated the effectiveness of QUS at the phalanx in detecting postmenopausal subjects with osteoporotic fractures (vertebra, hip), obtaining an OR for AD-SoS of 1.7 (95% CI 1.5–1.8)[46].

Comparison with DXA techniques has revealed no significant differences between the methods with regard to analysis of their diagnostic sensitivity, receiver operating characteristics (ROC)[46,60]. The Basel Osteoporosis Study demonstrated in subjects within an age range of 65–75 years that the performances of devices used at the calcaneus and phalanx were comparable to results obtained with axial DXA in discriminating subjects for vertebral fractures (Table 2)[61].

A recent European study carried out by Glüer and colleagues, the OPUS (Osteoporosis Prevention Using Soy) study, on the evaluation of vertebral fractures in postmenopausal women, concluded that all ultrasonometry variables (calcaneus) show a significant association with vertebral deformity, and forearm and clinical fracture[38]. The SEMOF (Schweizerische Evaluierung der Messmethode des osteoporotischen Frakturrisikos) multicenter study, involving over 6000 elderly women with a mean age > 70 years, demonstrated that QUS parameters at the phalanx and calcaneus were able to discriminate women with hip fracture[39].

Comparison of the results of these studies reveals an equal ability of QUS in comparison with DXA to predict future osteoporosis-related fracture.

One very important aspect deriving from the analysis of some of these large databases is the identification of appropriate diagnostic thresholds for osteoporosis, calculated on the basis of criteria selected by the WHO (Table 3)[1]. These values, confirmed by various studies[46,61], represent an important starting point for the use of such devices in screening of the postmenopausal female population.

Validation of the QUS technique for study of osteoporosis is now complete, and is supported by ample scientific documentation that has led to the following statement issued by the British National Osteoporosis Society (NOS)[40]:

(1) A low QUS value constitutes an independent risk factor for osteoporotic fracture in postmenopausal women;

(2) A low QUS value constitutes an indicator of low bone mass more important than clinical risk factors;

(3) Patients with low QUS values can be prescribed a further BMD test or a therapeutic regimen if other clinical risk factors are present.

Clinical interest relates to performing studies involving QUS to investigate further its ability to determine the rapidity of bone loss after the menopause. Early identification of postmenopausal women at higher risk of fracture by QUS today is already a very attractive option.

QUS can also monitor the effect of osteotropic treatments. This possibility has been repeatedly demonstrated in prospective studies for measurements at the phalanx and the calcaneus. Taking measurements at the phalanx, Mauloni and colleagues[48] performed a longitudinal study in subjects undergoing HRT, taking into consideration the precision of the method and the variations expected in time: they calculated that an interval of 18 months is required between one measurement and the following in order to reveal the effectiveness of the treatment. This interval confirms the estimates already reported from a large database, according to the precision of the instrument[62]. Also, treatment with alendronate can be monitored by phalanx QUS[63,64]. Similar studies using QUS of the calcaneus have shown the ability to display the effects of therapy with calcitonin[65], bisphosphonates[64] or HRT[34,41,42] already after 2 years. Table 4 reports the results of the most important longitudinal studies of the effectiveness of QUS at the phalanx and calcaneus in monitoring treatments.

Table 3 *T-score thresholds for diagnosis of osteoporosis calculated by Hartl and colleagues[61]*

Parameter	T-score threshold value
Achilles BUA	−1.0
Achilles SoS	−1.8
Achilles stiffness	−1.6
Sahara BUA	−1.6
Sahara SoS	−1.5
Sahara QUI	−1.5
Bone Profiler AD-SoS	−3.2
Bone Profiler UBPI	−3.1

BUA, broadband ultrasound attenuation; SoS, speed of sound; QUI, quantitative ultrasound index; AD-SoS, amplitude-dependent SoS; UBPI, ultrasound bone profile index

Table 4 Main studies performed to assess effectiveness of bone ultrasound in monitoring therapies

Authors	Site	Treatment	Follow-up time	QUS parameters	Percentage increase
Mauloni et al.[48]	phalanx	HRT	4 years	pSoS	1.5
				BTT	10.6
Machado et al.[63]	phalanx	alendronate	2 years	pSoS	1.0
				BTT	6.0
Giorgino et al.[41]	calcaneus	HRT	3 years	stiffness	5.3
Gonnelli et al.[42]	calcaneus	HRT	2 years	stiffness	2.9
Giorgino et al.[64]	calcaneus	bisphosphonates	3 years	stiffness	6.7
Gonnelli et al.[65]	calcaneus	salmon calcitonin	2 years	stiffness	2.12

HRT, hormone replacement therapy; QUS, qualitative ultrasonometry; pSoS, phalanx speed of sound, BTT, bone transmission time

QUS IN CLINICAL GYNECOLOGICAL PRACTICE

Studies carried out in recent years have clearly demonstrated the validity of QUS in evaluating bone health after the menopause; performances of the techniques are comparable with those obtained by DXA with regard to ability for fracture risk prediction. Large-scale cross-sectional and longitudinal studies have demonstrated the applicability of QUS in screening the female population at the climacteric and after the menopause.

Since bone demineralization is closely linked with hormone deficiency found after the menopause, the problem emerges in the gynecological context. The key role of the clinician is to investigate the state of bone tissue in the female population, shifting the perspective of reference towards a new biological zero: the menopause. Using the menopause reference curve, the clinician can compare the individual female biological zero in relation to normal values for the population and determine the loss of bone mass as a function of months since the menopause on the normative curve[20,56].

After the menopause, assessment of bone tissue with QUS could be a part of the routine management of gynecological screening and pre-vention. Conversely, the management of osteoporosis later in life and the treatment of established osteoporosis cannot be seen as part of routine gynecological practice: these topics are matters for the bone specialist. Using the QUS method, the clinician can also acquire specific information on bone tissue. Practical utilization of a first-level screening device for osteoporosis involves identifying a score threshold to classify the population into normal subjects with a low risk of osteoporosis, and subjects at higher risk. An effective screening device must be able to minimize the number of false negatives while restricting the number of subjects for second-level referral for DXA and/or spinal X-ray. It is therefore essential to identify the QUS values below which further referral is necessary.

From this perspective, in a population of 1597 women undergoing DXA and QUS at the phalanx, we evaluated the T-score threshold for AD-SoS that could identify the greatest number of subjects with DXA T-score < -2.5, while restricting the number of subjects examined with DXA. Figure 5 reports the values obtained with lumbar DXA and femoral neck DXA as a function of the different T-score thresholds for AD-SoS. The threshold value of T-score $= -2$ seems to offer the best compromise between the two parameters analyzed, keeping the subjects for

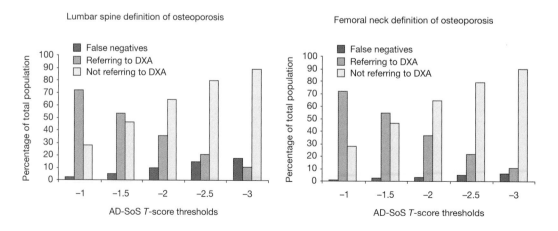

Figure 5 Dual-energy X-ray absorptiometry (DXA) referrals with selected amplitude-dependent speed of sound (AD-SoS) T-score values for osteoporosis screening (DXA T-score < -2.5) at spine (left) or hip (right) for all subjects. DXA referral: true positives + false positives; no DXA: true negatives; missed cases: false negatives

further referral at around 40% and maintaining the number of false negatives at 8.5% for lumbar DXA and 3.5% for femoral neck DXA. Table 5 reports the DXA *T*-score values as a function of the AD-SoS T-score values.

Hereby, two different strategies could be applied. The first strategy, the 'stand alone approach', employs the DXA-independent ability of QUS to identify women with a high risk of fracture. Here, a very low QUS result can directly lead to preventive treatment without any further DXA examination (Figure 6). The second strategy refers women with a very low QUS result to DXA measurement, and any treatment decision is based on DXA results (Figure 7).

Table 5 Densitometry values at the lumbar spine and femoral neck as a function of amplitude-dependent speed of sound (AD-SoS)

AD-SoS T-score	n	L2 : L4 BMD	T-score	Neck BMD	T-score
T-score ≤ −3.2	133	0.899 (0.135)	−2.51 (1.13)	0.743 (0.098)	−1.99 (0.82)
			$p < 0.001$		$p < 0.001$
−3.2 < T-score ≤ −2	447	0.961 (0.154)	−1.99 (1.28)	0.815 (0.132)	−1.39 (1.11)
			$p < 0.001$		$p < 0.001$
T-score > −2	1017	1.068 (0.170)	−1.10 (1.42)	0.869 (0.128)	−0.93 (1.08)

BMD, bone mineral density

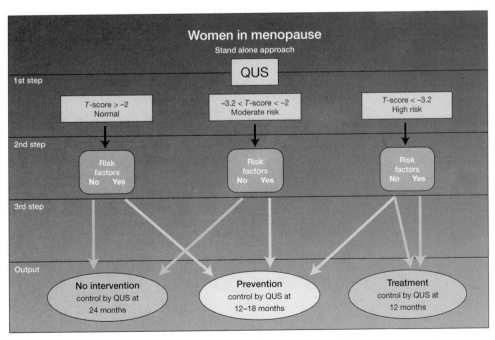

Figure 6 Scheme for the possible use of qualitative ultrasonometry (QUS) in a 'stand alone approach' for management of women in the menopause. The *T*-score values reported for QUS refer to measurements performed at the phalanx[66]

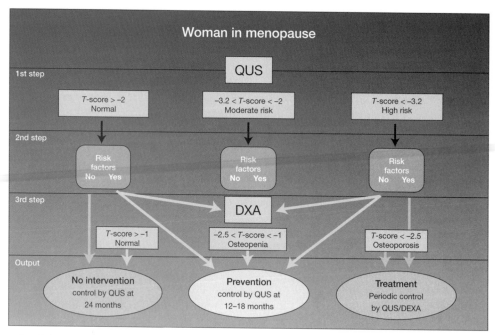

Figure 7 Scheme for the possible use of qualitative ultrasonometry (QUS) and dual-energy X-ray absorptiometry (DXA) for management of women in the menopause. The *T*-score values reported for QUS refer to measurements performed at the phalanx[66]

LEGAL ASPECTS OF OSTEOPOROSIS DETECTION IN THE EUROPEAN UNION

From this perspective, QUS examination represents a first assessment of the state of bone tissue; with this examination it is possible to select only a part of the population for further DXA referral, thus reducing costs and considerably restricting waiting lists, as well as limiting the amount of patients exposed to ionizing radiation. This is well in line with the European norm on regulating the use of X-rays in clinical practice, as per the directive to use ' ...available alternative techniques, having the same objective but not involving exposure to ionising radiation [...].' (European Directive 97/43/Euratom of 30/6/97 recently ratified in Italy by Legislative Decree.

'Implementation of directive 97/43 Euratom regarding health protection of persons against the hazards of ionising radiation connected with medical exposure' of *26/5/2000, no. 187* – art. 3.1.)

In this respect, it emerges that, if QUS is used in a systematic and rational manner in clinical practice, it is a valid device in the hands of the trained clinician for prevention of osteoporosis in postmenopausal women. QUS is already widely used, and, in Europe, the number of QUS devices exceeds that of DXA by far. It is therefore crucial to adopt guidelines for interpreting results that can be used by the clinician, such as those previously proposed. Likewise, it is necessary to offer training courses to enhance the clinical performance of an already established procedure for the study of bone health of climacteric women.

References

1. World Health Organization Study Group. Assessment of Fracture Risk and Its Application to Screening for Postmenopausal Osteoporosis. WHO Tech Rep Series: 1994: 843

2. Slemenda C, Hui SL, Longcope C, Johnston CC. Sex steroids and bone mass: a study of changes about the time of menopause. *J Clin Invest* 1987; 80: 1261–9

3. Riggs BL, Wahner HW, Dunn WL, et al. Differential changes in bone mineral density of the appendicular and axial skeleton with aging. *J Clin Invest* 1981; 67: 328–35

4. Noteloviz M. Osteoporosis: screening, prevention, and management. *Fertil Steril* 1993; 59: 707–25

5. Nilas L, Christiansen C. The pathophysiology of peri- and postmenopausal bone loss. *Br J Obstet Gynaecol* 1989; 96: 580–7

6. Gambacciani M, Spinetti A, de Simone L, et al. The relative contributions of menopause and aging to postmenopausal vertebral osteopenia. *J Clin Endocrinol Metab* 1993; 77: 1148–51

7. Gambacciani M, Spinetti A, de Simone L, et al. Postmenopausal bone loss of the proximal femur: estimated contribution of menopause and aging. *Menopause* 1995; 2: 169–74

8. Consensus Development Conference: Prophylaxis and Treatment of Osteoporosis. *Am J Med* 1993; 94: 646–50

9. Langton CM, Palmer SD, Porter RW. The measurement of broadband ultrasonic attenuation in cancellous bone. *Eng Med* 1984; 13: 89–91

10. Glüer CC for the International Quantitative Ultrasound Consensus Group. Quantitative ultrasound technique for the assessment of osteoporosis: expert agreement on current status. *J Bone Miner Res* 1997; 12: 1280–8

11. Hans D, Dargent-Molina P, Schott AM, et al. Ultrasonographic heel measurements to predict hip fracture in elderly women: the EPIDOS prospective study. *Lancet* 1996; 348: 511–14

12. Bauer DC, Glüer CC, Cauley JA, et al. Bone ultrasound predicts fractures strongly and independently of densitometry in older women: a prospective study. *Arch Intern Med* 1997; 157: 629–34

13. Hans D, Fuerst T, Lang T, et al. How can we measure bone quality? *Baillière's Clin Rheumatol* 1997; 11: 495–515

14. Sili Scavalli A, Marini M, Spadaro A, et al. Ultrasound transmission velocity of the proximal phalanxes of the non-dominant hand in the study of osteoporosis. *Clin Rheumatol* 1997; 16: 396–403

15. National Osteoporosis Society. The use of quantitative ultrasound in the management of osteoporosis in primary or secondary care. Position statement, 30 June 1998, NOS, London

16. Gambacciani A, Spinetti R, Gallo B, et al. Ultrasonographic bone characteristics during normal pregnancy: longitudinal and cross-sectional evaluation. *Am J Obstet Gynecol* 1995; 173: 890–3

17. Rubin CT, Pratt GW, Porter AL. The use of ultrasound in vivo to determine acute change in mechanical properties of bone following intense physical activity. *J Biomech* 1987; 20: 723–7

18. Cepollaro C, Agnusdei D, Gonnelli S, et al. Ultrasonographic assessment of bone in normal Italian males and females. *Br J Radiol* 1995; 68: 910–14

19. Gambacciani M, Benussi C, Cappagli B, et al. Quantitative bone ultrasonometry in climacteric women. *J Clin Densitometry* 1998; 3: 303–8

20. Ventura V, Mauloni M, Mura M, et al. Ultrasound velocity changes at the proximal phalanxes of the hand in pre-, peri- and postmenopausal women. *Osteoporos Int* 1996; 6: 368–75

21. Maalouf H, Hadji P. Age-associated changes in quantitative ultrasonomery (QUS) of the os calcis in Lebanese women – assessment of a Lebanese reference population. *J Musculoskel Neuron Interact* 2003; 3: 232–9

22. Hadji P, Kalder M, Backhus J, et al. Age-associated changes in bone ultrasonometry of the os calcis. Expanded data in healthy German women. *J Clin Densitometry* 2002; 5: 297–303

23. Hadji P, Hars O, Bock K, et al. The influence of serum leptin concentrations on bone mass assessed by quantitative ultrasound in pre- and postmenopausal women. *Maturitas* 2002; 44: 141–8

24. Hadji P, Ziller V, Kalder M, et al. Influence of pregnancy and breast-feeding on quantitataive

ultrasonometry of bone in postmenopausal women. *Climacteric* 2002; 5: 277–85

25. Murgia C, Cagnacci A, Paoletti AM, et al. Comparison between a new ultrasound densitometer and single-photon absorptiometry. *Menopause* 1996; 3: 149–53

26. Baran DT. Quantitative ultrasound: a technique to target women with low bone mass for preventive therapy. *Am J Med* 1995; 98: 48S–51S

27. De Aloysio D, Rovati LC, Cadossi R, et al. Bone effects of transdermal hormone replacement therapy in postmenopausal women as evaluated by means of ultrasound: an open one year prospective study. *Maturitas* 1997; 27: 61–8

28. Mautalen C, Vega E, Gonzales D, et al. Ultrasound and dual X-ray absorptiometry densitometry in women with hip fracture. *Calcif Tiss Int* 1995; 57: 165–8

29. Faulkner KG, McClung MR, Coleman LJ, Kingston-Sandahl E. Quantitative ultrasound of the heel: correlation with densitometric measurements at different skeletal sites. *Osteoporos Int* 1994; 4: 42–7

30. Gonnelli S, Cepollaro C, Agnusdei D, et al. Diagnostic value of ultrasound analysis and bone densitometry as predictors of vertebral deformity in postmenopausal women. *Osteoporos Int* 1995; 5: 413–18

31. Baran DT, Kelley AM, Karellas A, et al. Ultrasound attenuation of the os calcis in women with osteoporosis and hip fractures. *Calcif Tissue Int* 1988; 43: 138–42

32. Gregg EW, Kriska AM, Salamone LM, et al. The epidemiology of quantitative ultrasound: a review of the relationships with bone mass, osteoporosis and fracture risk. *Osteoporos Int* 1997; 7: 89–99

33. Benitez CL, Schneider DL, Barrett-Connor E, Sartoris DJ. Hand ultrasound for osteoporosis screening in postmenopausal women. *Osteoporos Int* 2000; 11: 203–10

34. Hadji P, Bock K, Wüster C, et al. Effect of hormone replacement therapy on ultrasonometric heel measurement. *Am J Obstet Gynecol* 2000; 182: 529–34

35. Hadji P, Hars O, Görke K, et al. Quantitative ultrasound of the calcaneus in postmenopausal women with spine and hip fracture. *J Clin Densitometry* 2000; 3: 233–9

36. Hadji P, Hars O, Wüster C, et al. Stiffness index identifies patients with osteoporotic fracture better than ultrasound velocity or attenuation alone. *Maturitas* 1999; 31: 221–6

37. Mele R, Masci G, Ventura V, et al. Three-year longitudinal study with quantitative ultrasound at the hand phalanx in a female population. *Osteoporos Int* 1997; 7: 550–7

38. Glüer C-C, Eastell R, Reid DM, et al. Association of quantitative ultrasound parameters and bone density with osteoporotic vertebral deformities in a population based sample: the OPUS study. Presented at the 23rd Annual Meeting of the American Society for Bone and Mineral Research, Phoenix, Arizona, USA, October 2001: F103

39. Krieg M, Cornuz J, Burckardt P and the SEMOF Study group. Comparison of three bone ultrasounds for determining hip fracture odds ratios. Results of the SEMOF study. Presented at the 23rd Annual Meeting of the American Society for Bone and Mineral Research, Phoenix, Arizona, USA, October 2001: F101

40. National Osteoporosis Society. The use of quantitative ultrasound in the management of osteoporosis. Position statement 31 January 2002, NOS, London

41. Giorgino R, Lorusso D, Paparella P. Ultrasound bone densitometry and 2-year hormonal replacement therapy efficacy in the prevention of early postmenopausal bone loss. *Osteoporos Int* 1996; 6 (Suppl 1): S341

42. Gonnelli S, Cepollaro C, Pondrelli C. Ultrasound parameters in the follow-up of osteoporotic women treated with oestrogen. *J Clin Densitometry* 1998; 1: 97

43. Siris ES, Miller PD, Barrett-Connor E, et al. Identification and fracture outcomes of undiagnosed low bone mineral density in postmenopausal women. Results from the National Osteoporosis Risk Assessment. *J Am Med Assoc* 2001; 286: 2815–21

44. Black DM, Cummings SR, Karpf DB, et al. Randomised trial of effect of alendronate on risk of fracture in women with existing vertebral fractures: Fracture Intervention Trial Research Group. *Lancet* 1996; 348: 1535–41

45. Ettinger B, Black DM, Mitlak B, et al: Reduction of vertebral fracture risk in postmenopausal women with osteoporosis treated with raloxifene.

Results from a 3-year randomized clinical trial. *J Am Med Assoc* 1999; 282: 637–45

46. Wüster C, Albanese C, de Aloysio D, et al. Phalangeal osteosonogrammetry study (PhOS): age related changes, diagnostic sensitivity and discrimination power. *J Bone Miner Res* 2000; 15: 1603–14

47. Luisetto G, Camozzi V, de Terlizzi F. Use of quantitative ultrasonography in differentiating osteomalacia from osteoporosis: preliminary study. *J Ultrasound Med* 2000; 19: 251–6

48. Mauloni M, Rovati LC, Cadossi R, et al. Monitoring bone effect of transdermal hormone replacement therapy by ultrasound investigation at the phalanx. A four year follow up study. *Menopause* 2000; 7: 402–12

49. Njeh CF, Hans D, Fuerst T, et al. *Quantitative Ultrasound: Assessment of Osteoporosis and Bone Status*. London: Martin Dunitz, 1999; 47–73

50. Hans D, Njeh CF, Genant HK, Meunier PJ. Quantitative ultrasound in bone status assessment. *Rev Rhum* 1998; 65: 7–9

51. de Terlizzi F, Battista S, Cavani F, et al. Influence of bone tissue density and elasticity on ultrasound propagation: an in vitro study. *J Bone Miner Res* 2000; 15: 2458–66

52. Hans D, Wu C, Njeh CF, et al. Ultrasound velocity of trabecular bones reflects mainly bone density and elasticity. *Calcif Tissue Int* 1999; 64: 18–23

53. Glüer C-C, Wu CY, Jergas M, et al. Three quantitative ultrasound parameters reflect bone structure. *Calcif Tissue Int* 1994; 55: 46–52

54. Battista S, de Terlizzi F, Müller R, Wüster C. Bone density and architecture: how do they affect ultrasound parameters? Presented at the 14th International Bone Densitometry Workshop, Warnemünde, Germany, September 2000

55. Barkmann R, Lüsse S, Stampa B, et al. Assessment of the geometry of human finger phalanges using quantitative ultrasound in vivo. *Osteoporos Int* 2000; 11: 745–55

56. Chaffai S, Peyrin F, Nuzzo S, et al. Ultrasonic characterization of human cancellous bone using transmission and backscatter measurements: relationships to density and microstructure. *Bone* 2002; 30: 229–37

57. Cadossi R, Canè V. Pathways of transmission of ultrasound energy through the distal metaphysis of the second phalanx of pigs: an in vitro study. *Osteoporos Int* 1996; 6: 196–206

58. Buckwalter JA, Glimcher MJ, Cooper RR, Recker R. Bone biology. *J Bone Joint Surg* 1995; 77-A:1256–89

59. Barkmann R, Kantorovich E, Singal C, et al. A new method for quantitative ultrasound measurements at multiple skeletal sites. *J Clin Densitometry* 2000; 3: 1–7

60. Reginster JY, Dethor M, Pirenne H, et al. Reproducibility and diagnostic sensitivity of ultrasonometry of the phalanges to assess osteoporosis. *Int J Gynecol Obstet* 1998; 63: 21–8

61 Hartl F, Tyndall A, Kraenzlin M, et al. Discriminatory ability of quantitative ultrasound parameters and bone mineral density in a population-based sample of postmenopausal women with vertebral fractures: result of the Basel Osteoporosis Study. *J Bone Miner Res* 2002; 17: 321–30

62. Gambacciani M, Benussi C, Cappagli B, et al. Quantitative bone ultrasonometry in climacteric women. *J Clin Densitometry* 1998; 3: 303–8

63. Machado ABC, Ingle BM, Eastell R. Monitoring alendronate therapy with QUS and dual X-ray absorptiometry (DXA). Presented at the American Society of Bone and Mineral Research meeting, September 1999

64. Giorgino R, Mancuso S. Oral alendronate and calcaneus ultrasound densitometry: a three-year prospective study. The Second International Conference on Osteoporosis. *Osteoporos Int* 1997; 7 (Suppl 2): 15

65. Gonnelli S, Cepollaro C, Pondrelli C. Ultrasound parameters in osteoporotic patients treated with salmon calcitonin: a longitudinal study. *Osteoporos Int* 1996; 6: 303–7

66. Gambacciani M. Hadji P. Quantitative ultrasound (QUS) of bone in the management of postmenopausal women. *Maturitas* 2003; 8: 1–12

Awareness of osteoporosis and related treatments

15

A. D. Woolf

The effective prevention and management of osteoporosis depend on awareness at a personal, professional and political level. Awareness needs to relate to an understanding of the impact of osteoporosis and fracture on the individual and society; who is at most risk; for whom prevention is a priority; what can be achieved in the prevention and treatment of osteoporosis and fracture; and, finally, how to gain priority and resources for this.

Osteoporosis is a skeletal disorder characterized by compromised bone and strength predisposing to an increased risk of fracture. Bone strength reflects the integration of two main features: bone density and bone quality[1]. Bone mass declines with age, and, as a result, an increasing number become osteopenic and osteoporotic. This is associated with changes in bone quality and an increase in fracture risk. The estimated lifetime risk of fracture for a woman aged 50 in the USA is 17.5% of the proximal humerus, 15.6% of the vertebra and 16% of the distal forearm, and two in five women will sustain one of these[2]. Osteoporosis, that is low bone mass, has little effect on the individual, but fracture results in loss of mobility of the affected limb and usually has a dramatic effect on self-care, domestic life, work and leisure. This may be short-lived, improving with fracture repair, but often there is some degree of long-term limitation of activities and restriction of participation. Those who have already sustained one fracture due to osteoporosis are at high risk of further fracture, which will result in even greater disability. In this way, osteoporosis can have a major effect on the lifespan of an individual. Vertebral fractures have been shown to have a major effect on health-related quality of life, increasing with the

number of fractures. Even subclinical fractures have been shown to impair quality of life. Hip fractures are associated with not only loss of function but also a significant excess mortality. Fear of sustaining another fracture can also have a further impact on the quality of life and restrict activities. This is a genuine concern as, following the first distal forearm fracture, it has been demonstrated that there is a 1.4-fold increase in risk of hip fracture in women and 2.7-fold increase in men, and the increased risk of vertebral fracture is 5.2-fold in women and 10.7-fold in men[3]. Prevalent vertebral fractures have also been shown to increase the risk of sustaining a new vertebral fracture over a 1-year period, with more than two prevalent fractures increasing the risk of a new vertebral fracture by 7.3-fold[4]. When women over 75 years, who had fallen during the last year, were given a description of what might have been the outcome if they had sustained a hip fracture, 80% said they would rather be dead than experience the loss of independence and impairment of quality of life. In a time trade-off study, on a scale between 0 equaling death and 1 equaling full health, a bad hip fracture was valued at 0.05 and a good hip fracture valued at 0.31, in contrast to breast cancer valued at 0.75 and myocardial infarct valued at 0.90[5]. Osteoporosis also has a major impact on society in utilization of health-care and social support.

The burden of osteoporosis and fracture on the individual and society is going to increase with the aging of the population worldwide. The greatest predicted increase is in Asia[6], but in Europe there is also expected to be a considerable increase with the anticipation that the over 65-year-old population will rise from 15.4% in 1995 to 22.4% by 2025. The greatest increase is going to be in the very elderly, and these are most at risk of sustaining fracture and of adverse outcome from fracture. Other reasons for increasing prevalence of osteoporosis and fracture are changes in life-style with less physical activity, smoking and excess alcohol and bad nutrition. In the USA, only 26% of adults undertake the recommended amount of leisure activity five times a week for 30 min or vigorous activity three times a week for 20 min; 46% take insufficient activity and 28% are considered physically inactive[7]. Globally, it is estimated that 17% of adults are physically inactive[8], and it is estimated that physical inactivity causes 1.9 million deaths and 19 million disability-adjusted life-years globally. Osteoporosis is considered within that.

Despite the great and growing burden, osteoporosis is not a priority in most countries. There is also a lack of individual awareness about personal risk and what should be done to reduce this. Public education campaigns are needed to enable people to recognize risk factors, such as by trying the 1-min test[9], and to know what to do to reduce this risk.

Access to evidence-based prevention and treatment is needed, and awareness is important to gain priority and resources for this. There is now a wealth of evidence for what can be achieved. There are a large number of randomized controlled trials, systematic reviews and evidence-based guidelines that demonstrate the effectiveness of interventions for the prevention and treatment of osteoporosis and the prevention of fracture. The European Bone & Joint Health Strategies Project reviewed the evidence base for what can be achieved in the prevention and treatment of osteoporosis and other musculoskeletal conditions, and clear recommendations have been made for the normal population, for those at risk and for those with osteoporosis[10]. The aim of these recommendations is that they not only benefit osteoporosis but also reduce the risk of other musculoskeletal conditions. To reduce the risk of osteoporosis and other musculoskeletal conditions, it is recommended that people of all ages should be encouraged to follow a healthy life-style and to avoid specific risks related to musculoskeletal health. They should keep physically active, maintain an ideal body weight, avoid injuries, have adequate dietary calcium and avoid tobacco use and excess alcohol. These have all been shown to benefit osteoporosis. However, it is known that the ability of such life-style changes to prevent osteoporosis is small, and a key strategy is to identify those at greatest risk and target them with more effective interventions. Not only should the at-risk population therefore follow the general life-style recommendations, but those individuals at highest risk of fracture, identified by case-finding strategies, will benefit from specific interventions aimed to increase bone strength. In older people, the risk of falling is greatly increased, and fall-prevention programs are a key part of preventing fractures. In those who have already sustained a fracture, then appropriate fracture management with multidisciplinary rehabilitation is essential, as well as interventions to prevent further fracture. The most important thing is to be able to identify those at most risk, and a simple 1-min osteoporosis risk test has been developed by the International Osteoporosis Foundation. This can help to identify those who need further assessment by bone density measurement. In this way, treatment can be targeted at those who will benefit most.

There are therefore strong arguments as to why there needs to be greater priority for the effective prevention and treatment of osteoporosis. There are evidence-based ways of achieving this. The present challenge is how to implement these strategies. The greatest barrier to effective prevention and treatment is lack of awareness, which leads to lack of priority and resources. There is still an attitude of inevitability about the development of osteoporosis with aging. In the European Commission 'Report on Osteoporosis in the European Community – Action for Prevention' in 1998 it was recommended that osteoporosis should be a governmental health-care target; that there should be routine collection of fragility fracture statistics; planning for appropriate resource allocation; advice on calcium and vitamin D nutrition; access to and reimbursement of bone densitometry; access to and reimbursement of proven therapies; governmental support to patients and scientific societies and priority for health-care and professional training; and, finally, greater support for research. For this to happen, all the key stakeholders need to become involved at the different levels – from the international political level down to members of the public. At the international level, the World Health Organization has produced two technical reports relevant to osteoporosis, one highlighting the burden[11], and the second making recommendations for the prevention and management of osteoporosis[12]. The European Community has supported several actions, including the European Bone & Joint Health Strategies Project, which has made recommendations for public policy for the prevention and treatment of osteoporosis, amongst other conditions[10]. The European Community has also supported the development of a set of indicators to monitor musculoskeletal health, including osteoporosis[13]. Action mainly happens at the local or national level, and several countries now have national policies and guidelines relevant to osteoporosis, such as the recently published Surgeon General's Report in the USA. Priority for osteoporosis has also been achieved in some countries. There is in general still a lack of routine data collection. Health-promotion campaigns are often focused on cardiovascular disease, but there are common messages with respect to the benefit of physical activity which are not voiced. The importance of adequate dietary calcium needs to be promoted. Bone densitometry is not widely available in all countries, either due to lack of provision of equipment or lack of reimbursement for measurement. The cost limits accessibility in many countries. Likewise, pharmacological therapies are limited by their cost, especially in developing and less developed countries where treatment costs can exceed average incomes. An important problem remains the lack of awareness and knowledge by health- and social-care professionals about osteoporosis and fracture, which leads to a negative attitude of many about what can be achieved, and therefore a lack of activity in case-finding and treatment. This is demonstrated by several studies which have shown the low percentage of those with osteoporosis being treated, even those who have sustained a low-trauma fracture[14–17]. This has been demonstrated in Denmark, Australia, Spain and China and many other countries. Specific high-risk groups are often ignored. Several studies have demonstrated the lack of identification and treatment of those at risk of steroid-induced osteoporosis. Those who have already sustained a fragility fracture are also frequently not recognized as at high risk, and consequently are not treated to prevent further fracture. This was clearly demonstrated by a recent survey of 3422 orthopedic surgeons from six countries treating 54 000 fragility fractures each month between them[18]. There are many medical educational programs to reverse this situation. There are also campaigns to raise awareness and knowledge of patients and carers as well as the general public about osteoporosis, and the need to identify one's own risk and then seek appropriate assessment and treatment if required. World Osteoporosis Day has been effective at raising awareness in many countries, as well as other high-profile media events organized by the International Osteoporosis Foundation and several national osteoporosis organizations. Such awareness is, however, readily counteracted by negative publicity, such as that received for hormone replacement therapy. In general, it has been found that public education needs to be targeted at the individual as much as possible for it to be effective, and for them to recognize their own risks and take responsibility for maintaining their bone health.

There has been significant advancement of knowledge and awareness of osteoporosis over the past few decades. There had been the concept that osteoporosis was just a natural part of aging, but now it is recognized that it is a preventable and treatable condition which has an enormous impact on the individual and society. The next step is moving from awareness and knowledge to action and better outcomes for those with or at risk of osteoporosis and fracture.

References

1. Rosen CJ. Issues facing bone densitometry in the new century: reflections from the National Institutes of Health Consensus Development Conference on Osteoporosis. *J Clin Densitometry* 2000; 3: 211–13

2. Cooper C, Atkinson EJ, O'Fallon WM, Melton LJ III. Incidence of clinically diagnosed vertebral fractures: a population-based study in Rochester, Minnesota, 1985–1989. *J Bone Miner Res* 1992; 7: 221–7

3. Cuddihy MT, Gabriel SE, Crowson CS, et al. Forearm fractures as predictors of subsequent osteoporotic fractures. *Osteoporos Int* 1999; 9: 469–75

4. Lindsay R, Silverman SL, Cooper C, et al. Risk of new vertebral fracture in the year following a fracture. *J Am Med Assoc* 2001; 285: 320–3

5. Salkeld G, Cameron ID, Cumming RG, et al. Quality of life related to fear of falling and hip fracture in older women: a time trade off study. *Br Med J* 2000; 320: 341–6

6. Cooper C, Campion G, Melton LJ III. Hip fractures in the elderly: a world-wide projection. *Osteoporos Int* 1992; 2: 285–9

7. Prevalence of physical activity, including lifestyle activities among adults – United States, 2000–2001. *Morbid Mortal Weekly Rep* 2003; 52: 764–9

8. The World Health Report 2002 – Reducing Risks, Promoting Healthy Life. Geneva: WHO, 2002

9. International Osteoporosis Foundation. *The One Minute Test*. http://www.osteofound.org/osteoporosis/risk_test.html (2005)

10. European Bone & Joint Health Strategies Project. Lund: *Bone and Joint Decade* 2004

11. World Health Organization. *The Burden of Musculoskeletal Diseases at the Start of the New Millenium*. Report of a WHO Scientific Group. WHO Technical Report Series, 919. Geneva: WHO, 2003

12. World Health Organization. *Osteoporosis: Prevention, Diagnosis and Treatment*. Geneva: WHO, 2003

13. Indicators for Monitoring Musculoskeletal Problems and Conditions. Musculoskeletal Problems and Functional Limitation. Oslo: University of Oslo, 2003

14. Eisman J, Clapham S, Kehoe L. Osteoporosis prevalence and levels of treatment in primary care: the Australian BoneCare Study. *J Bone Miner Res* 2004; 19: 1969–75

15. Ip TP, Lam CL, Kung AW. Awareness of osteoporosis among physicians in China. *Osteoporos Int* 2004; 15: 329–34

16. Perez-Edo L, Ciria RM, Castelo-Branco C, et al. Management of osteoporosis in general practice: a cross-sectional survey of primary care practitioners in Spain. *Osteoporos Int* 2004; 15: 252–7

17. Vestergaard P, Rejnmark L, Mosekilde L. Osteoporosis is markedly underdiagnosed: a nationwide study from Denmark. *Osteoporos Int* 2005; 16: 134–41

18. Dreinhofer KE, Feron JM, Herrera A, et al. Orthopaedic surgeons and fragility fractures. A survey by the Bone and Joint Decade and the International Osteoporosis Foundation. *J Bone Joint Surg Br* 2004; 86: 958–61

Intervention thresholds for osteoporosis 16

J. A. Kanis

INTRODUCTION

The internationally agreed description of osteoporosis is a progressive systemic skeletal disease characterized by low bone mass and microarchitectural deterioration of bone tissue, with a consequent increase in bone fragility and susceptibility to fracture[1]. The description captures the notion that low bone mineral density forms a central component, but that other skeletal factors and also non-skeletal factors such as liability to falls are also important in the pathogenesis of fracture. Notwithstanding, the operational definition of osteoporosis is on the basis of bone mineral density (BMD) values, since these can be measured with some accuracy and precision, whereas this is not the case for other determinants of osteoporotic fracture risk. In 1994, the World Health Organization[2] provided an operation definition in terms of bone mineral density. Osteoporosis was defined as a decrease in BMD in postmenopausal women that was equal to or greater than 2.5 standard deviations (SD) below the average value for young healthy women (a *T*-score of ″ −2.5 SD). With the development of more technologies and more epidemiological information in men, the reference standard has been set using dual-energy X-ray absorptiometry (DXA) at the proximal femur. The same criteria for osteoporosis are also applied to men[3].

The risk of fracture increases with decreasing BMD in a continuous manner. Because BMD decreases progressively with age, the incidence of osteoporosis increases in an exponential manner, and the risk of many fragility fractures increases in a similar fashion. Osteoporotic fracture is a major cause of morbidity and mortality in the aging population[4]. In the UK, approximately 270 000 fractures are attributable to osteoporosis every year, resulting in a total estimated cost of £1.5 billion[5]. The past 10 years have, however, witnessed a revolution in our ability to decrease fracture risk. A number of treatments have been developed which have been shown by double-blind randomized controlled studies to decrease the risk of vertebral fracture, and in some instances the risk of non-vertebral fracture in postmenopausal women[6]. Against this background, it has become necessary to devise strategies for the prevention and treatment of osteoporosis so that interventions can be directed to those most at need, and unnecessary interventions avoided. The most appropriate threshold of risk at which intervention should be considered, and how this is derived, has been the subject of some debate[7], and is briefly reviewed in this chapter.

SCREENING OF THE POPULATION WITH BONE MINERAL DENSITY

It seems intuitive that, because estrogen deficiency occurs at the time of the menopause and causes bone loss, the prevention of osteoporosis could be optimally achieved by screening women at this age to detect those women with the lowest bone mineral density, who might, therefore, be at highest risk for future fracture. This would provide an opportunity for hormone replacement therapy, the selective estrogen receptor modulators or indeed the many non-hormonal interventions that are available. Most authorities agree that this is not reasonable. One of the problems is that, at the age of 50 years, the short-term absolute fracture risk is very low, even though the lifetime risk may be high. Treatments, however, are not commonly given for a lifetime because of costs, unwanted effects and poor continuance. Another reason relates to the performance characteristics of the BMD test to predict fractures[2,8]. The ability of BMD tests to predict hip fracture is as good as the use of blood pressure to predict stroke[2]. For each standard deviation decrease in BMD, the risk of hip fracture is increased by approximately 2.6-fold[9]. Within the first few years of the menopause, hip fracture is rare, however, whereas other osteoporotic fractures are much more common. For the prediction of these fractures, the gradient of risk is a 1.5-fold increase in risk for each standard deviation decrease in BMD. Over most reasonable assumptions, the test has a detection rate that is too low to be of value for population screening[2,3]. For example, if a screening policy were devised in women at the age of 65 years, and if it was decided to select 10% of the population with the lowest BMD for treatment, the sensitivity of the test, i.e. the detection rate of individuals who will sustain a fracture in the next 10 years with a positive test, is approximately 18%. In other words, 82% of all osteoporotic fractures would occur within the next 10 years in those individuals who were characterized to be at low risk[8]. Because of the low absolute risk of those identified, the positive predictive value (the proportion of patients with a positive test who would sustain a fracture in a 10-year interval) is also low, at about 10%. If drugs were 50% effective, 1000 women would need to be screened to detect 100 individuals with low bone mineral density in whom 12 fractures would be prevented. Despite this, bone mineral testing is recommended in all women over the age of 65 years in the United States[10–12]. In most other countries, a case-finding strategy is adopted.

CASE-FINDING STRATEGIES

The general model for case-finding strategies is to identify in an opportunistic way individuals with strong clinical risk factors for fracture. Risk factors commonly used include long-term exposure to glucocorticoid treatment, a history of prior fragility fracture, a family history of fracture, particularly hip fracture, premature menopause or other causes of gonadal deficiency,

and, in some countries, weaker risk factors such as smoking or excess alcohol consumption[12–14].

Under European guidance[13], patients with strong risk factors are referred for densitometry, and treatment is offered to those in whom the World Health Organization criteria for the diagnosis of osteoporosis are satisfied. In the USA, a case-finding strategy is also utilized, but differs in several important respects. As mentioned, bone mineral density testing is recommended in all women over the age of 65 years. Second, in the absence of risk factors, a less stringent criterion is used as an intervention threshold (a T-score of -2.0 SD). A third important difference is that the intervention threshold differs for women with a strong risk factor. In women with risk factors, the intervention threshold recommended is a T-score of -1.5 SD. Thus, many more women would be offered treatment in the USA than in Europe.

The two positions are polarized. On the one hand, the justification for screening, particularly as a national policy, is not strong. At the other extreme, the European approach is ultraconservative, in the sense that patients need to have both the risk factor as well as a diagnosis of osteoporosis in order to be offered treatment.

FUTURE DEVELOPMENTS

At present, case-finding strategies are centered around the use of BMD. In recent years there has, however, been a growing appreciation that a number of risk factors contribute to fracture risk at least partially independently of BMD. Of these, the most important is age, and for any given T-score the fracture risk is higher in the elderly[7]. For example, with a T-score at the threshold of osteoporosis, the 10-year hip fracture probability for women in Sweden is approximately 2% at the age of 50 years, but exceeds 10% at the age of 80 years. This indicates that both BMD and age should be considered in determining intervention thresholds. A number of other important risk indicators have been identified that provide information on fracture risk independently of age and BMD. These include a prior fragility fracture, low body mass index, the long-term use of corticosteroids, parental history of fracture, cigarette smoking, excess alcohol use and some secondary causes of osteoporosis[7,12,15,16] (Table 1). Biochemical indices of bone turnover may also provide an independent risk indicator[17]. The impact of integrating these risks is shown in Table 2 for hip fracture and spine fracture risk[18]. For example, at the age of 50 years, the average 10-year probability of a spine fracture is 1.2%. With low BMD this might be further increased two-fold, giving a probability of 2.4%. With a family history, this might be increased to a relative risk of 3, and so on. Thus, it is clear that the integration of risk factors permits populations at high risk to be targeted more accurately.

The multiplicity of independent risk factors gives rise to the view that intervention thresholds for osteoporosis should be based on absolute risk (probability) of fracture, rather than solely on diagnostic thresholds provided by the T-score of bone mineral density[3,7]. A similar approach is used in cardiovascular disease, where absolute risk has been used to determine the intervention thresholds for primary prevention with lipid-lowering agents[19–23].

A consequence of this is that guidance needs to be given concerning the level of risk that is sufficiently high to merit an intervention. These issues are particularly important for health-care purchasers, who might wish to ensure an equitable distribution of resources across many disease categories. In this context, cost-utility analysis to evaluate treatment strategies takes account of not only fractures avoided, but also change in attendant morbidity and mortality. In addition, comparisons can be made between different diseases. The unit of measurement is the quality-adjusted life-year gained, where each year of life is valued according to its utility that ranges from 0, the least desirable health state, to 1, or perfect health. This is balanced against the cost of intervention and the cost of fractures avoided.

Cost-effectiveness analyses have determined intervention thresholds for Sweden and the UK[24,25]. The effects of treatment, based on a meta-analysis of bisphosphonate trials, assumed a relative risk reduction of 35%, treatment for 5 years and an offset of effect thereafter that dissipated over a further 5 years. The threshold at which treatment was considered to be cost-effective was £30 000 per quality of life-year gained as recommended by the National Institute of Clinical Excellence (NICE)[26]. The 10-year probability at which intervention became cost-effective is shown for women from the UK in Table 3. The thresholds are rather similar between Sweden and the UK, despite different costs and fracture risks. An important finding is that the threshold of hip fracture probability at which treatment becomes cost-effective is lower with decreasing age (see Table 3). For example, intervention at the age of 50 years is cost-effective

Table 1 Risk ratios (RR) for hip fracture associated with the clinical risk factors shown. Risk ratios are age-adjusted and additionally adjusted for bone mineral density (BMD)[15]

	Without BMD		With BMD	
Risk indicator	RR	95% CI	RR	95% CI
Body mass index (20 vs. 25 kg/m²)	1.95	1.71–2.22	1.42	1.23–1.65
(30 vs. 25 kg/m²)	0.83	0.69–0.99	1.00	0.82–1.21
Prior fracture after 50 years	1.85	1.58–2.17	1.62	1.30–2.01
Parental history of hip fracture	2.27	1.47–3.49	2.28	1.48–3.51
Current smoking	1.84	1.52–2.22	1.60	1.27–2.02
Ever-use of systemic corticosteroids	2.31	1.67–3.20	2.25	1.60–3.15
Alcohol intake > 2 units daily	1.68	1.19–2.36	1.70	1.20–2.42
Rheumatoid arthritis	1.95	1.11–3.42	1.73	0.94–3.20

CI, confidence interval

Table 2 10-year probability of hip fracture and clinical spine fracture (%) according to age-specific relative risk. Adapted from reference 18

Age (years)	Relative risk							
	1.0	1.25	1.50	2.0	2.5	3.0	4.0	5.0
Hip								
50	0.5	0.6	0.7	0.9	1.1	1.4	1.8	2.2
55	0.7	0.9	1.0	1.4	1.7	2.0	2.7	3.3
60	1.3	1.6	1.9	2.6	3.2	3.8	5.0	6.1
65	2.9	3.7	4.4	3.7	7.1	3.9	10.9	13.4
70	5.2	6.4	7.6	10.0	12.2	14.4	18.5	22.4
75	8.3	10.2	12.1	15.7	19.0	22.2	28.0	33.2
80	12.6	15.4	20.0	22.8	27.2	31.2	38.2	44.0
85	15.3	18.5	21.4	26.8	31.4	35.5	42.4	47.8
90	16.0	19.1	21.9	26.9	31.1	34.8	40.8	45.5
Spine								
50	1.2	1.5	1.8	2.4	3.0	3.5	4.6	5.7
55	1.4	1.7	2.0	2.7	3.3	4.0	5.2	6.4
60	1.9	2.4	2.8	3.8	4.6	5.5	7.2	8.8
65	3.9	4.8	5.7	7.5	9.2	10.8	13.9	16.8
70	5.3	6.5	7.7	10.0	12.1	14.2	17.9	21.3
75	5.4	6.6	7.8	10.0	12.0	13.9	17.3	20.3
80	6.1	7.3	8.6	10.8	12.7	14.4	17.3	19.6
85	6.5	7.8	9.0	11.1	12.9	14.4	16.7	18.6
90	6.2	7.4	8.5	10.4	11.9	13.3	15.4	17.1

Table 3 Relative risk (RR) and 10-year hip fracture probability (%) at which treatment becomes cost-effective[24]

Age (years)	10-year hip fracture probability (%)		
	RR	Threshold	General population*
50	3.77	1.10	0.30
55	2.627	1.81	0.70
60	1.887	2.64	1.42
65	1.419	3.70	2.64
70	1.114	5.24	4.73
75	0.905	6.87	7.59
80	0.767	8.52	10.83
85	0.646	8.99	13.0
90	0.533	7.12	12.25

*General population (RR = 1.0)

with a 10-year probability of hip fractures that exceeds 1.1% in women from the UK. By contrast, treatment becomes cost-effective at the age of 80 years with a 10-year hip fracture probability of 8.5%. This appears to be paradoxical, but arises because intervention decreases the risk of all osteoporotic fractures. In younger women, proportionately more fractures occur at sites other than the hip.

An important question is: what are the clinical scenarios for which treatment can be judged to be competitive with other chronic diseases? Several clinical scenarios have been considered in the analysis undertaken in the setting of the UK[24]. For postmenopausal women with established osteoporosis (a prior fragility fracture and a BMD of −2.5 SD), treatment is always cost-effective, irrespective of age. Indeed, cost-effective scenarios are found for women with a history of prior fracture, even without measurement of BMD. In such patients it is cost-effective to intervene from the age of 65 years. There are also cost-effective scenarios for the prevention of first fracture. It is cost-effective to intervene in women from the UK at the threshold of osteoporosis from the age of 60 years. From a population perspective, women rarely have a *T*-score of exactly -2.5 SD at the hip, and, in populations of women with osteoporosis, it is cost-effective to intervene irrespective of age.

Some caution must be exercised in applying these recommendations widely. First, the setting of intervention thresholds will depend critically upon fracture costs and willingness of different countries to pay for treatment. In addition, the estimate of efficacy and the cost of intervention are based on the bisphosphonates, and the costs of other interventions will vary. In addition, hormone replacement treatment and the selective estrogen receptor modulators have extraskeletal benefits and risks, which will affect intervention thresholds for these particular agents. The model used is, however, conservative in its assumption about the offset time, the length of treatment and the exclusion of morphometric fractures. In addition, the increase in risk of fracture associated with a prior fracture may be underestimated for patients with a prior vertebral fracture, where the risk of a subsequent vertebral fracture is particularly high[16]. Within these limitations, the treatment of established osteoporosis can now be justified from a health-economic perspective. There is also good news for the prevention of first fracture, and favorable health-economic scenarios can be devised once the inter-relationships of clinical risk factors and BMD are established.

References

1. Consensus Development Conference. Diagnosis, prophylaxis and treatment of osteoporosis. *Am J Med* 1993; 94: 646–50

2. World Health Organization. Assessment of fracture risk and its application to screening for postmenopausal osteoporosis. WHO Technical Report Series, 843. Geneva: WHO, 1994

3. Kanis JA, Gluer C-C, for the Committee of Scientific Advisors, International Osteoporosis Foundation. An update on the diagnosis and assessment of osteoporosis with densitometry. *Osteoporos Int* 2000; 11: 192–202

4. Cummings SR, Melton LJ. Epidemiology and outcomes of osteoporotic fractures. *Lancet* 2002; 359: 1761–7

5. Johansen A, Stone M. The cost of treating osteoporotic fractures in the United Kingdom female population. *Osteoporos Int* 2000; 11: 551–2

6. Delmas PD. Treatment of postmenopausal osteoporosis. *Lancet* 2002; 359: 2018–26

7. Kanis JA. Diagnosis of osteoporosis and assessment of fracture risk. *Lancet* 2002; 359: 1929–36

8. Kanis JA, Johnell O, Oden A, et al. Ten year risk of osteoporotic fracture and the effect of risk factors on screening strategies. *Bone* 2002; 30: 251–8

9. Marshall D, Johnell O, Wedel H. Meta-analysis of how well measures of bone mineral density predict occurrence of osteoporotic fractures. *Br Med J* 1996; 312: 1254–9

10. Lewiecki EM, Watts NB, McClung MR, et al. for the International Society for Clinical Densitometry. Physician statement: official positions of the International Society for Clinical Densitometry. *J Clin Endocrinol Metab* 2004; 89: 3651–5

11. US Preventive Services Task Force. Screening for osteoporosis in postmenopausal women; recommendations and rationale. *Ann Intern Med* 2002; 137: 526–8

12. National Osteoporosis Foundation. *Physicians guide to prevention and treatment of osteopororosis*. Washington, DC: National Osteoporosis Foundation, 1998

13. Kanis JA, Delmas P, Burckhardt P, et al. Guidelines for diagnosis and management of osteoporosis. *Osteoporos Int* 1997; 7: 390–406

14. European Commission. Report on osteoporosis in the European Community. Luxembourg: Office

for Official Publications of the European Community, 1998

15. Kanis JA, Borgstrom F, De Laet C, et al. Assessment of fracture risk. *Osteoporos Int* 2005; 16: 581–9

16. Klotzbuecher CM, Ross PD, Landsman PB, et al. Patients with prior fractures have an increased risk of future fractures: a summary of the literature and statistical synthesis. *J Bone Miner Res* 2000; 15: 721–39

17. Delmas PD, Eastell R, Garnero P, et al. for the Committee of Scientific Advisors of the International Osteoporosis Foundation. The use of biochemical markers of bone turnover in osteoporosis. *Osteoporos Int* 2000; 11 (Suppl 6); S2-17

18. Kanis JA, Johnell O, Oden A, et al. Risk of hip fracture derived from relative risks: an analysis applied to the population of Sweden. *Osteoporos Int* 2000; 11: 120–7

19. Anonymous. Statin therapy – what now? *Drugs Ther Bull* 2001; 39: 17–21

20. Ramsay LE, Haq IU, Jackson PR, Yeo WW. The Sheffield table for primary prevention of coronary heart disease. Corrected. *Lancet* 1996; 348: 1251–2

21. Ramsay LE, Haq IU, Jackson PR, et al. Targeting lipid-lowering drug therapy for primary prevention of coronary artery disease: an updated Sheffield table. *Lancet* 1996; 348: 387–8

22. Wood D, DeBacker G, Faergemon O, et al. Prevention of coronary heart disease in clinical practice: recommendations of the second joint task force of European and other societies on coronary prevention. *Atherosclerosis* 1998; 140: 199–270

23. Johannesson M. At what coronary risk level is it cost-effective to initiate cholesterol lowering drug treatment in primary prevention. *Eur Heart J* 2001; 22: 919–25

24. Kanis JA, Borgstrom F, Zethraeus N, et al. Intervention thresholds for osteoporosis in the UK. *Bone* 2005; 36: 22–32

25. Kanis JA, Johnell O, Oden A, et al. Intervention thresholds for osteoporosis in men and women. A study based on data from Sweden. *Osteoporos Int* 2005; 16: 6–14

26. Raftery J. NICE: faster access to modern treatments? Analysis of guidance on health technologies. *Br Med J* 2001; 323: 1300–3

Vitamin D and calcium supplements $\qquad$ 17

R. Nuti, L. Gennari, D. Merlotti and G. Martini

INTRODUCTION

Osteoporosis is one of the most prevalent diseases of aging. For Caucasians, the lifetime risk of an osteoporotic fracture at 50 years of age has been estimated to be approximately 40% for women and 13% for men[1]. Each year more than 1.5 million people suffer hip, vertebral and wrist fractures due to osteoporosis, a disease that can be prevented and treated. In European Community (EC) member states, the high incidence of osteoporotic fractures leads to considerable mortality, morbidity, reduced mobility and decreased quality of life. Actually, the annual number of hip fractures in 15 countries of the EC has been estimated to be 500 000, with a total care cost of about €4.8 billion per year[2]. Given the magnitude of the problem, public-health measures are important for preventive intervention. This burden will increase in absolute terms because of the aging of the population.

Skeletal bone mass is determined by a combination of endogenous (genetic, hormonal) and exogenous (nutritional, physical activity) factors. In adolescence, to attain the optimal peak bone mass, the main determinants are genetic, nutritional and behavioral (exercise). In adult and elderly populations, the main determinants of age-related bone loss are represented by gonadal status, by the influence of some nutrients and by physical activity. Both a low peak bone mass and a high rate of bone loss represent risk factors for osteoporosis and osteoporotic fractures. In adults, a low bone mass increases the risk of fragility fracture. It has been estimated that a 1 standard deviation (SD) decrease in hip bone mineral density (BMD) is associated with a 2.5-fold increased risk of hip fracture[3]. Nutrition plays an important role in bone health. The two nutrients essential for bone health are calcium and vitamin D. Reduced supplies of calcium may be associated with reduced bone mass and osteoporosis, whereas chronic and severe vitamin D deficiency leads to osteomalacia, a metabolic bone disease characterized by decreased mineralization of the bone matrix and increased osteoid volume. Vitamin D deficiency can be confirmed by measuring the serum concentration of 25-hydroxyvitamin D (25(OH)D), which is the major circulating metabolite and represents the storage form of vitamin D. In patients with osteomalacia, serum 25(OH)D levels are usually below 5–6 ng/ml and often undetectable[4,5]. Biochemically, osteomalacia is characterized by normal or low serum concentrations of calcium and phosphate, and increased activity of alkaline phosphatase. Vitamin D deficiency is common in the elderly, particularly in institutionalized subjects. The major causes of vitamin D deficiency are infrequent exposure to sunlight, a decline in the synthesis of vitamin D in the skin, poor nutrition and decreased renal hydroxylation of vitamin D[5]. Subclinical vitamin D deficiency, characterized by a circulating level of 25(OH)D comprising between 6 and 30 ng/ml, is also common with aging. This condition, which has been defined as vitamin D insufficiency[4,5], is increasingly being recognized as a distinct pathological skeletal entity, characterized by normocalcemia and normal bone mineralization and by an increase in circulating levels of parathyroid hormone (PTH). In the presence of osteoporosis, vitamin D insufficiency may amplify bone loss and thus enhance fracture risk. It follows that at any age, but particularly in postmenopause and in the elderly, an adequate intake of both calcium and vitamin D is important for the preservation of bone mass and prevention of osteoporosis[6].

CALCIUM

Calcium plays many important roles in the organism, but the most crucial is in creating and maintaining bone mass. In bone, calcium salts provide the structural integrity of the skeleton, while, in intracellular fluids and in the cytosol, calcium concentration is critically important in the maintenance and control of different biochemical processes. The calcium in the skeleton has the additional role of acting as a reserve supply of calcium to meet the body's metabolic needs in states of calcium deficiency. Several studies have shown that low calcium intake is associated with low bone mass, rapid bone loss and high fracture rates[6]. Importantly, different national surveys have recently indicated that many people, especially those over the age of 50, are not consuming enough calcium. The daily average calcium intake in Europe has been evaluated in the SENECA study (Survey in Europe on Nutrition and the Elderly; a Concentrated Action), concerning the diet of elderly people from 19 towns of ten European countries[7]. The study was performed in random samples of residents stratified for age and sex, age range 71–76 years. Dietary-intake data were collected by a validated dietary-history method. In about one-third of subjects, the dietary calcium intake results were very low, between 300 and 600 mg/day in women, and 350 and 700 mg/day in men. Adequate calcium intake is important because our body loses calcium every day, mainly via the bowel, kidneys and skin (Figure 1). This lost calcium must be replaced daily through the diet. When the diet does not contain enough calcium to support these functions, calcium is taken from bone. Dairy foods, particularly milk, cheese and yoghurt, are the best and most economical sources of calcium. In general, intestinal calcium absorption as well as absorption of other minerals (such as magnesium and phosphate) represents the sum of two transport processes, a saturable transcellular absorption, which is physiologically regulated, and a non-saturable paracellular absorption, which is dependent on mineral concentration within the lumen of the gut (Figure 2). On average, healthy adults require calcium intakes higher than 400 mg/day to maintain calcium balance. Vitamin D, and in particular its active metabolite 1,25-dihydroxyvitamin D (1,25(OH)$_2$D or calcitriol), represents the major recognized hormonal stimulus of active intestinal calcium absorption that occurs principally in the duodenum and jejunum. Importantly, calcium absorption from the gut becomes less efficient with aging (Figure 3). Calcium is more easily absorbed from foods during childhood, whereas an adult assimilates only about one-third of the dietary calcium taken in. Moreover, calcium conservation is at least in part dependent upon estrogen status. In fact, intestinal absorption and renal tubular reabsorption of calcium decline after the menopause and can be returned to premenopausal levels by estrogen replacement therapy[8–10]. It also seems that the more gradual impairment of calcium conservation in aging men is due to a decline in estrogen levels[10].

VITAMIN D

Vitamin D is important for bone, for its essential role in promoting intestinal calcium absorption and mineralization of bone matrix. The major source of vitamin D is the skin, where it is produced by the action of ultraviolet light on steroid precursors. Vitamin D is also present in a limited number of foods, and dietary sources of the vitamin can be important under circumstances of decreased sunlight exposure. Vitamin D is derived from plant (vitamin D$_2$ or ergocalciferol) and animal (vitamin D$_3$ or cholecalciferol) sources. The main dietary sources of vitamin D are fatty fish (salmon, sardines, tuna) and oils derived from them, some meat products (liver), eggs and wild mushrooms. Vitamin D (D$_3$ and D$_2$ collectively) is not a true vitamin, but a prosteroid hormone that is biologically inert until metabolized (Figure 4). It is transported to the liver bound to a specific α-globulin (vitamin D-binding protein), and to a small extent albumin and lipoproteins. In the liver, vitamin D is metabolized to 25(OH)D, which functions as the major storage form by virtue of its long half-life. In the kidney, 25(OH)D is further metabolized by a 1α-hydroxylase enzyme to 1,25(OH)$_2$D, the hormone responsible for the biological effects of

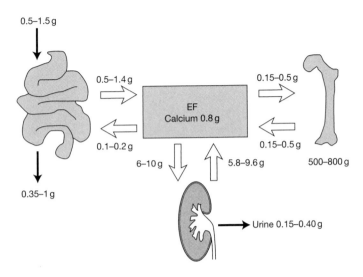

Figure 1 Schematic representation of calcium homeostasis. EF, extracellular fluid

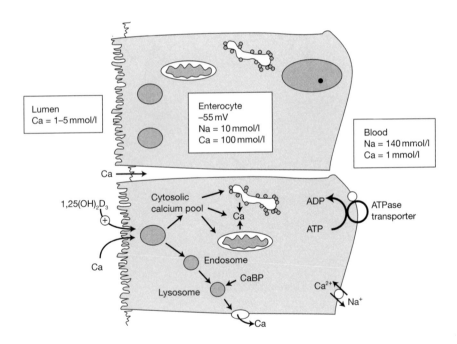

Figure 2 Schematic representation of intestinal calcium absorption. The two transport processes, a saturable transcellular absorption, which is mainly regulated by $1,25(OH)_2$ vitamin D, and a non-saturable paracellular absorption, which is dependent on mineral concentration within the lumen of the gut, are indicated. ADP, adenosine diphosphate; ATP, adenosine triphosphate; CABP, calcium binding protein

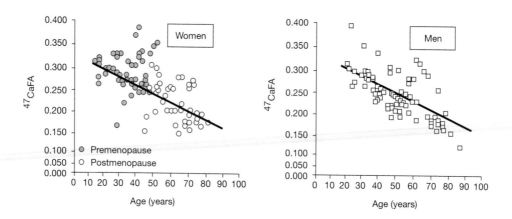

Figure 3 Intestinal calcium (^{47}CaFA) absorption according to age in 70 males and 97 females living in Siena District

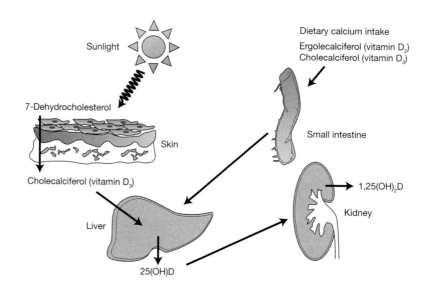

Figure 4 Schematic representation of vitamin D metabolism

vitamin D. The binding of calcitriol to the vitamin D receptor (VDR), a nuclear steroid hormone receptor, activates VDR to interact with retinoid X receptor (RXR) and form the VDR–RXR–cofactor complex, which binds to vitamin D response elements in the promoter region of target genes to regulate gene transcription.

As we age, the absorption of calcium and vitamin D declines, as does production of vitamin D by the skin from exposure to sunlight. This reduced ability to absorb calcium contributes to age-related and postmenopausal bone loss. Calcitriol is the major biologically active metabolite of vitamin D. The principal regulators of 1,25(OH)$_2$D production are PTH,

$1,25(OH)_2D$ itself, and dietary intake of calcium and phosphate. There are three primary target organs for circulating $1,25(OH)_2D$: intestine, parathyroid gland and bone. The overall effects of $1,25(OH)_2D$ on mineral metabolism may be summarized as:

(1) Increased intestinal calcium absorption, leading to an increase in serum calcium;

(2) Decreased serum PTH level (through both direct inhibition of PTH secretion from the parathyroid gland and indirect inhibition of PTH secretion by the raised serum calcium levels);

(3) Decreased bone resorption (mainly due to a reduction in PTH-mediated bone resorption);

(4) Under certain conditions, increased bone formation[11].

Usually, under normal vitamin D status, the small intestine absorbs about 30% of dietary calcium. In the absence of calcitriol, intestinal calcium absorption is solely by the passive, extracellular route, which limits gross calcium absorption to about 10–15% of intake.

The vitamin D status may be evaluated by measuring the serum concentration of 25(OH)D. Since 25(OH)D concentrations are mainly affected by sunlight exposure and intensity[12], the two major determinants of serum 25(OH)D levels are the season and the geographical location. In fact, the cutaneous synthesis of previtamin D is maximal in summer and minimal in winter (Figure 5), and an inverse association exists between mean 25(OH)D concentration and latitude. There is no general consensus on normal serum 25(OH)D values. In healthy adult subjects, the lower limit of the normal range for serum 25(OH)D is approximately 30 ng/ml[4]. When serum 25(OH)D values fall below this threshold, there is an increase in PTH secretion[4] that may increase bone resorption. A long-lasting and severe deficiency of vitamin D, as defined by a serum level of 25(OH)D lower than 6 ng/ml, is associated with defective mineralization resulting in rickets in children and osteomalacia in adults. Vitamin D insufficiency, the preclinical phase of vitamin D deficiency, as defined by a serum level of 25(OH)D comprising between 6 and 30 ng/ml, causes a reduced calcium supply and secondary hyperparathyroidism. If this state remains chronic, osteopenia results.

CALCIUM INTAKE, VITAMIN D AND OSTEOPOROSIS

In recent years, convincing evidence has been given that dietary calcium intake is positively related to bone mineral density in children and adolescents[14]. In adolescents, the higher is the calcium intake, the greater is the peak bone mass[15]. A positive correlation between bone mass and calcium intake has been demonstrated also in adults, particularly in premenopausal women[16,17]. The relationship between calcium intake and fracture rate is less certain. Some studies have reported an inverse correlation between dietary calcium intake and fracture (mainly of the hip), others have not demonstrated any significant correlation and some have even shown a positive correlation between calcium intake and hip fracture[18].

Although there are many factors that modulate the progression of age-related bone loss syndromes, the pathogenesis of this process has been attributed, at least in part, to decreased calcium absorption by an 'aging intestine', to an associated elevation in circulating PTH and to decreased synthesis of $1,25(OH)_2D$ (Figure 6). Decreased $1,25(OH)_2D$ synthesis by the aging kidney results from both age-related progressive loss in the capacity of the renal 1α-hydroxylase to respond to progressive elevation in PTH and an age-related decrease in the circulating 25(OH)D precursor[19]. Women with osteoporosis have often been demonstrated to be characterized by reduced intestinal calcium absorption when compared with age-matched control subjects[17,20]. This abnormality is particularly relevant in those women who have a low-calcium diet. Moreover, increments in serum osteocalcin levels observed in humans treated with $1,25(OH)_2D$, and animal studies demonstrating an increased number of bone marrow osteoblast

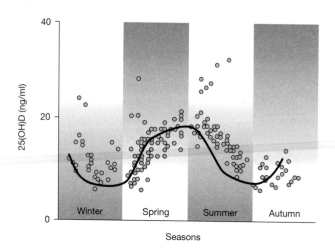

Figure 5 Annual variations of 25(OH)D serum levels in healthy subjects with age range between 66 and 95 years. Adapted from reference 13

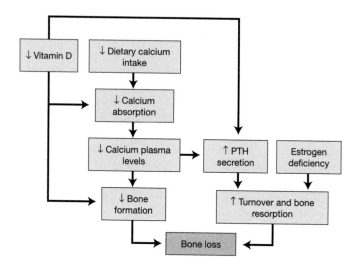

Figure 6 Schematic representation of the relationships between calcium, vitamin D endocrine system and bone loss. PTH, parathyroid hormone

precursors during 1,25(OH)$_2$D administration, are consistent with the hypothesis that abnormalities in the production and skeletal distribution of 1,25(OH)$_2$D may also contribute to the defects in osteoblast function and bone formation[21,22]. Both calcium and vitamin D deficiency and insufficiency are therefore important risk factors for osteoporosis and osteoporotic fractures. Importantly, both type I (postmenopausal) and type II (senile) osteoporosis appear to be, at least in part, related to primary and secondary abnormalities of the vitamin D endocrine system[23]. Recently, the observation that VDR genotypes are predictive of differences in bone mass and intestinal calcium absorption in postmenopausal women adds further complexity to this issue[24].

In the past decade, a positive association between serum 25(OH)D concentrations and bone mass has been reported in adult and elderly populations from North America and Europe. Several studies have shown a relationship between bone mineral density, vitamin D insufficiency and secondary hyperparathyroidism in the elderly[25,26], but also in postmenopausal and middle-aged women[27,28]. In a cross-sectional study conducted in the UK, a positive relationship between serum 25(OH)D values and BMD was observed in a group of middle-aged women[28]. In an American study performed in postmenopausal women with low vertebral bone mass, a relationship between vertebral BMD and PTH values was found only in subjects with low 25(OH)-vitamin D values[27]. In another study, a significant association between low femoral BMD and low 25(OH)D levels was described in normal women older than 60 years[25]. Finally, women with acute hip fracture showed markedly reduced bone levels of 1,25(OH)$_2$D as well as reduced circulating 25(OH)D levels (Figure 7) with respect to controls in different studies[29,30].

CALCIUM SUPPLEMENTATION

Of all the available preventive strategies for osteoporosis, calcium is the simplest and least expensive. Calcium is generally well tolerated and reports of significant side-effects are rare. The Food and Drug Administration in the United States has permitted a bone-health claim for calcium-rich foods, and the National Institutes of Health (NIH) in their Consensus Development Process approved a statement that high calcium intake reduces the risk of osteoporosis[31]. The best source of calcium is food; however, some dependence upon calcium supplements is usually necessary. Actually, there is no universal consensus on optimal calcium intake. In the USA, the National Academy of Sciences and the National Osteoporosis Foundation recommend a calcium intake of 1200 mg/day for men and women aged over 50 years, while for younger

adults 1000 mg/day is considered an adequate intake[32]. Recommendations within the EC are lower, at 700–800 mg/day for all ages and 800 mg for women aged 50–65 years[33]. In addition, the European Commission has set the tolerable upper-intake level for calcium in adults at 2500 mg/day[34]. Generally, all the chemical salts of calcium are about equivalently absorbed, even though differences have been reported in some studies (Figure 8). Choice among the various formulations should be based on convenience, cost and tolerability.

Effects of calcium supplementation on bone mass

There is good evidence that calcium intake influences bone mass in all age groups. In children and adolescents, a positive effect of calcium on bone mass has been reported in cross-sectional and intervention studies[35,36]. In a prospective study, the dietary calcium intake in childhood and adolescence was found to be positively related to bone mass in young women[14]. A recent meta-analysis of 33 studies showed that there was a significant association between calcium intake and bone mass in premenopausal women, while this relationship was not significant in young men[16]. Results from the four intervention studies included in the meta-analysis demonstrated that calcium supplementation of approximately 1000 mg/day in premenopausal women could prevent the annual loss of 1% of bone at all bone sites except the ulna[16].

In adults, calcium supplementation reduces the rate of age-related bone loss[37]. In elderly men and women, calcium supplementation also reduces bone loss, and the lower is the dietary calcium intake the better is the response in bone[38]. The majority of randomized controlled calcium-intervention trials examining change in bone mineral density have been performed in postmenopausal women[6,37]. Women with low to moderate calcium intakes benefit significantly from calcium supplementation[39]. Some studies suggest that recently estrogen-deficient women (within the first 5 years of the menopause) are generally less responsive to calcium than women who are 6 or more years past the menopause[39,40].

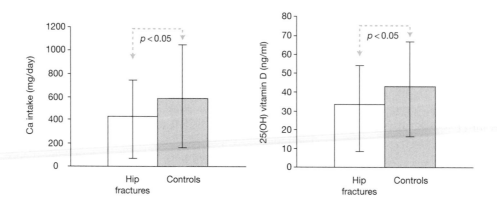

Figure 7 Calcium intake and 25(OH)D levels in women with and without acute hip fractures. Adapted from reference 30

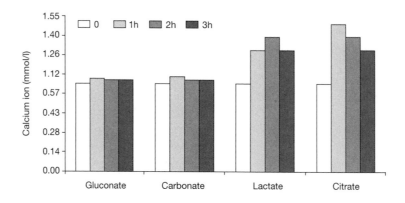

Figure 8 Calcium ion plasma levels in postmenopausal osteoporosis subjects after administration of different calcium salts

A review of 20 prospective calcium trials in postmenopausal women concluded that calcium supplementation reduced bone loss on average by about 1% per year[41]. Similar results have come from two recent meta-analyses of controlled trials in postmenopausal women that demonstrated calcium to be more effective than placebo in reducing rates of bone loss after 2 or more years of treatment[42,43]. The pooled difference in percentage change from baseline between calcium-treated and placebo groups was about 2% for total body BMD, 1.7% for the lumbar spine, 1.6% for the hip and 1.9% for the distal radius[42]. Moreover, a meta-analysis of studies concerning BMD responses to hormone replacement therapy in relation to calcium intake showed that the BMD gain at each skeletal site (spine, hip and forearm) was significantly greater in women who increased their calcium intake than in women who took hormonal replacement therapy alone[44].

The mechanism by which calcium supplementation slows bone loss is probably through a reduction in serum PTH. With age there is an increase in serum PTH and bone turnover[45] due to the combined effects of reduced calcium intake and absorption and to vitamin D insufficiency. Low calcium intakes rather than higher calcium intakes are associated with higher serum PTH levels[46]. The beneficial effects on bone of calcium supplements may therefore be mediated via an antiresorptive effect. In general, the most consistent effects of calcium are observed in the appendicular skeleton, while the positive effects on trabecular bone appear to be transient[47]. In a recent study, where citrate and calcium infusions were used to characterize the impact of age and gender on PTH secretion in normal subjects, aging was associated with an increase in PTH-secretory response to changes in serum calcium, in both women and men[48].

Although calcium alone is considered not sufficient to treat established osteoporosis, treatment with any of the bone-active hormonal or pharmacological agents will be less effective if attention is not given to ensuring an adequate intake of calcium[34]. Published clinical trials investigating the efficacy of antiresorptive agents, including estrogens, calcitonin and bisphosphonates, on bone mass have involved calcium supplementation in both the treatment and control groups. Therefore, the additional benefit, if any, of a calcium supplement with antiresorptive treatment for bone mass is not known. There is some evidence that a calcium supplementation may have a synergistic effect with antiresorptive agents. In a recent meta-analysis of patients treated with either estrogens or calcitonin, it was found that the treatment-induced improvement in bone density was two- to four-fold greater if calcium was combined with the active agent[44]. However, no studies have addressed the question of how much calcium may be required during treatment with bone-active agents. The optimal calcium intake in conjunction with antiresorptive therapy is unknown, although there is a general agreement to provide at least 1200 mg/day of calcium in patients receiving antiresorptive agents.

Both mechanical loading on the skeleton and adequate nutrition are essential for the maintenance of bone mass. Exercise and calcium intake are important determinants of peak bone mass during childhood and adolescence[6,14]. Later in life, some of the age-related bone loss results from a decline in physical activity. Studies evaluating the combined effect of increased calcium intake and increased exercise in young and postmenopausal women have shown more striking benefits than those produced by either modality alone[49].

Effects of calcium supplementation on osteoporotic fractures

Calcium supplements decrease bone turnover by suppressing PTH secretion and reducing the rate of bone loss in osteoporotic patients. Recently, some studies have reported a significant positive effect of calcium treatment not only on bone mass but also on fracture incidence. In the epidemiological case–control study performed in six European countries (Mediterranean Osteoporosis Study, MEDOS), calcium treatment has been reported to reduce the risk of hip fractures[50]. A few controlled trials have suggested that calcium supplementation may reduce fracture incidence in postmenopausal women (Figure 9). In one study, women with a mean age of 73.6 years and a low dietary calcium intake (mean 430 mg/day) were randomly treated with calcium (600 mg twice daily) or placebo[51]. After 4 years, women with prevalent fractures at the beginning of the study developed fewer fractures in the calcium group than in the placebo group. This study indicates that relatively high doses of calcium supplements given to calcium-deficient elderly women with vertebral fractures may reduce the incidence of new fractures. In another study, performed in osteoporotic women with low bone mass but without vertebral fractures, a significant reduction in first vertebral fracture was observed as a result of calcium supplementation[52]. In a smaller trial, women taking 1000 mg of supplemental calcium per day presented fewer vertebral fractures than women taking placebo[53]. In a more recent 4-year study of postmenopausal women, Riggs and colleagues did not demonstrate significant differences between the calcium-treated group (1600 mg/day as the citrate) and the placebo-treated group in the numbers of new vertebral and non-vertebral

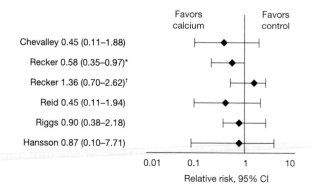

Figure 9 Relative risk (with 95% confidence interval (CI)) of vertebral fractures after treatment with calcium. Major randomized, double-blind, controlled studies have been considered[51–55]. *, Fracture group; †, non-fracture group

fractures[54]. Overall, these trials with fracture data, although performed in a limited number of patients, found reductions in fracture incidence ranging from 10 to 50% in patients with an initial low calcium intake (ranging from 400–700 mg/day). It remains to be determined whether calcium supplementation is able to reduce fractures in subjects with normal starting intakes of calcium (above 1000 mg/day). In a recent meta-analysis of all the published controlled trials[42], a non-significant trend of calcium supplementation alone toward a reduction in vertebral fractures was observed with a relative risk of 0.77 (95% confidence interval (CI) 0.54–1.09). However, all these studies should be interpreted with caution because they were not powered to assess the effects of calcium supplementation on fractures.

VITAMIN D AND ITS METABOLITES IN THE TREATMENT OF OSTEOPOROSIS

The observation in several studies of a seasonal variation in BMD may provide indirect evidence that relatively small changes in vitamin D status may have significant effects on bone mass. This justifies the use of vitamin D and its active metabolites in the treatment of osteoporosis, since vitamin D deficiency or insufficiency has been found to be frequent in the elderly as well as in postmenopausal women, particularly during low sun exposure.

Treatment with vitamin D

The most rational approach to reducing vitamin D insufficiency is supplementation. In the USA it has been shown that an intake of about 600 IU/day (15 mg/day) is needed, from all sources, to sustain serum 25(OH)D levels and avoid a condition of vitamin D insufficiency in adults[56]. This is substantially above the current recommended daily allowance in the USA of only 200 IU for adults[57]. In Europe, recommended dietary allowances (RDAs) for vitamin D were proposed in 1998 by a report on 'osteoporosis – action on prevention'[33]. The requirement for dietary vitamin D, based on European and Nordic recommendations, depends on the amount of sunshine exposure, according to a range where the higher limit is the estimated dietary requirement of an individual with minimal endogenous synthesis, whereas the lower limit indicates the intake of an individual able to produce adequate vitamin D. The RDA is 400 IU (10 μg) daily for people aged 65 years or over. However, the available evidence suggests that, in elderly and other high-risk populations, 800 IU (20 mg) daily should be advised[58]. This dose is safe and free of side-effects. Nevertheless, excess vitamin D intake should be avoided. Although the maximum safe dose is still unknown, intakes of 50 μg (2000 IU) daily should not be exceeded to avoid some harmful effects such as hypercalcemia and hypercalciuria[34,59]. Fortification of foods with vitamin D provides an alternative approach. Supplementation of food with vitamin D is common in the USA, where milk is fortified with vitamin D, but is not common in Europe with the exception of some Northern European countries (Belgium, The Netherlands and The United Kingdom), where fortification is compulsory only in margarines[33].

Although longitudinal data have suggested a role of vitamin D intake in modulating bone loss in peri- and postmenopausal women, most studies of vitamin D and calcium supplementation have failed to support a significant effect of vitamin D and calcium during the early menopause. In a 2-year double-blind study in early postmenopausal women (mean age 57 years) whose average baseline serum 25(OH)D concentration was well within the normal range, the addition of 10 000 U vitamin D weekly to calcium supplementation at 1000 mg/day did not confer benefits on BMD beyond those achieved with calcium supplementation alone[60]. In contrast, a more recent double-blind, randomized, 30-month controlled trial in 120 peri- (age range 45–50 years) and early postmenopausal women (age range 50–55 years) showed a positive effect of calcium and vitamin D supplementation (calcium 500 mg and vitamin D 200 IU, daily) on BMD change with respect to placebo[61]. There is a clearer benefit of vitamin D and calcium supplementation in older postmenopausal women. Vitamin D intake between 500 and 800 IU daily, with or without calcium supplementation, has been shown to increase BMD in women with a mean age of approximately 60–65 years. A prospective study showed that supplementation with small doses of vitamin D is able to prevent the fall in BMD that occurs during the winter in postmenopausal women[62]. In women older than 65 as well as in elderly men, there is even more benefit. This latter point has been clearly addressed by a number of studies of the effects of vitamin D supplementation on bone loss in the elderly. Some studies have been performed with vitamin D alone, some others with vitamin D and calcium supplementation[6,34,38]. It appears from these studies that supplementations with daily doses of 400–800 IU of vitamin D, given alone or in combination with calcium (1200–1500 mg daily), are able to reverse vitamin D insufficiency, reduce secondary hyperparathyroidism, prevent bone loss and improve bone density in the elderly.

Some randomized controlled prospective studies[38,63] and a retrospective study[50] have examined the effects of calcium and vitamin D supplementation on osteoporotic fracture incidence (Figure 10). In the epidemiological case–control study conducted in six European Mediterranean countries (MEDOS), treatment with vitamin D has been reported to be associated with a reduced incidence of hip fracture[50]. The first prospective, large, multicenter, randomized, double-blind, placebo-controlled study was performed in a French cohort of over 3000 institutionalized elderly women (mean age 84 years) during treatment with either vitamin D (800 IU/day) and calcium (1.2 g/day) or placebo for 3 years[63]. Active treatment significantly reduced the incidence of new hip fractures by 29% and that of all non-vertebral fractures by 24%[63]. Similar results for hip fracture prevention (relative risk (RR) 1.6, 95% CI 0.96–3.0) were obtained in a multicenter, randomized, double-masked, placebo-controlled confirmatory study in 583 French ambulatory institutionalized women (mean age 85.2 years)[64]. Of particular interest are the results of a placebo-controlled trial on the effect of calcium (500 mg/day) and vitamin D (700 IU/day) in healthy community-based men and women older than 65 years, with a mean dietary calcium intake of about 700 mg/day[38]. After 3 years, 12.9% of subjects treated with placebo and 5.9% of those treated with vitamin D and calcium sustained non-vertebral fractures, a statistically significant difference[38].

Recent meta-analyses confirmed the role of calcium and vitamin D supplementation in the prevention of postmenopausal osteoporosis, even though they did not take into account baseline calcium and vitamin D status or the multiplicity

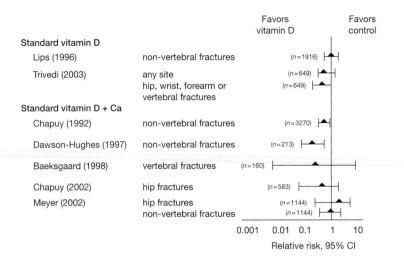

Figure 10 Relative risk (with 95% confidence interval) of vertebral fractures after treatment with standard vitamin D compounds (with and without calcium supplementation). Major randomized, double-blind, controlled studies have been considered[38,63–68]

of study designs[69,70]. Moreover, as concluded by a recent Cochrane review[70], the relative contribution of vitamin D and calcium to these benefits was less clear. In a Dutch study, the administration of 400 IU daily of vitamin D to elderly subjects with a high calcium intake produced no reduction in fracture rate[65]. Similarly, intervention with 10 µg daily of vitamin D₃ failed to prevent either hip or vertebral fractures over a 2-year period in a nursing-home population[68]. On the other hand, an open randomized study of a single annual injection of 150 000–300 000 IU of vitamin D each autumn in an elderly Finnish population showed a significant reduction in overall fracture rate but not in the rate of hip fractures[71]. Recently, Trivedi and colleagues, in a large randomized, double-blind, placebo-controlled trial in 2686 people aged 65–85 years and living in the UK in the general community, demonstrated that vitamin D₃ treatment alone (100 000 IU every 4 months) was safe and effective in decreasing the incidence of all osteoporotic fractures[66]. When analysis was restricted to specific sites, however, a significant reduction was observed only at the forearm in men, but not at the spine and the hip. Thus, the problem of whether vitamin D supplementation

alone is able to prevent vertebral and/or hip fractures remains to be confirmed in larger trials.

Although the effects of calcium and vitamin D in fracture prevention are generally attributed to increases in BMD, it has also been hypothesized that supplementation might increase muscular strength, thereby reducing the risk of falls. In a study involving a group of 122 elderly institutionalized women, 50% of whom had vitamin D insufficiency, musculoskeletal function was shown to improve significantly after 3 months' therapy with calcium and vitamin D, while there was no significant improvement in women treated with calcium alone[72]. The incidence of falls in the women who received calcium and vitamin D was reduced by 49%. Likewise, Pfeifer and colleagues observed a reduction in body sway and a reduction in falls with short-term calcium and vitamin D supplementation as compared with calcium alone in a sample of 148 elderly women[73].

Taken together, these studies underline the need for adequate vitamin D and calcium nutrition in the elderly, particularly in populations at risk of osteoporotic fractures, such as individuals living indoors in nursing-homes, who have a high prevalence of vitamin D deficiency or insufficiency.

Treatment with active vitamin D metabolites

The 1α-hydroxylated forms of vitamin D, 1,25-dihydroxycholecalciferol or calcitriol, and 1α-hydroxycholecalciferol or alfacalcidol, have been proposed as possible therapies for osteoporosis[74,75]. Both compounds strongly stimulate intestinal calcium absorption, and the response is dose-dependent (Figure 11). This leads to a suppression of PTH secretion and a decrease in bone turnover. Over the past two decades, several clinical trials have been performed in osteoporotic patients using calcitriol or alfacalcidol, at doses from 0.25 to 2.0 µg/day. A positive effect of both compounds on BMD was seen in some clinical trials, whereas in others there was no change in BMD[23,77]. In addition, there is not yet a definite answer as to whether these compounds decrease the incidence of osteoporotic fractures. A meta-analysis of published randomized controlled trials showed a consistent, statistically significant effect of hydroxylated vitamin D in all BMD sites for doses above 0.43 µg, with an overall effect that was higher than that of standard vitamin D treatment[69]. A more recent meta-analysis revised the overall effect of active vitamin D metabolites (alfacalcidol and calcitriol) on BMD and fracture rate[78]. A global effect in preventing bone loss in patients not exposed to corticosteroids was demonstrated. Moreover, active vitamin D metabolites significantly reduced the overall fracture rate (RR 0.52, 95% CI 0.46–0.59), and both vertebral (RR 0.53, 95% CI 0.47–0.60) and non-vertebral (RR 0.34, 95% CI 0.16–0.71) fracture rates, respectively[78]. The therapeutic effects seem to be pharmacological rather than physiological, and some concern exists about the potential side-effects of this treatment. Hypercalcemia and impairment of renal function are rare with lower doses (up to 0.5 µg/day) but more frequent with higher doses (1–2 µg/day). For these reasons, treatment with calcitriol or alfacalcidol necessitates monitoring of serum calcium and renal function, unlike treatment with vitamin D.

A number of clinical trials have been conducted over the past few years with the aim of verifying the efficacy of calcitriol in postmenopausal and involutional osteoporosis[23,74,75,77–81].

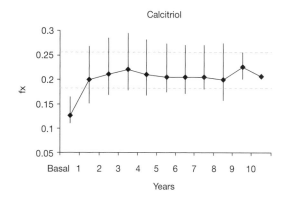

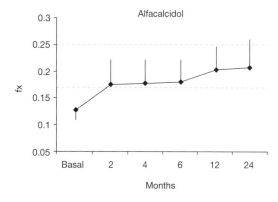

Figure 11 Fractional radiocalcium absorption (fx) during long-term treatment with calcitriol or alfacalcidol in postmenopausal osteoporotic patients. Dotted lines indicate the normal range. Adapted from reference 76

Due to differences in study design and dosage used, these studies led to conflicting results, with bone mass and vertebral fracture rate reported as improving in some studies but remaining unchanged or worsening in others. One of the most likely explanations for the negative results is that these studies used ineffective doses, because it seems that the efficacy of 1α-hydroxylated vitamin D_3 compounds is dose-related. It is now more widely appreciated that the window of efficacy for calcitriol is quite narrow[74,77]. Whereas 0.4 µg/day may be insufficient for increasing calcium absorption in many patients, a dose of 0.5 µg/day or higher is effective in nearly all patients with an appropriate supply of intestinal as dietary calcium (not higher than 0.8 µg/day so as not to increase the risk of

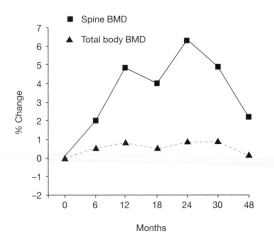

Figure 12 Mean percentage lumbar and total body bone mineral density (BMD) change after treatment with calcitriol (0.5 μg/day) for 48 months in patients with established osteoporosis. Adapted from reference 23

hypercalcemia). Using doses ranging from 0.5 to 0.8 μg/day, calcitriol has been shown to increase total body and spine BMD (Figure 12), and to reduce the incidence of new vertebral fractures[77]. There are few data yet on the effect of calcitriol on fracture incidence (Figure 13). A significant effect on vertebral fracture rate was obtained in one study[79], while another showed a positive but not significant trend[80]. In the former study, 0.5 μg calcitriol per day decreased the incidence of vertebral fractures in women with post-menopausal osteoporosis and with fewer than five fractured vertebrae, but not in those with more than five fractured vertebrae[79]. A more recent double-blind randomized trial investigated the effect of calcitriol or estrogen therapy on BMD and the incidence of falls and fractures[81]. A reduced incidence of falls and non-vertebral fractures over a 3-year period was demonstrated in the calcitriol and estrogen plus calcitriol groups with respect to placebo.

In addition to its role in postmenopausal and involutional osteoporosis, calcitriol has an important role in the treatment of secondary osteoporosis, especially corticosteroid-induced osteoporosis and post-transplantation bone loss[78]. Corticosteroids result in impaired gastrointestinal

absorption of calcium and increased urinary calcium loss, leading to secondary hyperparathyroidism with enhanced bone resorption, as well as having direct inhibitory effects on osteoblasts and bone formation. Calcitriol has recently been shown to be able to prevent and significantly reduce bone loss after cardiac, lung and liver transplantation[77,89]. The mechanism of action of calcitriol in preventing transplant osteoporosis may be related to effects on either corticosteroid or cyclosporine pathways, especially secondary hyperparathyroidism, or to its immunomodulatory properties with consequent immunosuppressive-agent sparing[89]. Recent clinical trials also suggest an important future role of calcitriol as adjunctive therapy to bisphosphonates and estrogen in the treatment of involutional osteoporosis. In particular, a significant benefit of calcitriol treatment combined with HRT on BMD at different skeletal sites has been demonstrated in postmenopausal women[90].

Alfacalcidol is a synthetic precursor of $1,25(OH)_2D_3$ that has to be converted into $1,25(OH)_2D_3$ predominantly by vitamin D 25-hydroxylase before exerting its biological effects. This activation takes places even with advanced liver disease. Because of these pharmacokinetic aspects, alfacalcidol is characterized by a more safe profile, with respect to calcidiol, regarding the risk of developing hypercalcemia or hypercalciuria. This vitamin D analog is a pharmacologically active compound, which acts independently of vitamin D status[74,75,78]. Alfacalcidol was initially synthesized in order to treat the bone disease of patients with chronic renal disease more effectively, since renal 1α-hydroxylation of $25(OH)D_3$ was compromised in these individuals[91]. Subsequently, observations showed that osteoblasts contain a 25-hydroxylase enzyme which converts $1\alpha\text{-}(OH)D_3$ into $1,25(OH)_2D_3$, and that there are higher skeletal concentrations of $1,25(OH)_2D_3$ after $1\alpha\text{-}(OH)D_3$ administration than after $1,25(OH)_2D_3$, despite the fact that serum levels of $1,25(OH)_2D_3$ are lower after $1\alpha\text{-}(OH)D_3$ than after $1,25(OH)_2D_3$ administration[92]. Thus, a small proportion of administered alfacalcidol may be directly activated in bone by 25-hydroxylase expressed by osteoblasts, suggesting a localized autocrine or paracrine effect in

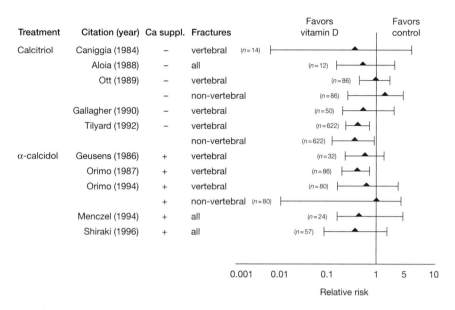

Figure 13 Relative risk (with 95% confidence interval) of vertebral fractures after treatment with active vitamin D metabolites (calcitriol or alfacalcidol with and without calcium supplementation). Major randomized, double-blind, controlled studies have been considered[19,79,80,82–88]

bone tissue, in addition to the systemic effects. *In vivo* experimental evidence suggests that alfacalcidol not only suppresses bone resorption but also simultaneously stimulates bone formation[93]. Alfacalcidol was demonstrated to improve intestinal calcium absorption in osteoporotic women, and has been utilized to treat osteoporosis for more than 20 years in Japan. In different studies, this compound was demonstrated to maintain BMD, and prevent the occurrence of osteoporotic fractures[74,75,78] (Figure 13). Moreover, clinical studies suggest an increased efficacy of alfacalcidol over vitamin D in the treatment of glucocorticoid-induced osteoporosis[94]. Among the multiple pleiotropic effects of alfacalcidol and other vitamin D analogs, their positive action on muscle strength and neuromuscular coordination may exert an important role in fracture risk reduction[95]. The effect of alfacalcidol in increasing the number and diameter of type 2 fiber muscles was demonstrated in elderly women with osteoporosis, after 3 months of treatment[96].

Recently, vitamin D analogs have been developed that retain the suppressive action on PTH and parathyroid gland growth, but have less

calcemic and phosphatemic activity. Currently, two analogs, 19-nor-1,25(OH)$_2$D$_2$ and 1α-(OH)D$_2$, are being used for the treatment of secondary hyperparathyroidism in the United States, and two are being used in Japan, 22-oxa-calcitriol and 1,25(OH)$_2$-26,27F6D$_3$[97]. Elucidation of the mechanism of action for the different vitamin D analogs in the near future will enhance our understanding of the vitamin D pathway and improve their therapeutic use in osteoporosis.

CONCLUSIONS

Vitamin D and calcium are important for normal skeletal growth and for maintaining the mechanical and structural integrity of the skeleton. Even though secure inferences from randomized controlled trials on the prevention of osteoporotic fracture with calcium and vitamin D supplementation are very limited, especially in women within the first years of the menopause, these compounds have been demonstrated to be pharmacologically active, safe and cost-effective for the prevention and treatment of osteoporosis. Their use should therefore be encouraged, particularly in the elderly, as well as in other conditions of dietary deficiency. There is also consistent evidence that calcium and vitamin D supplementation exert a synergistic effect with antiresorptive agents on bone, and, certainly, most patients will derive further benefit in terms of fracture prevention from the addition of an antiresorptive agent. Further studies will be needed to evaluate the relative impact of different vitamin D formulations as well as the relative contribution of calcium and vitamin D compounds on fracture prevention.

References

1. Melton LJ III, Chrischilles EA, Cooper C, et al. Perspective. How many women have osteoporosis? *J Bone Miner Res* 1992; 7: 1005–10
2. International Osteoporosis Foundation. Survey by Helmut Minne, November 1999, IOF. www.osteofound.org
3. Cummings SR, Black DM, Nevitt MC, et al. Bone density at various sites for prediction of hip fractures. The Study of Osteoporotic Fractures Research Group. *Lancet* 1993; 341: 72–5
4. Chapuy MC, Preziosi P, Maamer M, et al. Prevalence of vitamin D insufficiency in an adult normal population. *Osteoporos Int* 1997; 7: 439–43
5. Sahota O, Masud T, San P, et al. Vitamin D insufficiency increases bone turnover markers and enhances bone loss at the hip in the patients with established vertebral osteoporosis. *Clin Endocrinol* 1999; 51: 217–21
6. Gennari C. Calcium and vitamin D nutrition and bone disease of the elderly. *Public Health Nutr* 2001; 4: 547–59
7. Amorin Cruz JA, Moreiras O, Brzozowska A. Longitudinal changes in the intake of vitamins and minerals of elderly Europeans. *Eur J Clin Nutr* 1996; 50: S577–85
8. Gennari C, Agnusdei D, Nardi P, et al. Estrogen preserves a normal intestinal responsiveness to 1,25-dihydroxyvitamin D3 in oophorectomized women. *J Clin Endocrinol Metab* 1990; 71: 1288–93
9. Heaney RP. Estrogen–calcium interactions in the postmenopause: a quantitative description. *Bone Miner* 1990; 11: 67–84
10. Riggs BL, Khosla S, Melton LJ III. A unitary model for involutional osteoporosis: estrogen deficiency causes both type I and type II osteoporosis in postmenopausal women and contributes to bone loss in aging men. *J Bone Miner Res* 1998; 13: 763–73
11. Reichel H, Koeffler PH, Norman AW. The role of the vitamin D endocrine system in health and disease. *N Engl J Med* 1989; 320: 980–91
12. Webb AR, Pilbeam C, Hanafin N, et al. An evaluation of the relative contributions of exposure to sunlight and of diet to the circulating concentrations of 25-hydroxyvitamin D in an elderly nursing home population in Boston. *Am J Clin Nutr* 1990; 51: 1075–81
13. Loré F, Di Cairano G, Manasse G, et al. *Ital J Miner Electrolyte Metab* 1988; 2: 93–106
14. Valimaki MJ, Karkkainen M, Lamberg-Allardt C, et al. Exercise, smoking, and calcium intake during adolescence and early adulthood as determinants of peak bone mass. Cardiovascular Risk in Young Finns Study Group. *Br Med J* 1994; 309: 230–5
15. Jackman LA, Millane SS, Martin BR, et al. Calcium retention in relation to calcium intake and postmenarcheal age in adolescent females. *Am J Clin Nutr* 1997; 66: 327–33
16. Welten DC, Kemper HC, Post GB, et al. A meta-analysis of the effect of calcium intake on bone mass in young and middle aged females and males. *J Nutr* 1995; 25: 2802–13
17. Caniggia A, Gennari C, Bianchi V, et al. Intestinal absorption of 45Ca in senile osteoporosis. *Acta Med Scand* 1963; 173: 613–17
18. Kanis JA. The use of calcium in the management of osteoporosis. *Bone* 1999; 24: 279–90
19. Caniggia A, Nuti R, Loré F, et al. The hormonal form of vitamin D in the pathophysiology and

therapy of postmenopausal osteoporosis. *J Endocrinol Invest* 1984; 7: 373–8

20. Gallagher JC, Riggs BL, Eisman J, et al. Intestinal calcium absorption and serum vitamin D metabolites in normal subjects and osteoporotic patients: effect of age and dietary calcium. *J Clin Invest* 1979; 64: 729–36

21. Caniggia A, Loré F, Di Cairano G, et al. Main endocrine modulators of vitamin D hydroxylase in human pathophysiology. *J Steroid Biochem* 1987; 27: 815–24

22. De Luca HF. 1,25-Dihydroxyvitamin D3 in the pathogenesis and treatment of osteoporosis. *Osteoporos Int* 1997; 7: S24–9

23. Nuti R, Martini G. The role of vitamin D and its metabolites in osteomalacia and involutional osteoporosis. *Ital J Miner Electrolyte Metab* 1994; 8: 225–32

24. Gennari L, Becherini L, Falchetti A, et al. Genetics of osteoporosis: role of steroid hormone receptor gene polymorphisms. *J Steroid Biochem Mol Biol* 2002; 81: 1–24

25. Martinez ME, Delcampo MJ, Sanchez-Cabezudo MJ, et al. Relations between calcidiol serum levels and bone mineral density in postmenopausal women with low bone density. *Calcif Tissue Int* 1994; 55: 253–6

26. Rosen CJ, Morrison A, Zhou H, et al. Elderly women in northern New England exhibit seasonal changes in bone mineral density and calciotropic hormones. *Bone Miner* 1994; 2: 83–92

27. Villareal DT, Civitelli R, Chines A, et al. Subclinical vitamin D deficiency in postmenopausal women with low vertebral bone mass. *J Clin Endocrinol Metab* 1991; 72: 628–34

28. Khaw KT, Sheyd MJ, Compston J. Bone density, parathyroid hormone and 25-hydroxyvitamin D concentrations in middle-aged women. *Br Med J* 1992; 305: 273–7

29. Lidor C, Sagiv P, Amdur B, et al. Decrease in bone levels of 1,25-dihydroxyvitamin D in women with subcapital fracture of the femur. *Calcif Tissue Int* 1993; 52: 146–8

30. Nuti R, Martini G, Valenti R, et al. Vitamin D status and bone turnover in women with acute hip fracture. *Clin Orthop* 2004; 422: 208–13

31. NIH Consensus Conference. Optimal calcium intake. NIH Consensus Development Panel on Optimal Calcium Intake. *J Am Med Assoc* 1994; 272: 1942–8

32. Yates AA, Schlicker SA, Suitor CW. Dietary reference intakes: the new basis for recommendations for calcium and related nutrients, B vitamins, and choline. *J Am Diet Assoc* 1998; 98: 699–706

33. European Commission. Report on osteoporosis in the European Community – action on prevention. Luxembourg: Office of Official Publications of the European Communities, 1998: 112

34. Boonen S, Rizzoli R, Meunier PJ, et al. The need for clinical guidance in the use of calcium and vitamin D in the management of osteoporosis: a consensus report. *Osteoporos Int* 2004; 15: 511–19

35. Johnston CC, Miller JZ, Slemenda CW, et al. Calcium supplementation and increases in bone mineral density in children. *N Engl J Med* 1992; 327: 82–7

36. Dawson-Hughes B. Calcium insufficiency and fracture risk. *Osteoporos Int* 1996; 3: S37–41

37. Dawson-Hughes B. Calcium supplementation and bone loss: a review of controlled clinical trials. *Am J Clin Nutr* 1991; 54: S274–80

38. Dawson-Hughes B, Harris SS, Krall EA, et al. Effect of calcium and vitamin D supplementation on bone density in men and women 65 years of age or older. *N Engl J Med* 1997; 337: 670–6

39. Dawson-Hughes B, Dallal GE, Krall EA, et al. A controlled trial of the effect of calcium supplementation on bone density in postmenopausal women. *N Engl J Med* 1990; 323: 878–83

40. Elders PJ, Lips P, Netelenbos JC, et al. Long-term effect of calcium supplementation on bone loss in perimenopausal women. *J Bone Miner Res* 1994; 9: 963–70

41. Nordin BE. Calcium and osteoporosis. *Nutrition* 1997; 3: 664–86

42. Shea B, Wells G, Cranney A, et al. Osteoporosis Methodology Group and The Osteoporosis Research Advisory Group. Meta-analyses of therapies for postmenopausal osteoporosis. VII. Meta-analysis of calcium supplementation for the prevention of postmenopausal osteoporosis. *Endocr Rev* 2002; 23: 552–9

43. Shea B, Wells G, Cranney A, et al. Osteoporosis Methodology Group; Osteoporosis Research Advisory Group. Calcium supplementation on

bone loss in postmenopausal women. *Cochrane Database Syst Rev* 2004: CD004526

44. Nieves JW, Komar L, Cosman F, et al. Calcium potentiates the effect of estrogen and calcitonin on bone mass: review and analysis. *Am J Clin Nutr* 1998; 67: 18–24

45. Eastell R, Yergey AL, Vieira NE, et al. Interrelationships among vitamin D metabolism, true calcium absorption, parathyroid function, and age in women: evidence of an age-related intestinal resistance to 1,25-dihydroxyvitamin D action. *J Bone Miner Res* 1991; 6: 125–32

46. McKane WR, Khosla S, Egan KS, et al. Role of calcium intake in modulating age-related increases in parathyroid function and bone resorption. *J Clin Endocrinol Metab* 1996; 81: 1699–703

47. Compston J. The role of vitamin D and calcium supplementation in the prevention of osteoporosis fractures in the elderly. *Clin Endocrinol* 1995; 43: 393–405

48. Haden ST, Brown EM, Hurwitz S, et al. The effects of age and gender on parathyroid hormone dynamics. *Clin Endocrinol* 2000; 52: 329–38

49. Prince R, Devine A, Dick I, et al. The effects of calcium supplementation (milk powder or tablets) and exercise on bone density in postmenopausal women. *J Bone Miner Res* 1995; 10: 1068–75

50. Kanis JA, Johnell O, Gullberg B, et al. Evidence for the efficacy of drugs affecting bone metabolism in preventing hip fracture. *Br Med J* 1992; 305: 1124–8

51. Recker RR, Hinders S, Davies KM, et al. Correcting calcium nutritional deficiency prevents spine fractures in elderly women. *J Bone Miner Res* 1996; 11: 1961–6

52. Chevalley T, Rizzoli R, Nydegger V, et al. Effects of calcium supplements on femoral bone mineral density and vertebral fracture rate in vitamin-D-replete elderly patients. *Osteoporos Int* 1994; 5: 245–52

53. Reid IR, Ames RW, Evans MC, et al. Long-term effect of calcium supplementation on bone loss and fractures in postmenopausal women; a randomized controlled trial. *Am J Med* 1995; 4: 331–5

54. Riggs BL, O'Fallon WM, Muhs J, et al. Long-term effects of calcium supplementation on serum parathyroid hormone level, bone turnover, and bone loss in elderly women. *J Bone Miner Res* 1998; 13: 168–74

55. Hansson T, Roos B. The effect of fluoride and calcium on spinal bone mineral content: a controlled, prospective (3 years) study. *Calcif Tissue Int* 1987; 40: 315–17

56. Food and Nutrition Board, Institute of Medicine. Dietary reference intakes for calcium, magnesium, phosphorus, vitamin D, and fluoride. Washington, DC: National Academy Press, 1997

57. NIH. Recommended Dietary Allowances, 10th edn. Washington, DC: National Academic Press, 1989

58. Compston JE. Vitamin D deficiency: time for action. *Br Med J* 1998; 317: 1466–7

59. European Commission Scientific Committee on Food. Opinion of the Scientific Committee on Food on the tolerable upper intake level of vitamin D. Brussels: European Commission, 2002

60. Cooper L, Clifton-Bligh PB, Nery ML, et al. Vitamin D supplementation and bone mineral density in early postmenopausal women. *Am J Clin Nutr* 2003; 77: 1324–9

61. Di Daniele N, Carbonelli MG, Candeloro N, et al. Effect of supplementation of calcium and vitamin D on bone mineral density and bone mineral content in peri- and post-menopausal women; a double-blind, randomized, controlled trial. *Pharmacol Res* 2004; 50: 637–41

62. Dawson-Huges B, Dallal GE, Krall EA, et al. Effect of vitamin D supplementation on overall bone loss in healthy postmenopausal women. *Ann Intern Med* 1991; 115: 505–12

63. Chapuy MC, Arlot ME, Duboeuf F, et al. Vitamin D3 and calcium to prevent hip fractures in elderly women. *N Engl J Med* 1992; 327: 1637–42

64. Chapuy MC, Pamphile R, Paris E, et al. Combined calcium and vitamin D3 supplementation in elderly women: confirmation of reversal of secondary hyperparathyroidism and hip fracture risk: the Decalyos II study. *Osteoporos Int* 2002; 13: 257–64

65. Lips P, Graafmans WC, Ooms ME, et al. Vitamin D supplementation and fracture incidence in elderly persons – a randomized, placebo-controlled clinical trial. *Ann Intern Med* 1996; 124: 400–6

66. Trivedi DP, Doll R, Khaw KT, et al. Effect of four monthly oral vitamin D3 (cholecalciferol)

supplementation on fractures and mortality in men and women living in the community: randomised double blind controlled trial. *Br Med J* 2003; 26: 469–72

67. Baeksgaard L, Andersen KP, Hyldstrup L. Calcium and vitamin D supplementaion increases spinal BMD in healthy postmenopausal women. *Osteoporos Int* 1998; 8: 255–60

68. Meyer HE, Smedshaug GB, Kvaavik E, et al. Can vitamin D supplementation reduce the risk of fracture in the elderly? A randomized controlled trial. *J Bone Miner Res* 2002; 17: 709–15

69. Papadimitropoulos E, Wells G, Shea B, et al. Metaanalysis of the efficacy of vitamin D treatment in preventing osteoporosis in postmenopausal women. *Endocr Rev* 2002; 23: 560–9

70. Gillespie WJ, Avenell A, Henry DA, et al. Vitamin D and vitamin D analogues for preventing fractures associated with involutional and postmenopausal osteoporosis. *Cochrane Database Syst Rev* 2001; 1: CD000227

71. Heikinheimo RJ, Inkovaara JA, Harjv EJ, et al. Annual injections of vitamin D and fractures of aged bone. *Calcif Tissue Int* 1992; 51: 105–10

72. Bischoff HA, Stahelin HB, Dick W, et al. Effects of vitamin D and calcium supplementation on falls: a randomized controlled trial. *J Bone Miner Res* 2003; 18: 343–51

73. Pfeifer M, Begerow B, Minne HW, et al. Effects of a short-term vitamin D and calcium supplementation on body sway and secondary hyperparathyroidism in elderly women. *J Bone Miner Res* 2000; 15: 1113–18

74. Burckhardt P, Lamy O. Vitamin D and its metabolites in the treatment of osteoporosis. *Osteoporos Int* 1998; 8: S40–4

75. Avioli LV. Vitamin D and the D-hormones, alfacalcidol and calcitriol, as therapeutic agents for osteoporotic populations. *Calcif Tissue Int* 1999; 65: 292–4

76. Nuti R, Lore F, et al. Total body absorptiometry in postmenopausal osteoporosis patients treated with 1 alpha-hydroxylated vitamin D metabolites. *Osteoporos Int* 1993; 3: S181–5

77. Nuti R, Bonucci E, Brancaccio D, et al. The role of calcitriol in the treatment of osteoporosis. *Calcif Tissue Int* 2000; 66: 239–40

78. Richy F, Ethgen O, Bruyere O, et al. Efficacy of alphacalcidol and calcitriol in primary and corticosteroid-induced osteoporosis: a meta-analysis of their effects on bone mineral density and fracture rate. *Osteoporos Int* 2004; 15: 301–10

79. Tilyard MW, Spears GF, Thomson J, et al. Treatment of postmenopausal osteoporosis with calcitriol or calcium. *N Engl J Med* 1992; 326: 357–62

80. Gallagher JC, Goldgar D. Treatment of postmenopausal osteoporosis with high doses of synthetic calcitriol. A randomized controlled study. *Ann Intern Med* 1990; 113: 649–55

81. Gallagher JC. The effects of calcitriol on falls and fractures and physical performance tests. *J Steroid Biochem Mol Biol* 2004; 89–90: 497–501

82. Aloia JF, Vaswani A, Yeh JK, et al. Calcitriol in the treatment of postmenopausal osteoporosis. *Am J Med* 1988; 84: 401–8

83. Ott SM, Chesnut CH III. Calcitriol treatment is not effective in postmenopausal osteoporosis. *Ann Intern Med* 1989; 110: 267–74

84. Geusens P, Dequeker J. Long-term effect of nandrolone decanoate, 1 alpha-hydroxyvitamin D3 or intermittent calcium infusion therapy on bone mineral content, bone remodelling and fracture rate in symptomatic osteoporosis: a double-blind controlled study. *Bone Miner* 1986; 1: 347–57

85. Orimo H, Shiraki M, Hayashi Y, et al. Effects of 1 alpha (OH)-vitamin D3. *Bone Miner* 1987; 3: 47–52

86. Orimo H, Shiraki M, Hayashi Y, et al. Effects of 1 alpha-hydroxyvitamin D3 on lumbar bone mineral density and vertebral fractures in patients with postmenopausal osteoporosis. *Calcif Tissue Int* 1994; 54: 370–6

87. Menczel J, Foldes J, Steinberg R, et al. Alfacalcidol (alpha D3) and calcium in osteoporosis. *Clin Orthop Relat Res* 1994; 300: 241–7

88. Shiraki M, Kushida K, Yamazaki K, et al. Effects of 2 years' treatment of osteoporosis with 1 alpha-hydroxyvitamin D3 on bone mineral density and incidence of fracture: a placebo-controlled, double-blind prospective study. *Endocr J* 1996; 43: 211–20

89. Shane E, Addesso V, Namerow PB, et al. Alendronate versus calcitriol for the prevention of bone loss after cardiac transplantation. *N Engl J Med* 2004; 350: 767–76

90. Gutteridge DH, Holzherr ML, Retallack RW, et al. A randomized trial comparing hormone

replacement therapy (HRT) and HRT plus calcitriol in the treatment of postmenopausal osteoporosis with vertebral fractures: benefit of the combination on total body and hip density. *Calcif Tissue Int* 2003; 73: 33–43

91. Barton DH, Hesse HR, Pechet MM, et al. A convenient synthesis of 1α-vitamin D3. *J Am Chem Soc* 1973; 95: 2748–9

92. Civitelli R. Role of vitamin D metabolites in treatment of osteoporosis. *Calcif Tissue Int* 1995; 57: 409–14

93. Shiraishi A, Takeda S, Masaki T, et al. Alfacalcidol inhibits bone resorption and stimulates formation in an ovariectomized rat model of osteoporosis: distinct actions from estrogen. *J Bone Miner Res* 2000; 15: 770–9

94. Ringe JD, Dorst A, Faber H, et al. Superiority of alfacalcidol over plain vitamin D in the treatment of glucocorticoid-induced osteoporosis. *Rheumatol Int* 2004; 24: 63–70

95. Pfeifer M, Begerow B, Minne HW. Vitamin D and muscle function. *Osteoporos Int* 2002; 13: 187–94

96. Sorenson OH, Lund B, Saltin B. Myopathy in bone loss of aging: improvement by treatment with 1-alphahydroxycholecalciferol and calcium. *Clin Sci (Colch)* 1979; 56: 157–61

97. Slatopolsky E, Finch J, Brown A. New vitamin D analogs. *Kidney Int Suppl* 2003; 85: S83–7

Estrogen dose response in bone density and bone histology

18

E. Horner and J. Studd

The many guidelines[1,2] following the Women's Health Initiative (WHI) study have strongly suggested that the lowest possible dose of estrogens[3–8] should be used for postmenopausal women and that estrogens should not be first-line therapy for osteoporosis as the risks outweigh the benefits[9,10]. The American College of Obstetricians and Gynecologists recommends the smallest effective dose in the shortest possible duration, as well as a discontinuation attempt after 5 years of estrogen therapy, for menopausal symptoms in general. The British Menopause Society has issued one of the few recommendations currently supporting the use of estrogens for first-line therapy for the prevention and treatment of osteoporosis in women. There also remains a continuing debate about the value of ultra-low doses.

It has been shown that low-dose estrogen preparations increase lumbar bone mineral density in healthy early-menopausal women, and this seems to slow down between the second year and third year of use[11]. Evans and Davie[12] reported in their study of older symptomatic women that transdermal low-dose estrogen is effective in preventing bone loss in the spine and femoral neck over 3 years. There was no evidence in this study of a higher transdermal estrogen dose being associated with a greater response of bone mass.

It seems that estrogen stops bone loss in early- and late-menopausal women by inhibition of bone resorption, with an increase of 5–10% in bone density over a period of 1–3 years[13]. Nevertheless, when hormone replacement therapy (HRT) is discontinued, bone loss resumes at the same rate as without HRT in the menopause, approximately 2% per year for the first 5 years after the menopause and 1% per year subsequently[14,15].

A number of other treatment options (alendronate, risedronate, raloxifene, parathyroid hormone, calcitonin) for the prevention of osteoporosis are already well established, but estrogens will still remain a valuable option to treat symptomatic pre- and early-postmenopausal women[16,17].

The realization that increased side-effects of estrogen–progestogen therapy in the WHI trial occurred in older women either over the age of 70 on commencement of estrogens, or who started estrogen therapy 20 years after their menopause, calls for a review of the above advice.

For the early-postmenopausal woman (aged 50–59), when the use of HRT is most prevalent, there would appear to be no evidence of an increased incidence of coronary heart disease or strokes, and very contested evidence about an increase of breast cancer[18,19]. Cardiovascular disease becomes more important over the age of 70 after long-term HRT use[20,21].

There is an annual bone loss in postmenopausal women of about 3–5%[22]. We know of the efficacy of estrogen therapy in preserving bone mass and preventing osteoporosis around the menopause. Nevertheless, it is time to reconsider the prohibition of estrogens for the prevention and treatment of osteoporosis and to re-evaluate evidence, if any, that the risks of HRT are dose-dependent. Even with very low doses of estrogen, bone mineral density (BMD) can be maintained and increased[23,24]. However, in the light of successful prevention of osteoporosis with HRT, compliance is important, as bone loss has been reported to occur soon after the therapy has ceased[25]. Long-term experience of the effect of low-dose HRT on BMD is lacking. A short-term study from Mizunuma and colleagues[26] showed a positive overall efficacy in increasing lumbar

BMD with low-dose HRT over a period of 2 years. Crandall[27] searched the Medline database (1966–2003) for randomized controlled trials of low-dose estrogen therapy for menopausal women, and reported that the low-dose preparations should not yet be emphasized as being more efficacious. Especially, bone preservation is less effective, and protection of bone with low-dose estrogen will only be achieved with additional calcium.

Ettinger and colleagues reported in the latest study of ultra-low-dose estradiol (0.014 mg/day transdermal estradiol) for menopausal women aged 60–80 years an increase in lumbar spine and femoral neck bone density of 2.6% and 0.4%, respectively, over a period of 2 years[28]. They also measured the endogenous estradiol levels prior to therapy. The median estradiol level was 5 pg/ml, and after 2 years increased to 8.5 pg/ml. With this level, well below the premenopausal range, bone density was increased.

The risks of HRT are clearly duration-dependent[3], but evidence of increased risk with a higher dose, or a greater plasma estradiol level, is not easy to find. Banks and associates[29] have stated that there is no evidence of a dose-related risk, as well as only weak evidence of heterogeneity between the different routes of administration.

Much of the confusion about the response of osteoporotic bone to estrogens is because the majority of publications relate to the use of Premarin® (conjugated equine estrogens, CEE), where plasma estradiol levels have not been measured or reported. This is for obvious technical reasons of the inability at a clinical or even research level to measure the estrogenicity of a compound that contains at least ten estrogens in their sulfate ester form, progestogens and androgens[30].

There is a need to study the effects of different HRT regimens, including different doses and different combinations. HRT as a class cannot be dismissed on the basis of the findings of one specific regimen[31]. A systematic review of 2-year trials over the past decade, assessing changes in BMD according to different estrogen regimens, reported surprisingly that there seems to be no apparent difference between the various estrogen compounds (oral, non-oral, human and non-human estrogens)[32].

Thus, there are about 20 years of literature relating to the response of bone density to estrogens without a mention of plasma estradiol levels. It is as fundamental an error as writing about diabetes and insulin without reference to blood glucose levels.

One of the earliest studies to consider plasma estradiol levels was treatment with 2 mg estradiol valerate and 75 μg levonorgestrel over periods of 1 and 2 years, which showed, respectively, a 5.1% and 6.1% increase in the density of the lumbar spine, and a 3.5% and 4.5% increase, respectively, in the femoral neck, with a median plasma estradiol level of 310 pmol/l being obtained[33]. A dose-related study of subcutaneous estradiol over 1 year[34] investigated the relationship of plasma estradiol to incremental increase in bone density, with estradiol levels of 358 pmol/l producing an increase in 4.1% at the hip and 6.5% at the lumbar spine. A higher dose produced plasma estradiol levels of 500 pmol/l and an increase in femoral neck BMD of 5.45% and lumbar spine BMD of 10%. The increase in bone mass with higher doses is most evident at the spine, which contains a greater amount of trabecular bone compared with the hip. Similarly, study of older women showed this clear correlation after 1 year of therapy of plasma estradiol level and incremental increase in bone density. The increase in BMD was greatest in older women furthest into the menopause.

There remains a question whether this substantial increase in bone density is due to the production of healthy new bone, or whether the increase is merely the thickening of the trabeculae without any repair of the myriad of microfractures in the skeleton. Estrogen has been shown to stimulate the differentiation and activity of osteoblasts[35]. Estrogen has also been shown to increase bone formation and bone mass in animal models[36].

Histomorphometric studies of bone biopsies have helped to clarify this.

Khastgir and colleagues[37] studied bone biopsies in older women who were a mean of 17 years past the menopause with a low bone density, having 75-mg estradiol implants every 6 months for 6 years. This was the first report confirming histological evidence for an increase in cancellous bone volume together with an increase in wall thickness. The results after 6 years showed an increase in the bone density of every patient, the median being 31.4% at the lumbar spine and 15.1% at the proximal femur. Both T- and Z-scores improved from osteoporotic levels before therapy to normal levels 6 years after therapy. The bone histomorphometric results showed an increase in mean wall thickness from 31.2 to 38.3 μm, and there was an increase in cancellous bone volume from 10.75 to 17.31%. There were also few trabecular ends and more trabecular nodes, indicating growth and repair of the broken bone. There was a direct correlation between serum estradiol levels and cancellous bone volume, wall thickness and trabecular number, but inverse correlation with trabecular ends and trabecular separation.

In a similar study conducted in healthy postmenopausal women, the effects of conventional HRT and high-dose estradiol on cortical bone were investigated[38]. There was a definite trend toward higher cortical width with increasing dose of estrogen. Estrogen-induced effects on bone remodeling were similar in cancellous and cortical bone. High doses of estrogen stimulate anabolic skeletal effects. This was reported by Wahab and co-workers[39] for long-term estradiol-implant patients (15–21 years), as bone mass was significantly elevated to a degree that had never been documented before. The mean difference in absolute bone mass between the implanted and the untreated women was 39.5% at the femoral neck and 45.5% at the lumbar spine.

The role of the collagen matrix is often understated, but collagen is responsible for the strength of bone. It constitutes 90% of the organic matrix of bone. The collagen content of bone falls with aging, but decreases significantly more in the postmenopausal period due to estrogen deficiency[40]. Further studies showed that the total collagen in cortical and cancellous bone rose by a median percentage change of 6.7–25.6% with an increase in intermediate cross-links at both types of bone and mature cross-links increasing in cortical bone only[41]. Both the estradiol levels and bone mineral density correlated with cortical bone collagen levels. The long-term use of high-dose estradiol had an anabolic effect on bone in older women suffering from severe osteoporosis.

What about the anabolic effect of estrogens before the menopause? A similar picture is seen in the osteopenic bones of young women with Turner's syndrome, or other forms of premature ovarian failure. A recent study in 21 women aged 20–40 years with Turner's syndrome, given 50-mg estradiol implants over 3 years, reported a significant increase in cancellous bone volume from 13.4 to 18.8%[42]. This regimen also achieved estradiol levels at the higher end of the physiological range, and therefore exerted an anabolic effect on the skeleton of these young women. There is evidence that low-dose estradiol therapy leads to lower estradiol plasma levels, and this will only be sufficient to suppress bone resorption[43].

Will low-dose HRT with its minimal side-effects be our future regimen to prevent and reverse bone loss and to reduce menopausal symptoms? Clinical research should focus on the efficacy of low-dose HRT in women with severe osteoporosis, and its increased risks and side-effects. Large, long-term trials are needed in the future to determine the potential benefits of low-dose HRT.

References

1. North American Menopause Society. Management of postmenopausal osteoporosis: position statement of the North American Menopause Society. *Menopause* 2002; 2: 84–101

2. Royal College of Physicians. Edinburgh Consensus Conference on Hormone Replacement Therapy. London: Royal College of Physicians, 2003

3. Naftolin F, Schneider HP, Sturdee DW. Executive Committee of the International Menopause Society. Guidelines for the hormone treatment of women in the menopausal transition and beyond. *Climacteric* 2004; 1: 8–11

4. Haas JS, Kaplan CP, Gerstenberger EP, et al. Changes in the use of postmenopausal hormone therapy after the publication of clinical trial results. *Ann Intern Med* 2004; 3: 184–8

5. Rossouw JE, Anderson GL, Prentice RL, et al. Risks and benefits of estrogen plus progestin in healthy postmenopausal women: principal results from the Women's Health Initiative randomized controlled trial. *J Am Med Assoc* 2002; 288: 321–33

6. Stevenson JC, Teter P, Lees B. 17beta-estradiol (1 mg/day) continuously combined with dydrogesterone (5, 10 or 20 mg/day) increases bone mineral density in postmenopausal women. *Maturitas* 2001; 38: 197–203

7. Heikkinen J, Vaheri R, Kainulainen P, et al. Long-term continuous combined hormone replacement therapy in the prevention of postmenopausal bone loss: a comparison of high- and low-dose estrogen–progestin regimens. *Osteoporos Int* 2000; 11: 929–37

8. Archer DF. Low-dose hormone therapy for postmenopausal women. *Clin Obstet Gynecol* 2003; 46: 317–24

9. Royal College of Physicians. Osteoporosis: clinical guidelines for prevention and treatment. Update on pharmacological interventions and algorithm for management. London: Royal College of Physicians, 2000

10. Seeman E, Eisman JA. Treatment of osteoporosis: why, whom, when and how to treat. *Med J Aust* 2004; 180: 298–303

11. Delmas PD, Pornel B, Felsenberg D, et al. Three-year follow-up of the use of transdermal 17beta-estradiol matrix patches for the prevention of bone loss in early postmenopausal women. *Am J Obstet Gynecol* 2001; 184: 32–40

12. Evans SF, Davie MW. Low and conventional dose transdermal oestradiol are equally effective at preventing bone loss in spine and femur at all post-menopausal ages. *Clin Endocrinol (Oxf)* 1996; 44: 79–84

13. The Writing Group for the PEPI. Effects of hormone therapy on bone mineral density: results from the Postmenopausal Estrogen/Progestin Interventions (PEPI) trial. *J Am Med Assoc* 1996; 276: 1389–96

14. Dennison E, Cooper C. The epidemiology of osteoporosis. *Br J Clin Pract* 1996; 50: 33–6

15. Thomsen K, Riis BJ, Johansen JS, et al. Bone turnover in postmenopausal women after withdrawal of estrogen/gestagen replacement therapy. *Gynecol Endocrinol* 1987; 1: 169–75

16. Delmas PD. Treatment of postmenopausal osteoporosis. *Lancet* 2002; 359: 2018–26

17. Compston JE, Watts NB. Combination therapy for postmenopausal osteoporosis. *Clin Endocrinol (Oxf)* 2002; 5: 565–9

18. Beral V, Banks E, Reeves G. Evidence from randomised trials on the long-term effects of hormone replacement therapy. *Lancet* 2002; 360: 942–4

19. Manson JE, Hsia J, Johnson KC, et al. Estrogen plus progestin and the risk of coronary heart disease. *N Engl J Med* 2003; 349: 523–34

20. Hulley SB, Grady D, Bush T, et al. Randomized trial of estrogen plus progestin for secondary prevention of coronary heart disease in postmenopausal women. Heart and Estrogen/progestin Replacement Study (HERS) Research Group. *J Am Med Assoc* 1998; 280: 605–13

21. Anderson GL, Limacher M, Assaf AR, et al. Effects of conjugated equine estrogen in postmenopausal women with hysterectomy: the Women's Health Initiative randomized controlled trial. *J Am Med Assoc* 2004; 291: 1701–12

22. Slipman CW, Whyte II W. Consensus development conference. Diagnosis, prophylaxis and treatment of osteoporosis. *Am J Med* 1993; 94: 646–50

23. Recker RR, Davies KM, Dowd RM, et al. The effect of low-dose continuous estrogen and progesterone therapy with calcium and vitamin D on bone in elderly women. A randomized, controlled trial. *Ann Intern Med* 1999; 130: 897–904

24. Gambacciani M, Ciaponi M, Cappagli B, et al. Postmenopausal femur bone loss: effects of a low dose hormone replacement therapy. *Maturitas* 2003; 45: 175–83

25. The Swedish Hip Fracture Study Group. Hormone replacement therapy and risk of hip fracture: population based case–control study. The Swedish Hip Fracture Study Group. *Br Med J* 1998; 316: 1858–63

26. Mizunuma H, Okano H, Soda M, et al. Prevention of postmenopausal bone loss with minimal uterine bleeding using low dose continuous estrogen/progestin therapy: a 2-year prospective study. *Maturitas* 1997; 27: 69–76

27. Crandall C. Low-dose estrogen therapy for menopausal women: a review of efficacy and safety. *J Women's Health* 2003; 12: 723–47

28. Ettinger B, Ensrud KE, Wallace R, et al. Effects of ultralow-dose transdermal estradiol on bone mineral density: a randomized clinical trial. *Obstet Gynecol* 2004; 104: 443–51

29. Banks E, Beral V, Reeves G, et al. Million Women Study Collaborators: fracture incidence in relation to the pattern of use of hormone therapy in postmenopausal women. *J Am Med Assoc* 2004; 291: 2212–20

30. Bhavnani BR. Pharmacokinetics and pharmacodynamics of conjugated equine estrogens: chemistry and metabolism. *Proc Soc Exp Biol Med* 1998; 217: 6–16

31. Stevenson JC. Long-term effects of hormone replacement therapy. *Lancet* 2003; 361: 253–4

32. Doren M, Nilsson JA, Johnell O. Effects of specific post-menopausal hormone therapies on bone mineral density in post-menopausal women: a meta-analysis. *Hum Reprod* 2003; 18: 1737–46

33. Holland EF, Leather AT, Studd JW, et al. The effect of a new sequential oestradiol valerate and levonorgestrel preparation on the bone mineral density of postmenopausal women. *Br J Obstet Gynaecol* 1993; 100: 966–7

34. Studd JW, Holland EF, Leather AT, et al. The dose-response of percutaneous oestradiol implants on the skeletons of postmenopausal women. *Br J Obstet Gynaecol* 1994; 101: 787–91

35. Ernst M, Schmid C, Froesch ER. Enhanced osteoblast proliferation and collagen gene expression by estradiol. *Proc Natl Acad Sci USA* 1988; 85: 2307–10

36. Takano-Yamamoto T, Rodan GA. Direct effects of 17 beta-estradiol on trabecular bone in ovariectomized rats. *Proc Natl Acad Sci USA* 1990; 87: 2172–6

37. Khastgir G, Studd J, Holland N, et al. Anabolic effect of estrogen replacement on bone in postmenopausal women with osteoporosis: histomorphometric evidence in a longitudinal study. *J Clin Endocrinol Metab* 2001; 86: 289–95

38. Vedi S, Bell KL, Loveridge N, et al. The effects of hormone replacement therapy on cortical bone in postmenopausal women. A histomorphometric study. *Bone* 2003; 33: 330–4

39. Wahab M, Ballard P, Purdie DW, et al. The effect of long-term oestradiol implantation on bone mineral density in postmenopausal women who have undergone hysterectomy and bilateral oophorectomy. *Br J Obstet Gynaecol* 1997; 104: 728–31

40. Smith R. Collagen and disorders of bone. *Clin Sci (Lond)* 1980; 59: 215–23

41. Khastgir G, Studd J, Holland N, et al. Anabolic effect of long-term estrogen replacement on bone collagen in elderly postmenopausal women with osteoporosis. *Osteoporos Int* 2001; 12: 465–70

42. Khastgir G, Studd JW, Fox SW, et al. A longitudinal study of the effect of subcutaneous estrogen replacement on bone in young women with Turner's syndrome. *J Bone Miner Res* 2003; 18: 925–32

43. Hall JM, McDonnell DP. The estrogen receptor beta-isoform (ERbeta) of the human estrogen receptor modulates ERalpha transcriptional activity and is a key regulator of the cellular response to estrogens and antiestrogens. *Endocrinology* 1999; 140: 5566–78

Effects of oral contraceptive preparation on bone health   19

M. Gambacciani

INTRODUCTION

Ovarian steroids play key roles in bone metabolism and the accumulation and retention of normal bone mineral density (BMD). Therefore, the use of hormonal contraception may interfere with bone mineral density and metabolism in all periods of a woman's life[1]. Estrogen deficiency is associated with a substantial decrease in bone density in adolescents and young women who develop estrogen-deficiency amenorrhea, as well as in the perimenopausal period[1–3]. Amenorrhea is a marker for conditions that have been associated with osteopenia, such as eating disorders, stress-induced hypothalamic hypogonadism, premature ovarian failure, hyperprolactinemia and gonadal dysgenesis. In functional hypothalamic amenorrhea (FHA), the marked reduction in estradiol production is related to a decreased BMD (Figure 1). BMD is further reduced in young amenorrheic women suffering from severe amenorrhea in addition to eating disorders such as anorexia nervosa (Figure 2).

The correlation between ovarian steroid production and bone metabolism and density has led to questions regarding the possible impact of hormonal contraception. Among combined hormonal methods, data are available primarily for oral contraceptives. Newer methods of hormone delivery, such as the contraceptive patch and vaginal ring, have not been evaluated. Among progestin-only methods, data are available primarily for depot medroxyprogesterone acetate (DMPA). Few data exist regarding progestin-only oral contraceptives or the levonorgestrel intrauterine system.

DEPOT MEDROXYPROGESTERONE ACETATE

The relationship between the injectable progestin DMPA and bone mineral density is uncertain. DMPA suppresses ovulation by inhibiting pituitary gonadotropins. With continued use, ovarian estradiol production decreases, and the majority of women become amenorrheic. Estradiol levels are as low as during the early follicular phase of the menstrual cycle, leading to questions regarding bone density in a constant, relatively hypoestrogenic state. In 1991, a cross-sectional study first drew attention to the issue of DMPA and bone loss[4]. DMPA users had significantly lower bone density than premenopausal controls at both the lumbar spine (-8%) and the femoral neck (-7%)[4]. Later, other investigators reported conflicting results showing no or little effect of DMPA in adult women[5,6]. Investigators reported a weak correlation between degree of bone loss and duration of use. Potential reductions in bone density with DMPA use appear to be reversible in adult women after stopping the drug. A recent cross-sectional study by the World Health Organization examined bone mineral density in nearly 2500 women aged 30–34 years, and concluded that hormonal contraceptive use by young adult women is associated with a significant decrease in bone mineral density that occurs early after initiation of use and is reversible[7]. The negative effect of DMPA on bone density and metabolism in adult women seems to be transient and parallel to the amenorrheic state[8–11].

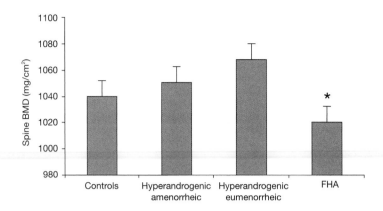

Figure 1 Spine bone mineral density (BMD) measured in normal menstruating women (n = 19), hyperandrogenic amenorrheic (n = 15) and eumenorrheic (n = 12) subjects and in functional hypothalamic amenorrhea (FHA) (n = 21) patients. $^*p$ < 0.05 vs. the other groups

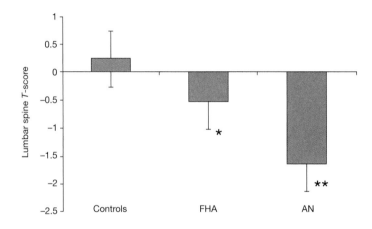

Figure 2 Osteopenia in young women with functional hypothalamic amenorrhea (FHA) and anorexia nervosa (AN). T-scores for lumbar spine bone mineral density in normal controls (n = 30) and patients with FHA (n = 23) and AN (n = 15). $^*p$ < 0.01 vs. controls; $^{**}p$ < 0.001 vs. controls and FHA

DEPOT MEDROXYPROGESTERONE ACETATE IN ADOLESCENTS

The potential negative effect of DMPA use on bone density raises particular concerns in adolescents. The long-term consequences of slowing or reversing bone mass acquisition during early adolescence could be greater than in adult women who have reached their peak bone mass. Few studies have examined bone density among adolescent DMPA users. In a prospective study[12], the investigators determined lumbar vertebral bone density in adolescents using DMPA, combined oral contraceptives (OCs) and levonorgestrel subdermal implants, and controls receiving no hormonal treatment. After 2 years, DMPA users had a 3% loss of bone density versus a 10% increase in controls (p < 0.001). DMPA is associated with about a 1–2% per year loss in bone, regardless of age. For a 40-year-old woman, who by virtue of her age is losing 1–2%

per year anyway, this can be an issue. In adolescents, however, this DMPA effect on bone health can be even more relevant.

Adolescents experience large increases in bone density (from 2 to 10% annually, according to age). Comparing the normal pattern of attainment of peak bone mass with the 1–2% loss induced by DMPA, the considerable differences may have relevant clinical consequences.

Estrogen supplementation helps to prevent the bone loss incurred by adolescents receiving DMPA[13]. In a randomized trial, 123 adolescents received DMPA injections every 12 weeks, associated with monthly injections of estradiol cypionate or placebo. During the 24-month study period, the change in BMD at both lumbar spine and femoral neck was significantly different between women receiving estradiol (2.8% and 4.7%) and those given placebo (–1.8% and –5.1%)[13]. This study clearly confirmed that the deleterious effect of DMPA on bone density is related to the decrease in endogenous estradiol production. In adolescents, the potential lack of normal increase in bone density warrants cautious use of DMPA. Since the majority of bone mass is accrued during adolescence, the greatest and potentially permanent impact could occur with DMPA use at that point. Research must be focused on bone-sparing strategies in adolescents who use DMPA for contraception.

ORAL CONTRACEPTIVES

The impact of combined oral contraceptives (OCs) on bone mineral density has been a matter of debate. Some studies have reported a positive effect; others have found no association. Evidence-based reviews of the literature, however, have concluded that OCs likely provide bone-sparing effects for premenopausal women. The positive effect of OCs on bone is present even with low-dose formulations (20 μg ethinylestradiol). With the exception of a few reports[14–17], the use of OCs containing estrogen and a progestin have been associated with postitive effects on bone density and metabolism[18–23]). A review[24] examined the relationship between low-dose OCs and bone and concluded that the

evidence supporting a positive association between OC use and increased bone mineral density is level II, and that fair evidence (category B) supports the position that OC use has a favorable effect on bone[24].

The effects of low-dose OCs are particularly relevant in hypoestrogenic young women experiencing a decrease in BMD. Women suffering from hypoestrogenic amenorrhea associated with eating disorders (excessive, compulsive reduction of food intake, increased use of fiber in order to reduce body weight) can most benefit from OC administration (Figure 3). However, the OC effect on bone density and metabolism can be optimized only with relevant changes in nutritional life-style (Figure 3). Even lower-dose OCs, particularly the formulation containing 15 μg ethinylestradiol, can be of benefit for bone in amenorrheic young women (Figure 4).

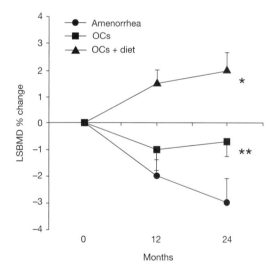

Figure 3 Effect of oral contraceptives (OCs; 20 μg ethinylestradiol-containing products) in osteopenic young women (mean age 23.5 years; body mass index < 22) with functional hypothalamic amenorrhea associated with eating disorders. OC administration is associated with significant increase in bone mineral density at the lumbar spine (LSBMD) in comparison with women remaining amenorrheic. Data are expressed as percentage change over baseline levels. $n = 15$ in each group. $*p < 0.01$ vs. amenorrhea and OCs group; $**p < 0.05$ vs. amenorrhea

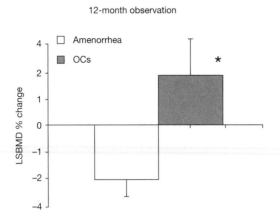

Figure 4 Effect of low-dose oral contraceptives (OCs; 15 μg ethinylestradiol plus 60 μg gestodene) in osteopenic young women (mean age 20.5 years) with functional hypothalamic amenorrhea. OC administration is associated with significant increase in bone mineral density at the lumbar spine (LSBMD) in comparison with women remaining amenorrheic. Data are expressed as percentage change over baseline levels. $n = 21$ in each group. $^*p < 0.01$ vs. amenorrhea

In premenopausal oligomenorrheic women, progressive ovarian failure is associated with a decrease of estradiol production. During the menopausal transition, a progressive impairment in bone metabolism and significant bone loss can occur, particularly in women suffering from hypoestrogenic oligomenorrhea[2,3,25]. OC administration is able to prevent the perimenopausal increase in bone turnover observed in untreated oligomenorrheic women, and to prevent the decrease in radial[26], vertebral[27] and femoral[28] BMD. The activation of bone turnover characterizes the perimenopausal woman suffering from hypoestrogenic oligomenorrhea[26–28]. In fact, no evidence of increased bone resorption was observed in age-matched, normally menstruating perimenopausal women[26–28]. Conversely, progressive impairment of ovarian function corresponded to an increase in markers of bone turnover, which was accompanied by a progressive decrease in BMD at all tested skeletal sites[26–28]. Calcium supplementation, at the dose of at least 500 mg/day, was unable to block the

bone remodeling that occurs in perimenopausal oligomenorrheic women[26–28]. The extent of bone loss can vary at different sites depending on the relative trabecular/cortical ratio, but a definite decline in femur bone density has been clearly correlated with involutional osteoporosis[29]. As reviewed by Rico[30], in involutional osteoporosis, cortical bone loss is greater than trabecular bone loss. The cortical bone compartment represents 80% of the total bone mass, and is the major determinant of bone strength. The individualization of early changes in cortical bone mass can help achieve the final goal of preventing osteoporosis-related, mainly hip, fractures.

The relationship between ovarian function and bone turnover suggests that, during the perimenopausal transition, oligomenorrheic subjects with low estrogen production may lose substantial BMD before entering the menopause. Thus, a long menopausal transition can represent a risk factor for future osteoporosis. Conversely, the maintenance of normal ovarian function or the administration of low-dose (20 μg ethinylestradiol) OC preparation can protect against perimenopausal osteopenia.

Recently, it has been reported that not only postmenopausal hormone replacement[31–37] but also oral contraceptive use can reduce the risk of hip fracture[38]. The protective effect of oral contraceptives on the risk of hip fracture is evident when OCs are used late in reproductive life, after age 40[38]. These data suggest that oral contraceptives might balance the deleterious effect of gonadal impairment on bone. The observation of a protective effect of oral contraceptives on the risk of hip fracture[38] is supported by the results of longitudinal studies[26–28], showing that, in perimenopausal oligomenorrheic women, bone density exhibits a significant decrease that is negated by the administration of a low-dose OC preparation.

The bone-sparing effects of OCs in all hypoestrogenic states is relevant also for women treated with gonadotropin-releasing hormone analogs (GnRH-a)[39]. GnRH-a are effective in relieving the symptoms of endometriosis and symptomatic uterine fibroids. Unfortunately, the induced low-estrogen state is associated with adverse effects, including a decrease in BMD.

Either danazol or progesterone plus estrogen add-back is protective of BMD at the lumbar spine during GnRH-a treatment[39]. A consensus on add-back therapy has already been reached, showing that progesterone plus estrogen therapy does not reduce the effectiveness of GnRH-a on endometriosis treatment, while it can provide effective relief of vasomotor symptoms and decrease or eliminate BMD loss[40]. Thus, the efficacy of GnRH agonists may be preserved, and treatment extended, while overcoming hypo-estrogenic side-effects with the use of appropriate add-back regimens. The use of low-dose OCs in these particular cases can be of value. In a pilot study, low-dose OCs have been administered to GnRH-a-treated women suffering from severe endometriosis and uterine fibroids (Figure 5). The effects of these treatments were evaluated after 6 and 12 months by dual-energy X-ray absorptiometry (DXA) at the lumbar spine. Administration of only calcium supplement was ineffective in terms of bone protection in young premenopausal women given GnRH-a. Conversely, a low-dose (15 µg ethinylestradiol plus 60 µg gestodene) OC preparation was able to negate the reduction of BMD induced by GnRH-a-generated hypoestrogenism. Thus, the combination of a GnRH agonist and low-dose OC administered to symptomatic endometriosis and fibroid patients can provide extended BMD preservation.

CONCLUSION

Administration of OCs in normal eumenorrheic women has no effect on bone mineral density and bone metabolism. Conversely, DMPA is associated with bone loss in normal women, and blocks the attainment of peak bone mass in adolescents.

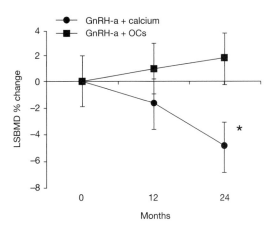

Figure 5 Effect of gonadotropin-releasing hormone analog (GnRH-a) administration in young women (mean age 35.5 years) given calcium (500 mg/day, $n = 21$) or the same calcium supplement associated with low-dose oral contraceptives (OCs; 15 µg ethinylestradiol plus 60 µg gestodene, $n = 11$). GnRH-a administration is associated with a significant (*$p < 0.05$) decrease in lumbar spine bone mineral density (LSBMD) in comparison with women given OCs. Data are expressed as percentage change over baseline levels

Women with functional hypothalamic amenorrhea may have lower BMD than age-matched eumenorrheic women, and the administration of an OC is effective in increasing BMD. In the menopausal transition, low-dose OCs prevent the increase in bone turnover and subsequent bone loss. The prevention of bone loss is one of the recognized non-contraceptive benefits of OCs, when administered in different pathophysiological conditions characterized by a reduction of endogenous estrogen production.

References

1. Ott SM. Attainment of peak bone mass. *J Clin Endocrinol Metab* 1990; 71: 1082a–c

2. Nilas L, Christiansen C. The pathophysiology of peri- and postmenopausal bone loss. *Br J Obstet Gynaecol* 1989; 96: 580–7

3. Gambacciani M, Spinetti A, Taponeco F, et al. Bone loss in perimenopausal women: a longitudinal study. *Maturitas* 1994; 18: 191–7

4. Cundy T, Evans M, Roberts H, et al. Bone density in women receiving depot medroxyprogesterone acetate for contraception. *Br Med J* 1991; 303: 13–16

5. Taneepanichskul S, Intaraprasert S, Theppisai U, et al. Bone mineral density in long-term depot medroxyprogesterone acetate acceptors. *Contraception* 1997; 56: 1–3

6. Gbolade B, Ellis S, Murby B, et al. Bone density in long-term users of depot medroxyprogesterone acetate. *Br J Obstet Gynaecol* 1998; 105: 790–4

7. Petitti DB, Piaggio G, Mehta S, et al. Steroid hormone contraception and bone mineral density: a cross-sectional study in an international population. The WHO Study of Hormonal Contraception and Bone Health. *Obstet Gynecol* 2000; 95: 736–44

8. Paiva LC, Pinto-Neto AM, Faundes A. Bone density among long-term users of medroxyprogesterone acetate as a contraceptive. *Contraception* 1998; 58: 351–5

9. Scholes D, Lacroix AZ, Ott SM, et al. Bone mineral density in women using depot medroxyprogesterone acetate for contraception. *Obstet Gynecol* 1999; 93: 233–8.

10. Scholes D, Lacroix AZ, Ichikawa LE, et al. Injectable hormone contraception and bone density: results from a prospective study. *Epidemiology* 2002; 13: 581–7

11. Bahamondes L, Perrotti M, Castro S, et al. Forearm bone density in users of Depo-Provera as a contraceptive method. *Fertil Steril* 1999; 71: 849–52

12. Cromer BA, Blair JM, Mahan JD, et al. A prospective comparison of bone density in adolescent girls receiving depot medroxyprogesterone acetate (Depo-Provera), levonorgestrel (Norplant), or oral contraceptives. *J Pediatr* 1996; 129: 671–6

13. Cromer BA, Lazebnik R, Rome E, et al. Double-blinded randomized controlled trial of estrogen supplementation in adolescent girls who receive depot medroxyprogesterone acetate for contraception. *Am J Obstet Gynecol* 2005; 192: 42–7

14. MacDougall J, Davies MC, Overton CE, et al. Bone density in a population of long term oral contraceptive pill users does not differ from that in menstruating women. *Br J Fam Plann* 1999; 25: 96–100

15. Murphy S, Khaw KT, Compston JE. Lack of relationship between hip and spine bone mineral density and oral contraceptive use. *Eur J Clin Invest* 1993; 23: 108–11

16. Polatti F, Perotti F, Filippa N, et al. Bone mass and long-term monophasic oral contraceptive treatment in young women. *Contraception* 1995; 51: 221–4

17. Recker RR, Davies KM, Hinders SM, et al. Bone gain in young adult women. *J Am Med Assoc* 1992; 268: 2403–8

18. Mazess RB, Barden HS. Bone density in premenopausal women: effects of age, dietary intake, physical activity, smoking, and birth-control pills. *Am J Clin Nutr* 1991; 53: 132–42

19. Kritz-Silverstein D, Barrett-Connor E. Bone mineral density in postmenopausal women as determined by prior oral contraceptive use. *Am J Public Health* 1993; 83: 100–2

20. Kleerekoper M, Brienza RS, Schultz LR, Johnson CC. Oral contraceptive use may protect against low bone mass. *Arch Intern Med* 1991; 151: 1971–6

21. Garnero P, Sornay-Rendu E, Delmas PD. Decreased bone turnover in oral contraceptive users. *Bone* 1995; 16: 499–503

22. Volpe A, Amram A, Cagnacci A, Battaglia C. Biochemical aspects of hormonal contraception: effects on bone metabolism. *Eur J Contracept Reprod Health Care* 1997; 2: 123–6

23. DeCherney A. Bone-sparing properties of oral contraceptives. *Am J Obstet Gynecol* 1996; 174: 15–20

24. Kuohung W, Borgatta L, Stubblefield P. Lowdose oral contraceptives and bone mineral density: an evidence-based analysis. *Contraception* 2000; 61: 77–82

25. Rodin A, Murby B, Smith MA, et al. Perimenopausal bone loss in the lumbar spine and neck of femur: a study of 225 Caucasian women. *Bone* 1990; 11: 1–5

26. Gambacciani M, Spinetti A, Cappagli B, et al. Hormone replacement therapy in perimenopausal women with a low dose oral contraceptive preparation: effects on bone mineral density and metabolism. *Maturitas* 1994; 19: 125–31

27. Gambacciani M, Spinetti A, Taponeco F, et al. Longitudinal evaluation of perimenopausal vertebral bone loss: effects of a low-dose oral contraceptive preparation on bone mineral density and metabolism. *Obstet Gynecol* 1994; 83: 392–6

28. Gambacciani M, Ciaponi M, Cappagli B, et al. Longitudinal evaluation of perimenopausal femoral bone loss: effects of a low-dose oral contraceptive preparation on bone mineral density and metabolism. *Osteoporos Int* 2000; 11: 544–8

29. Gambacciani M, Spinetti A, Taponeco F, et al. Longitudinal evaluation of perimenopausal vertebral bone loss: effects of a low-dose oral contraceptive preparation on bone mineral density and metabolism. *Obstet Gynecol* 1994; 83: 392–6

30. Rico H. The therapy of osteoporosis and the importance of cortical bone. *Calcif Tissue Int* 1997; 61: 431–2

31. Kiel DP, Felson DT, Anderson JJ, et al. Hip fracture and the use of estrogen in postmenopausal women: the Framingham Study. *N Engl J Med* 1987; 317: 1169–74

32. Altman DG. A meta-analysis of hormone replacement for fracture prevention. *J Am Med Assoc* 2001; 286: 1096–7

33. Michaelsson K, Baron JA, Farahmand BY, et al. Hormone replacement therapy and risk of hip fracture: population based case–control study. The Swedish Hip Fracture Study Group. *Br Med J* 1998; 20: 1858–63

34. Torgerson DJ, Bell-Syer SEM. Hormone replacement therapy and prevention of non vertebral fractures. A meta-analysis of randomized trials. *J Am Med Assoc* 2001; 285: 2891–7

35. Torgerson DJ, Bell-Syer SEM. Hormone replacement therapy and prevention of vertebral fractures. A meta-analysis of randomized trials. *BMC Musculoskeletal Disord* 2001; 2: 7

36. Rossouw JE, Anderson GL, Prentice RL, et al. Risks and benefits of estrogen plus progestin in healthy postmenopausal women: principal results from the Women's Health Initiative randomized controlled trial. *J Am Med Assoc* 2002; 288: 321–33

37. Cauley JA, Robbins J, Chen Z, et al. Effects of estrogen plus progestin on risk of fracture and bone mineral density. The Women's Health Initiative randomized trial. *J Am Med Assoc* 2003; 290: 1729–38

38. Michaelsson K, Baron JA, Farahmand BY, et al. Oral-contraceptive use and risk of hip fractures: a case–control study. *Lancet* 1999; 1: 1481–4

39. Sagsveen M, Farmer JE, Prentice A, Breeze A. Gonadotropin-releasing hormone analogues for endometriosis: bone mineral density. *Cochrane Database Syst Rev* 2003; (4): CD001297

40. Surrey ES. Add-back therapy and gonadotropin-releasing hormone agonists in the treatment of patients with endometriosis: can a consensus be reached? Add-Back Consensus Working Group. *Fertil Steril* 1999; 71: 420–4

Hormone replacement therapy 20

L. B. Tankó and C. Christiansen

INTRODUCTION

Ever since the early reports by Fuller Albright in the 1940s[1], major efforts have been dedicated to research aiming towards a better understanding of the role of estrogens in the regulation of bone turnover. The sudden and pronounced drop in circulating estrogens of ovarian origin after the menopause is by now unequivocally recognized as a major risk factor for osteoporosis. By using specific biomarkers of bone cell function, numerous follow-up studies have demonstrated the rapid and marked acceleration of osteoclast-mediated bone resorption unmatched by simultaneous bone formation as the major cause underlying the negative calcium balance characteristic of osteoporotic postmenopausal women (e.g. references 2–4).

SCREENING

As with most primary prevention, the best results and cost/benefit ratios can be achieved if treating those who benefit the most from clinical management countering the adverse trends accompanying the menopause. The *sine qua non* of finding these individuals is effective screening. Below is a list of criteria that should be satisfied before large-scale screening is undertaken:

(1) The disease should be common and serious regarding its outcomes;

(2) The natural disease history should be understood;

(3) Good screening tests should be available;

(4) Acceptable treatment should be available.

Ideally, it would be desirable to distinguish those women in their 50s who are most likely to develop osteoporosis by old age, and who are at the greatest risk of long-term complications such as vertebral and hip fracture(s). Emerging evidence suggests that combined measures of bone mass and bone turnover using tomoabsorptiometry and biomarkers, respectively, offer useful proxies of risk (e.g. references 5–7). Showing an example from our own results, Table 1 illustrates the baseline characteristics of participants of a long-term follow-up study that monitored bone loss in early-postmenopausal women. Fast losers

Table 1 Baseline characteristics of 'fast losers' versus 'normal losers'. Values are expressed as mean ± SD

	Fast losers	Normal losers
Baseline BMC (g)	3.09 ± 0.56	3.15 ± 0.48
Height (m)	161.6 ± 5.8	160.2 ± 5.6
Weight (kg)	62.9 ± 12.5[*]	67.3 ± 12.7
CrossLaps (ng/ml)	0.43 ± 0.17[**]	0.33 ± 0.14
Osteocalcin (ng/ml)	11.0 ± 4.8[**]	9.0 ± 4.8
Bone loss/15 years (%)	22.4 ± 8.5[***]	13.5 ± 9.4

[*]$p < 0.1$; [**]$p < 0.01$; [***]$p < 0.001$; BMC, bone mineral content

were leaner and had significantly elevated levels of bone formation and bone resorption markers, indicating accelerated bone turnover.

When assessing bone markers 15 years later, 'fast losers' still had ~30% higher levels compared with 'normal losers' ($p < 0.001$).

This finding also illustrates that body fat-derived endogenous estradiol plays an important compensatory role in the modulation of bone turnover in postmenopausal women lacking ovarian estradiol. Figure 1 shows bone turnover characteristics measured by bone markers as a function of total body fat mass, emphasizing that the more pronounced is body fatness, the smaller is the negative calcium balance.

Figure 2 indicates the decrease in bone mineral density (BMD) at different skeletal sites over the 15-year observation period. 'Fast losers', by definition, lost significantly more BMD at all sites compared with 'normal losers' ($p < 0.01$)

Figure 3a indicates the relative risk of vertebral fractures in women with low bone mass and accelerated bone turnover compared with controls and those with high bone mass and slow bone loss. Figure 3b indicates that the risk of fractures increases exponentially with increasing rate of bone loss.

The conclusions relevant to screening can be summarized as follows:

(1) Fast losers had increased bone turnover, which persisted over the 15-year follow-up period;

(2) Fast losers had approximately 1 standard deviation less bone mass after 15 years;

(3) Fast bone loss may predispose to fractures almost to the same extent as low bone mass;

(4) Low bone mass and fast rate of bone loss are additive risk factors;

(5) Rate of loss should be included in the risk stratification of postmenopausal women.

These findings also emphasize the need to combine bone mass and bone turnover assessments, which facilitates the prediction of bone status of the elderly, and thus the selection of individuals who can benefit most from preventive measures (Figure 4).

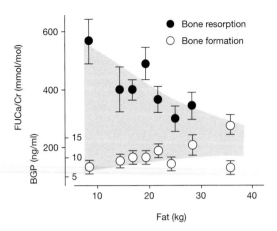

Figure 1 Bone resorption and formation in postmenopausal women as a function of total body fat mass. BGP, bone Gla protein; FUCa/Cr, fasting urinary calcium corrected for creatinine

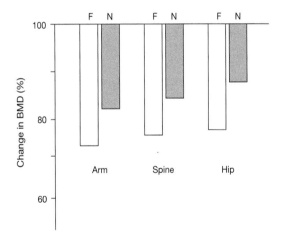

Figure 2 Changes in bone mineral density (BMD) (%) in 'fast losers' and 'normal losers' during a 15-year follow-up. F, fast loser (> 3% change in BMD per year); N, normal loser (< 3% change in BMD per year)

WHY THE SKELETAL EFFECTS OF HRT SHOULD NOT BE NEGLECTED

Currently, there are numerous antiresorptive therapies available on the market for the reversal of postmenopausal bone loss. Most, if not all,

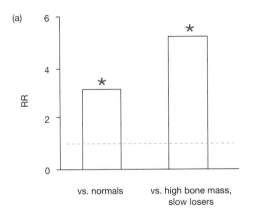

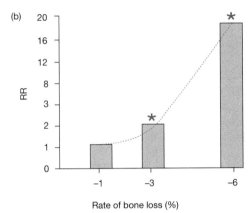

Figure 3 (a) Relative risk (RR) of osteoporotic fractures in women with low bone mass and accelerated bone loss versus normal controls and those with high bone mass and slow bone loss. (b) Relative risk (RR) of osteoporotic fractures as a function of the rate of bone loss. $^*p < 0.001$

Woman at 50 years	+	BONE MASS measurement	=	BONE MASS STATUS at 50 years
Woman at 50 years	+	Measurement of BIOCHEMICAL MARKERS	=	Prediction of RATE OF BONE LOSS
Woman at 50 years	+	Measurement of BONE MASS and BIOCHEMICAL MARKERS	=	Prediction of BONE MASS STATUS at 70 years

Figure 4 The value of combined bone mass and biomarker measurements in early-postmenopausal women for long-term prediction of bone status

Table 2 The relative effect of bisphosphonates on trabecular and cortical bone tissue. Extrapolating from these results, 2 years of treatment would increase 100% trabecular bone by 8.0% and 100% cortical bone by 0.8%

	Trabecular/ cortical	% Change in BMD
Spine	60/40	4.5
Hip	30/70	2.5
Total body	20/80	1/5
Arm	10/90	1/0
New ROI arm	65/35	5/0

ROI, regions of interest; BMD, bone mineral density

approved medications act sufficiently in bone compartments comprising mainly trabecular bone, but the effect at skeletal sites with cortical bone is less impressive. As an example, Table 2 illustrates the effect of bisphosphonate treatment at skeletal sites with different ratios of trabecular to cortical bone. Extrapolating from these results, the effect of 2 years of treatment would be to increase trabecular bone by 8% and cortical bone by 0.8%.

In other words, many therapeutic options are available for the prevention of vertebral fractures, but the prevention of non-vertebral fractures remains a weak point of osteoporosis therapy. This is seemingly least true for hormone replacement therapy (HRT). Historically, support for the use of estrogen replacement therapy for the prevention of bone loss and fractures comes from three lines of evidence. First, randomized clinical trials consistently show that this choice of therapy prevents postmenopausal bone loss (e.g. references 8 and 9). Second, observational studies consistently suggest that postmenopausal HRT reduces the risk of vertebral, hip and other types of osteoporotic fractures[10,11]. Third, early analyses of risk–benefit studies of

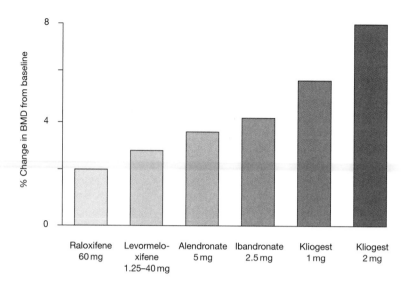

Figure 5 The relative potentials of different antiresorptive treatments for increasing bone mass. Kliogest® is estradiol + norethisterone acetate. BMD, bone mineral density

HRT for postmenopausal women indicated an increase in life-expectancy for most post-menopausal women, since protection against hip fracture and coronary heart disease would out-weigh the increase in the risk of breast cancer[10,12]. This latter perception was recently challenged by the Women's Health Initiative (WHI) study[13,14], yet, from the skeletal point of view, this study was the largest randomized setting that provided ultimate evidence for the ability of HRT to protect against hip fracture, the most feared complication of osteoporosis due to its significant contribution to morbidity and mortality in the elderly. No comparable evidence suggests that selective estrogen receptor modulators (SERMs) or bisphosphonates currently available can provide this therapeutic benefit.

Figure 5 summarizes percentage changes in spine BMD during treatment with effective doses of antiresorptive agents, clearly demonstrating the potentials of HRT (estradiol plus norethisterone acetate).

Figure 6 indicates that the relative benefits of HRT were greater at all skeletal sites when compared with an effective daily dose of alendronate in the Early Postmenopausal Intervention Cohort (EPIC) trial[15].

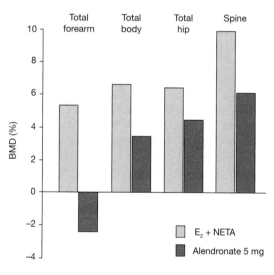

Figure 6 Changes in bone mineral density (BMD) with hormone replacement therapy (estradiol (E_2) plus norethisterone acetate (NETA)) versus alendronate at different skeletal sites[15]

Another critical issue is the percentage of women who respond to HRT. As shown in Figure 7, summarizing data from six different trials, the number of non-responders was very small.

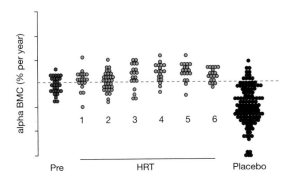

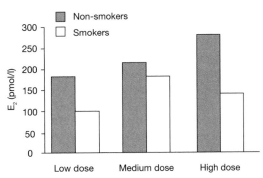

Figure 7 Changes in bone mineral content (BMC) in premenopausal and postmenopausal women treated with either placebo or hormone replacement therapy (HRT) (six different trials). Pre, premenopausal women

Figure 8 Serum estradiol (E_2) during oral hormone replacement therapy in non-smokers and smokers[16]

Who are typically the non-responders? We and others have repeatedly pointed out that smoking considerably attenuates the efficacy of oral HRT[16]. In smokers, the increase in serum estradiol during oral HRT is approximately half that in non-smokers, which can be explained by accelerated hepatic degradation of the sex steroid entering the portal circulation (first-pass effect). Figure 8 illustrates the phenomenon.

Thus, being a non-responder as a smoker can be effectively bypassed by prescribing transdermal HRT to women who smoke[16]. When in doubt, measurements of bone turnover may be informative regarding adequate response to the applied antiresorptive therapy.

IMPLICATIONS OF THE PROGESTIN COMPONENT FOR OVERALL EFFICACY

In women with an intact uterus, HRT means estrogen plus a progestin therapy. The primary role of the progestin is to protect the endometrium from chronic estrogen exposure, which may promote carcinogenesis and lead to endometrial cancer. However, observations suggest that selection of the progestin may have critical implications for overall benefits in terms of increasing bone mass. Figure 9 illustrates the

effects of different progestins and estradiol either alone or in combination on BMD during a 2-year treatment period[17-19].

Whereas medroxyprogesterone acetate (MPA) by itself tended to accelerate bone loss compared with placebo[17,18], norethisterone acetate (NETA) tended to decelerate bone loss[20]. Figure 10 shows results reported by Abdalla and colleagues illustrating that NETA by itself provided effective prevention of postmenopausal bone loss during a 12-month treatment period.

Estrogen alone increases BMD, which can be further enhanced by NETA but not by MPA[21]. This phenomenon can be attributed to the slight androgenic properties of NETA. Whereas oral estrogen increases sex hormone-binding globulin secretion from the liver that limits the bioavailability of estradiol, the androgenic properties of NETA may inhibit this response, ensuring sustained high bioavailability of estradiol. In addition, androgenic effects may also result in the stimulation of bone formation[22].

During conventional HRT there is a rapid decrease in bone resorption, followed by a slowly progressive decrease in bone formation (coupling). After 2–3 years of therapy, the increase in BMD may reach a maximum level[23]. Although this gain may provide a considerable relative protection against fractures, in certain cases further increases would be desirable. The application of androgenic progestins may maintain a relative 'uncoupling' between bone resorption and

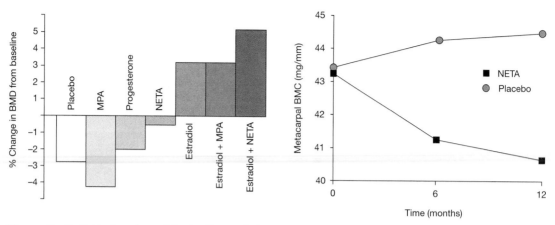

Figure 9 Individual and combined effects of the two components of hormone replacement therapy. BMD, bone mineral density; MPA, medroxyprogesterone acetate; NETA, norethisterone acetate

Figure 10 Changes in bone mineral content (BMC) during 12-month treatment with norethisterone acetate (NETA)

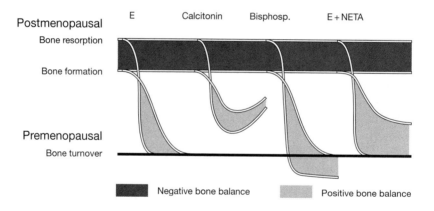

Figure 11 The relative impact of different antiresorptive therapies on bone resorption and formation in postmenopausal women. E, estrogen; NETA, norethisterone acetate; Bisphosph., bisphosphonate

formation, thereby opening up a wider range of positive calcium balance (i.e. therapeutic window). The relative impact of conventional HRT and some other antiresorptive agents versus estradiol plus NETA is illustrated in Figure 11.

This extra benefit can be particularly beneficial for preserving or increasing hip BMD. In other words, due consideration should be given to this therapeutic option when the aim of therapy is to counter rapid bone loss from the hip and prevention of hip fracture. Androgenic effects

can potentially facilitate preservation of skeletal muscle mass, which may have indirect implications for the prevention of hip fracture (by decreasing the risk of falls).

KEY CONCLUSIONS

(1) Early-postmenopausal women with low bone mass and elevated bone turnover are candidates for HRT;

190

(2) HRT provides effective protection not only for vertebral but also for non-vertebral bone;

(3) Smokers should be treated with transdermal HRT to avoid limited efficacy;

(4) Progestins with androgenic properties such as NETA may be preferential, especially when intending to protect the hip.

References

1. Albright F. The effect of hormones on osteo-genesis in man. *Rec Prog Horm Res* 1947; 1: 293–353

2. Hoshino H, Kushida K, Takahashi M, et al. Changes in levels of biochemical markers and ultrasound indices of os calcis across the menopausal transition. *Osteoporos Int* 2000; 11: 128–33

3. Seifert-Klauss V, Mueller JE, Luppa P, et al. Bone metabolism during the perimenopausal transition: a prospective study. *Maturitas* 2002; 41: 23–33

4. Nordin BE, Wishart JM, Clifton PM, et al. A longitudinal study of bone-related biochemical changes at the menopause. *Clin Endocrinol (Oxf)* 2004; 61: 123–30

5. Garnero P, Dargent-Molina P, Hans D, et al. Do markers of bone resorption add to bone mineral density and ultrasonographic heel measurement for the prediction of hip fracture in elderly women? The EPIDOS prospective study. *Osteoporos Int* 1998; 8: 563–9

6. Meier C, Nguyen TV, Center JR, et al. Bone resorption and osteoporotic fractures in elderly men: the Dubbo osteoporosis epidemiology study. *J Bone Miner Res* 2005; 20: 579–87

7. Garnero P, Hausherr E, Chapuy MC, et al. Markers of bone resorption predict hip fracture in elderly women: the EPIDOS Prospective Study. *J Bone Miner Res* 1996; 11: 1531–8

8. The Writing Group for the PEPI. Effects of hormone therapy on bone mineral density: results from the postmenopausal estrogen/progestin interventions (PEPI) trial. *J Am Med Assoc* 1996; 276: 1389–96

9. NIH Consensus Development Panel on Osteoporosis Prevention, Diagnosis, and Therapy, March 7–29, 2000: highlights of the conference. *South Med J* 2001; 94: 569–73

10. Grady D, Rubin SM, Petitti DB, et al. Hormone therapy to prevent disease and prolong life in postmenopausal women. *Ann Intern Med* 1992; 117: 1016–37

11. Lindsay R. Estrogen deficiency. In Riggs BL, Melton LJ III, eds. *Osteoporosis: Etiology, Diagnosis, and Management*, 2nd edn. Philadelphia: Lippincott-Raven, 1995: 133–60

12. Burkman RT, Collins JA, Greene RA. Current perspectives on benefits and risks of hormone replacement therapy. *Am J Obstet Gynecol* 2001; 185: S13–23

13. Rossouw JE, Anderson GL, Prentice RL, et al. Risks and benefits of estrogen plus progestin in healthy postmenopausal women: principal results from the Women's Health Initiative randomized controlled trial. *J Am Med Assoc* 2002; 288: 321–33

14. Anderson GL, Limacher M, Assaf AR, et al. Effects of conjugated equine estrogen in postmenopausal women with hysterectomy: the Women's Health Initiative randomized controlled trial. *J Am Med Assoc* 2004; 291: 1701–12

15. Ravn P, Bidstrup M, Wasnich RD, et al. Alendronate and estrogen–progestin in the long-term prevention of bone loss: four-year results from the Early Postmenopausal Intervention Cohort study. A randomized, controlled trial. *Ann Intern Med* 1999; 131: 935–42

16. Tanko LB, Christiansen C. An update on the antiestrogenic effect of smoking: a literature review with implications for researchers and practitioners. *Menopause* 2004; 11: 104–9

17. Hosking DJ. *J Bone Miner Res* 1996; 11 (Suppl 1): 133

18. Ishida Y, Ishida Y, Heersche JN. Pharmacologic doses of medroxyprogesterone may cause bone loss through glucocorticoid activity: an hypothesis. *Osteoporos Int* 2002; 13: 601–5

19. Clark MK, Sowers MR, Nichols S, Levy B. Bone mineral density changes over two years in first-time users of depot medroxyprogesterone acetate. *Fertil Steril* 2004; 82: 1580–6

20. Abdalla HI, Hart DM, Lindsay R, et al. Prevention of bone mineral loss in postmenopausal women by norethisterone. *Obstet Gynecol* 1985; 66: 789–92

21. Riis BJ, Lehmann HJ, Christiansen C. Norethisterone acetate in combination with estrogen: effects on the skeleton and other organs. A review. *Am J Obstet Gynecol* 2002; 187: 1101–16

22. Notelovitz M. Androgen effects on bone and muscle. *Fertil Steril* 2002; 77: S34–41

23. Komulainen M, Kroger H, Tuppurainen MT, et al. Prevention of femoral and lumbar bone loss with hormone replacement therapy and vitamin D3 in early postmenopausal women: a population-based 5-year randomized trial. *J Clin Endocrinol Metab* 1999; 84: 546–52

New physiologic approach to prevention of postmenopausal osteoporosis

21

B. Ettinger and J. S. Lee

INTRODUCTION

The purpose of this review is to summarize the epidemiologic and clinical trial evidence for estrogen's physiologic role in skeletal health among aging women. Emerging data from these studies indicate a need to redefine the levels at which estrogen physiologic adequacy is achieved, and support the use of much lower estrogen doses than are currently prescribed.

EPIDEMIOLOGIC STUDIES

Multiple epidemiologic studies have shown a relationship between low endogenous estradiol levels and low bone mineral density in postmenopausal women. In the Study of Osteoporotic Fractures (SOF) cohort of US women over age 65 years, estradiol was undetectable (< 5 pg/ml) in about one out of four. Compared with these women, those whose endogenous serum estradiol levels were 10–25 pg/ml had 4.9% higher bone mineral density (BMD) at the hip and 6.8% higher BMD at the lumbar spine[1]. In the Rotterdam Study of Dutch women aged 55 years and older, one-third of women had estradiol levels below 5 pg/ml, and again spinal BMD was about 6% higher among women whose serum estradiol levels exceeded 7 pg/ml, compared with those with very low levels[2]. In another US cohort of women aged 65–75 years, one-third had serum estradiol levels less than 9 pg/ml; their hip BMD was 14% lower and spine BMD was 9% lower than in those women whose estradiol levels exceeded 13.3 pg/ml[3].

In these same studies, an inverse relationship between BMD and sex hormone-binding globulin (SHBG) was also seen. Estradiol circulates bound to SHBG, and levels of SHBG determine in large part the amount of bioavailable estradiol. Higher levels of SHBG lowered bioavailable circulating estradiol, and this was linked to lower BMD. These substantial BMD differences persisted after adjustment for multiple risk factors including body mass index[1–3].

Bone turnover appears to be an independent risk factor for fracture[4]. Endogenous estradiol and bioavailable estradiol are inversely related to bone turnover; compared with those with higher levels of endogenous estradiol, women with levels in the lower one-third showed 10–20% higher levels of bone turnover markers[1,3].

As expected from these key physiologic differences in BMD and bone turnover, women with very low estradiol levels have been uniformly shown to have higher risks for fracture[1,2,4,5]. In the SOF cohort, very low estradiol was associated with more than twice the risk of hip or spine fracture (Figure 1), and adjustment for estradiol binding to SHBG further strengthened the associations between estradiol and fracture risk (Figure 2)[5]. Associations between serum estradiol and fracture risk have now been confirmed in two European cohorts[2,4]. In the OFELY observational study (Os des Femmes de Lyon) of postmenopausal French women aged 50–89 years (mean age 64 years), during 5 years of follow-up, women with low endogenous serum estradiol levels had twice the risk of any fracture than did women with higher levels of serum estradiol (Figure 3)[4]. In the Rotterdam Study, compared with women with estradiol levels > 7 pg/ml, those with levels < 5 pg/ml showed twice the risk of incident vertebral fracture during 6.5 years of follow-up (Figure 4)[2]. This latter study also confirmed the importance of SHBG, finding that women in the upper one-third level of SHBG had twice the risk of those in the lower one-third. Moreover, those women with both low estradiol and high SHBG levels were at considerably increased risk of fracture, compared with those without these characteristics.

CLINICAL TRIALS OF LOW-DOSE ESTROGEN

For the purpose of this review, 0.625 mg conjugated estrogens/day or its equivalent is considered standard dosage; 0.3 mg conjugated estrogens or its equivalent (e.g. 0.5 mg/day oral micronized estradiol or 25 μg/day transdermal estradiol) is considered low dosage; and half this amount (0.25 mg/day oral micronized estradiol or 14 μg/day transdermal estradiol) is considered very low or microdosage. Currently, the only microdosage estrogen marketed for osteoporosis prevention is the transdermal 14 μg/day product.

Recent studies designed to test various doses of estrogen have uniformly shown a linear dose response of the skeleton from the lowest to the highest doses tested[6–12]. This dose effect extends down to very low levels of plasma estradiol (10–20 pg/ml), and has been shown for various estrogen formulations and routes of administration. Similar results are seen with lower doses in the elderly to those in the early postmenopause[7,13]. *In toto*, these studies indicate that there is no threshold level for estrogen activity on the skeleton, but rather a small incremental effect with each increment in dose.

Estrogen's skeletal benefit is mediated by its antiresorptive effect, and thus can be measured by reductions in biochemical markers of bone turnover. Typically, standard doses of estrogens

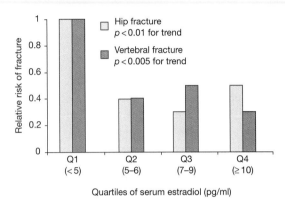

Figure 1 Age-adjusted relative risk of fracture in postmenopausal women ≥ 65 years of age versus quartile of baseline serum estradiol levels. *p* for trend < 0.01 for hip fracture and < 0.005 for vertebral fracture. Hip fracture analysis included 317 women; vertebral fracture analysis included 282 women. Reproduced with permission from reference 5

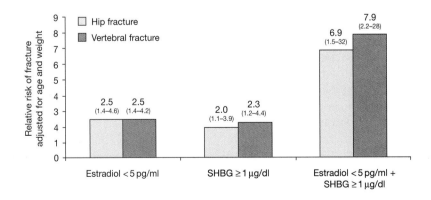

Figure 2 Age- and weight-adjusted relative risks (95% confidence intervals) of hip or vertebral fracture in postmenopausal women with undetectable serum estradiol levels (< 5 pg/ml), high serum sex hormone-binding globulin (SHBG) levels (≥ 1 μg/dl) or both, compared with women without these factors. Adapted from reference 5

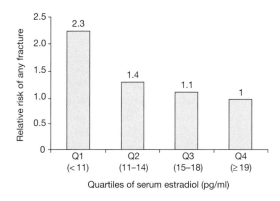

Figure 3 Relative risk of any fracture in 435 postmenopausal women (mean age 64 years) by quartile of baseline serum estradiol: the OFELY (Os des Femmes de Lyon) study. Reproduced with permission from reference 4

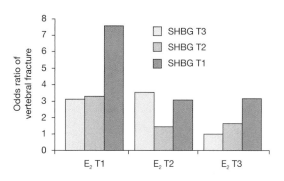

Figure 4 Odds ratios for incident vertebral fracture based on tertiles of serum estradiol (E_2) and sex hormone-binding globulin (SHBG) in 454 postmenopausal women ≥ 55 years old: the Rotterdam Study. Reproduced with permission from reference 2

reduce turnover by 40–50%[11], while low doses of oral estrogens[11,13] or transdermal estradiol[14] suppress bone turnover markers by about 25–30%.

The ultimate measure of estrogen's skeletal protection is reduction in fracture risk. The Women's Health Initiative showed that an average of 5.2 years of standard-dose estrogen combined with 2.5 mg medroxyprogesterone acetate reduced the risk of hip and clinical spine fractures by one-third[15]. In a parallel study of unopposed standard-dose estrogen lasting 7 years, similar fracture risk reductions were observed[16]. No similar clinical trial of low-dose estrogen on fracture risk has been conducted. One case–control study, with relatively small numbers of subjects, was not able to show that the use of lower doses of estrogen was associated with lower hip fracture risk[17]. Thus, while the links between antiresorptive effect, preservation of bone density and fracture risk reduction are well understood, clinical trial evidence is lacking for fracture risk reduction with the use of low-dose estrogen.

CLINICAL TRIALS OF VERY LOW ESTROGEN

In a short-term study, delivery of 7.5 μg/day by a transvaginal ring system showed modest suppression of bone turnover and small increments in radial BMD[18]; this route and formulation causes, at most, a few pg/ml rise in serum estradiol. Among women 65 years and older, relative to placebo, 0.25 mg oral micronized estradiol increased spine BMD by 2% and hip BMD by 4% over 3 years of study[19]. Unfortunately, the immunoassay used in this study did not provide accurate assessment of estradiol levels produced by this treatment.

Further proof of the concept that levels of about 10 pg/ml are linked to bone benefit in the elderly comes from a 2-year clinical trial of 417 women aged 60–80 years who received either placebo or 14 μg estradiol/day via a transdermal estradiol patch system[20]. Transdermal delivery of 14 μg/day estradiol raised median serum estradiol levels from 4.8 to 8.6 pg/ml during the ultralow-dosage transdermal estradiol assessment (ULTRA) study. Bone mineral density measured at the lumbar spine and total hip showed statistically significant increases from baseline; relative to those receiving placebo, the mean increase in BMD in women receiving the 14 μg patch was 2.0% and 1.2% at spine and hip, respectively (Figure 5). The improvement in BMD was linked to a 22% suppression of bone turnover markers. Thus, levels of plasma estradiol that would be considered inconsequentially

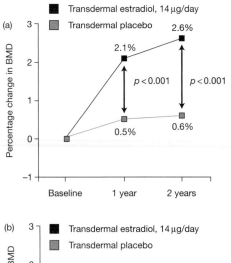

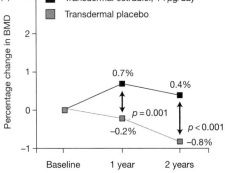

Figure 5 Percentage change from baseline lumbar spine bone mineral density (BMD) (a) and total hip BMD (b) over 2 years in postmenopausal women (60–80 years old) using transdermal estradiol 14 μg ($n = 208$) or placebo patch ($n = 209$). Reproduced with permission from reference 20

low in premenopausal women prevented bone loss.

Furthermore, the observed BMD increases and bone turnover decreases in the ULTRA study were related to the baseline level of endogenous estradiol[21]. Women who began the 2-year study with serum estradiol below the median (< 5 pg/ml) showed substantially greater skeletal response to estradiol treatment compared with those with higher levels of endogenous estradiol (Figure 6).

There is controversy over the ideal level of bone turnover to be achieved by antiresorptive therapy, many supporting the goal of reducing bone turnover to a level at or below the mean of

healthy premenopausal women but not to excessively low levels. Mean bone turnover reductions seen with very low oral[22] or transdermal[20] estrogens (about 20–25%) are similar in magnitude to those reported in women who received raloxifene, a drug that reduces risk of vertebral fracture by 36% during 3 years of treatment[23].

Some limited fracture data suggest that very low estrogen reduces the risk of clinical fractures. In the oral very-low-estradiol study, after 3 years, six fractures occurred among women receiving placebo while two were noted in the estradiol-treated group[19]. A similar ratio was observed during 2 years in the ULTRA study (ten in the placebo-treated group and four in the estradiol-treated group)[20]. Although neither study alone had sufficient statistical power for fracture outcomes, combining the results of both studies yields a significant reduction in risk (relative risk 0.4, $p < 0.05$).

Larger, long-term trials are needed to determine fracture risk reductions accurately as well as other potential benefits and harms of very-low-dosage estradiol therapy.

WHO SHOULD RECEIVE VERY LOW ESTROGEN?

Women who have continued to take hormone therapy

Despite the high rate of discontinuation in hormone therapy (HT) since publication of the Women's Health Initiative (WHI) study, about half of prior users remain on HT[24]. Most of these continuing users remain on standard estrogen doses in combination with daily progestin[24]. A large body of clinical trial data show that low- and very-low-estrogen therapies have far greater tolerability[7,9,11,20] than standard regimens; this is particularly important for achieving the lowest incidence of bleeding and breast tenderness, the major reasons for women's discontinuation of HT[25]. These data, coupled with emerging efficacy data, suggest that providers should consider changing a woman's hormone regimen over time. Whereas standard dosages are often required for troublesome symptoms at the time

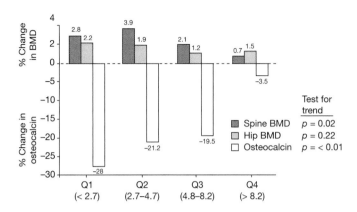

Figure 6 Mean differences in lumbar spine bone mineral density (BMD), total hip BMD and serum osteocalcin levels between women receiving transdermal estradiol 14 μg (*n* = 208) or placebo patch (*n* = 209) by quartile of baseline estradiol. Adapted from reference 21

of the menopausal transition, switching to lower dosages may become acceptable after some months of therapy. Half-strength regimens appear to be adequate to control vasomotor symptoms[26–28] as well as prevent bone loss[7–13]. Low-dosage estrogen is likely to become the preferred HT option because of its superior tolerability and because of greater potential for patient acceptance and continuation. Health-care providers should now make every attempt to reduce the dosage to the lowest that is acceptable (i.e. controls menopausal symptoms) and is likely to promote health. A trial of reducing dosage in long-term users of standard HT to half-strength estrogen dosage found that only 6.5% returned to the standard dosage because of unacceptable vasomotor symptoms[29]. This same study showed that long-cycle progestin (14 days every 6 months) was adequate to protect the endometrium. Gradual tapering of the dose can be accomplished by alternate-day oral therapy or by reduction in transdermal patch strength.

Women who have recently stopped using hormone therapy

Approximately one in five women who stopped HT after learning of the Women's Health Initiative results report persisting and troublesome vasomotor symptoms[30]. These women have made the choice to live with the symptoms and lose bone density rather than return to HT. It is not known how many of them have been given counseling about low- and very-low-dosage HT. Adequate proof exists for the efficacy of low-dose estrogen in the relief of hot flushes and other menopausal symptoms, but only anecdotal evidence is thus far available for symptom relief using very low doses.

New starts for very low estrogen

In today's climate of increased concern about adverse effects of HT, many women would rather avoid starting standard HT. Lower doses of estrogen may not be effective in the control of severe vasomotor symptoms, especially in young oophorectomized women. However, for women well beyond the menopausal transition, who are not very troubled by vasomotor symptoms and who are at risk for osteoporosis, very low estrogen may be acceptable. The otherwise healthy woman who is at increased risk for osteoporosis can be identified by using the easily obtained National Osteoporosis Foundation (NOF) key risk factors: thinness, smoking, mother or sister with hip fracture and personal history of fracture[31]. Given the choice between bisphosphonates, raloxifene and the three levels of estrogen therapy, many women meeting these NOF criteria would choose very low estrogen.

HOW SHOULD UNOPPOSED VERY LOW ESTROGEN BE MONITORED?

Use of serum estradiol

Ideally, serum estradiol measurement could be used to guide initiation and follow-up of very-low-dose estrogen therapy, but only a few laboratories use the sensitive radioimmunoassay capable of accurately measuring very low levels of estradiol. Most clinical laboratories in the USA use the automated enzyme-linked immunosorbent assay (ELISA), for which the Food and Drug Administration (FDA)-approved lower limit of sensitivity is 15 pg/ml[32].

For skeletal effects

Ideally, antiresorptive therapy should be monitored for its effects using biochemical measures of bone turnover; usually, after 3–6 months of therapy, turnover markers reach a nadir. If the marker level is not at or below the premenopausal mean, then adjustment in dosage could be considered.

For endometrial safety

Endometrial proliferation is exceedingly rare among women aged 60 years and older because the production of estradiol in these women yields levels below the stimulation threshold for the endometrium. At the end of 2 years of 14 µg transdermal estradiol given *unopposed*, < 2% of women showed evidence of endometrial proliferation[33]. In this same study, the incidence of vaginal bleeding was not significantly increased by this dosage of estradiol. Thus, physiologic estrogen replacement should not require progestin opposition and, consistent with this, the US FDA has not required that concomitant daily or monthly progestin be used; they have, however, recommended the use of long-cycle progestin (14 days every 6–12 months) as a precaution against the development of endometrial abnormalities.

CONCLUSIONS

The foregoing review supports redefining estrogen deficiency among elderly women – not in comparison with premenopausal levels, but considering the physiologic effects of estradiol in this age group. In premenopausal women, serum estradiol ranges from about 50 to 200 pg/ml, depending on the menstrual cycle phase; standard HT increases levels of estradiol into this range. In marked contrast, most older postmenopausal women have levels below 10 pg/ml[1,2,5,12,20]. Those below the mean (e.g. 5–9 pg/ml, depending on the assay) have lower BMD, higher bone turnover and greater fracture risk compared with their peers whose levels are above the mean. Physiologic enhancement aimed at increasing serum estradiol to an age-appropriate level is able to reduce bone turnover and prevent bone loss. Given the remarkable new research showing that a small amount of circulating estradiol is needed for bone health, and having the means to restore levels to those appropriate for age, providers can add microdosage estradiol to their osteoporosis prevention armamentarium.

WHAT IS THE FUTURE FOR VERY-LOW-ESTROGEN THERAPY?

Further studies of very low estradiol will help to provide additional long-term safety and efficacy information. Both a head-to-head comparison of BMD effects against raloxifene and a trial of effectiveness for relief of hot flushes are under way. A 3–5-year study is planned to examine its effect on fracture risk and long-term endometrial safety. Beyond these, a new generation of low-dose estrogen studies will be required to document adequately the risks and benefits.

ADDENDUM

This addendum is intended for readers of this chapter interested in knowing more about methodologies used to measure serum estradiol in very low concentrations, 0–20 pg/ml.

Differences in reported postmenopausal serum levels should be considered by those intending to use these assays for research or clinical applications. Without a practical method for standardizing assays, measuring low levels of estradiol using such assays and interpreting results of epidemiological studies[1–5,20] remain a challenge. The purpose of this review is to compare results of various estradiol assay methods and suggest a means for standardization.

In an immunoassay system, measurement of an analyte is generally based on the analyte binding the detection antibody and preventing the antibody from binding to either a solid phase or a tagged reporter molecule. The matrix is defined as everything other than the analyte in the immunoassay sample. Ill-defined matrix effects can be due to substances interfering with different aspects of the immunoassay, such as inhibiting signaling detection or affecting binding of the labeled antibody to the solid phase, to the analyte itself or to both. Thus, matrix effects may falsely under- or overestimate the true concentration of the analyte[34].

Estradiol immunoassays typically use either a radioactive or a non-radioactive detection marker, work by an excess-antigen/limited-antibody system (competitive immunoassay) and are performed with (extraction-type) or without (direct-type) purification steps. Extraction-type assays employ initial solvent extraction and subsequent chromatographic separation of estradiol from other steroids; they typically use radioactive estradiol as a marker. Direct immunoassays use either chemiluminescent or colorimetric markers and are typically faster and less labor-intensive (automated) than extraction-type assays. The presence of serum sex hormone-binding globulin and the difficulty in obtaining appropriate buffers have contributed to interference and matrix effects, leading to greater inaccuracy (higher or lower estradiol measurements) by direct immunoassays than by extraction-type assays. New methods are being developed to characterize better and reduce sample matrix effects in estradiol assays[34]. Extraction-chromatography may better remove estradiol from sex hormone-binding globulin and minimize potential cross-reacting steroids.

Estradiol measurements from different assays produce varying results at low estradiol levels[35–39]. For example, the mean of 20 postmenopausal women's estradiol levels using different direct assays ranged from 8 to 43 pg/ml, while an indirect assay measured a mean level < 3 pg/ml[36]. Newer direct assays and rapid extraction methods report improved accuracy and precision at postmenopausal estradiol levels[40,41].

The assays used in the epidemiologic and clinical studies reviewed in this chapter all share excellent sensitivities (ability to distinguish differences between a few pg/ml and none) as well as excellent precision (coefficient of variation on the order of 10% at levels of 10 pg/ml). The Rotterdam Study, STOP/IT study (Sites Testing Osteoporosis Prevention/Intervention) and ULTRA study all measured estradiol by direct immunoassays, while the OFELY and SOF studies used extraction-based radioimmunoassay (Table 1)[1–5,20]. Characteristic of direct immunoassays, the direct assays used by the Rotterdam Study, the ULTRA study and the STOP/IT study all report very low limits of detection, 1.3 pg/ml, 1.4 pg/ml and 2.2 pg/ml, respectively, which are lower than those of indirect radioimmunoassays (3 pg/ml and 5 pg/ml in the OFELY and SOF studies, respectively)[1–5,20].

The key issue is accuracy: are results obtained by the various assays really true? Examining the estradiol cut-off point for clinical outcomes is a useful way to compare these assays. Table 1 shows the lowest tertile or quartile cut-off points that, in these studies, were associated with either greater fracture risk or greater response to treatment; note the critical values differ four-fold, from < 2.7 pg/ml to < 11 pg/ml.

We conclude that there is substantial variability in measurements of low serum estradiol concentrations across different estradiol immunoassay methods. For estradiol to be clinically useful for discriminating risks of osteoporosis and predicting response to therapy, assay methods should be standardized. Mass spectrometry, using gas or liquid chromatography, has been suggested as a gold standard for measuring low estradiol levels; this method is capable of measuring to 0.1 pg/ml, but is not yet widely

Table 1 Characteristics of estradiol (E_2) assays used in large epidemiologic studies of bone health in post-menopausal women

Study	Assay type[*]	Manufacturer	E_2 detection limit (pg/ml)[†]	Lowest E_2 tertile or quartile (pg/ml)[†]
Cummings et al.[5], 1998 Ettinger et al.[1], 1998 SOF	extraction	Endocrine Sciences, Inc.	5	< 5 (quartile)
Garnero et al.[4], 2000 OFELY study	extraction	radioimmunoassay (in-house method)	3	< 11 (quartile)
Goderie-Plomp et al.[2], 2004 Rotterdam Study	direct	Diagnostic Systems Laboratories	1.3	< 11 (tertile)
Rapuri et al.[3], 2004 STOP/IT study	direct	Diagnostic Systems Laboratories	2.2	7.1 ± 0.14 (tertile)[‡]
Ettinger et al.[20], 2004 ULTRA study	direct	Diagnostic Products Corporation	1.4	< 2.7 (quartile)

[*]Extraction-type assay consists of an initial extraction step; [†]multiply pg/ml by 3.67 to convert to pmol/l; [‡]mean ± standard deviation of lowest tertile; SOF, Study of Osteoporotic Fractures; OFELY, Os des Femmes de Lyon; STOP/IT, Sites Testing Osteoporosis Prevention/Intervention; ULTRA, ultralow-dosage transdermal estradiol assessment

available[42]. Just as manufacturers of cholesterol assays have agreed to standardize their assays to results obtained by ultracentrifugation, those measuring estradiol could use mass spectrometry to provide this much needed standardization.

References

1. Ettinger B, Pressman A, Sklarin P, et al. Associations between low levels of serum estradiol, bone density, and fractures among elderly women: the study of osteoporotic fractures. *J Clin Endocrinol Metab* 1998; 83: 2239–43

2. Goderie-Plomp HW, Van Der Klift M, De Ronde W, et al. Endogenous sex hormones, sex hormone-binding globulin, and risk of vertebral fractures in elderly men and women: the Rotterdam Study. *J Clin Endocrinol Metab* 2004; 89: 3261–9

3. Rapuri PB, Gallagher JC, Haynatzi G. Endogenous levels of serum estradiol and sex hormone-binding globulin determine bone mineral density, bone remodeling, the rate of bone loss, and responses to treatment with estrogen in elderly women. *J Clin Endocrinol Metab* 2004; 89: 4954–62

4. Garnero P, Sornay-Rendu E, Claustrat B, et al. Biochemical markers of bone turnover, endogenous hormones and risk of fractures in postmenopausal women: the OFELY study. *J Bone Miner Res* 2000; 15: 1526–36

5. Cummings SR, Browner WS, Bauer D, et al. Endogenous hormones and the risk of hip and vertebral fractures among older women. Study of Osteoporotic Fractures Research Group. *N Engl J Med* 1998; 339: 733–8

6. Ettinger B, Genant HK, Steiger P, et al. Low-dosage micronized 17 beta-estradiol prevents bone loss in postmenopausal women. *Am J Obstet Gynecol* 1992; 166: 479–88

7. Evans SF, Davie MW. Low and conventional dose transdermal oestradiol are equally effective at preventing bone loss in spine and femur at all postmenopausal ages. *Clin Endocrinol (Oxf)* 1996; 44: 79–84

8. Genant HK, Lucas J, Weiss S, Akin M, et al. Low-dose esterified estrogen therapy: effects on bone, plasma estradiol concentrations, endometrium, and lipid levels. Estratab/Osteoporosis Study Group. *Arch Intern Med* 1997; 157: 2609–15

9. Delmas PD, Pornel B, Felsenberg D, et al. Three-year follow up of the use of transdermal 17 beta-estradiol matrix patches for the prevention of bone loss in early postmenopausal women. *Am J Obstet Gynecol* 2001; 184: 32–40

10. Notelovitz M, John VA, Good WR. Effectiveness of Alora estradiol matrix transdermal delivery system in improving lumbar bone mineral density in healthy, postmenopausal women. *Menopause* 2002; 9: 343–53

11. Lindsay R, Gallagher JC, Kleerekoper M, et al. Effect of lower doses of conjugated equine estrogens with and without medroxyprogesterone acetate on bone in early postmenopausal women. *J Am Med Assoc* 2002; 287: 2668–76

12. Weiss SR, Ellman H, Dolker M. A randomized controlled trial of four doses of transdermal estradiol for preventing postmenopausal bone loss. Transdermal Estradiol Investigator Group. *Obstet Gynecol* 1999; 94: 330–6

13. Recker RR, Davies KM, Dowd RM, et al. The effect of low-dose continuous estrogen and progesterone therapy with calcium and vitamin D on bone in elderly women. A randomized, controlled trial. *Ann Intern Med* 1999; 130: 897–904

14. Sharp CA, Evans SF, Risteli L, et al. Effects of low- and conventional-dose transcutaneous HRT over 2 years on bone metabolism in younger and older postmenopausal women. *Eur J Clin Invest* 1996; 26: 763–71

15. Rossouw JE, Anderson GL, Prentice RL, et al. Writing Group for the Women's Health Initiative Investigators. Risks and benefits of estrogen plus progestin in healthy postmenopausal women: principal results from the Women's Health Initiative randomized controlled trial. *J Am Med Assoc* 2002; 288: 321–33

16. Anderson GL, Limacher M, Assaf AR, et al. Women's Health Initiative Steering Committee. Effects of conjugated equine estrogen in postmenopausal women with hysterectomy: the Women's Health Initiative randomized controlled trial. *J Am Med Assoc* 2004; 291: 1701–12

17. Michaëlsson K, Baron JA, Farahmand BY, et al. On behalf of the Swedish Hip Fracture Study Group. Hormone replacement therapy and risk of hip fracture: population-based case–control study. *Br Med J* 1999; 316: 1858–63

18. Naessen T, Berglund L, Ulmsten U. Bone loss in elderly women prevented by ultralow doses of parenteral 17 beta-estradiol. *Am J Obstet Gynecol* 1997; 177: 115–19

19. Prestwood KM, Kenny AM, Kleppinger A, et al. Ultralow-dose micronized 17 beta-estradiol and bone density and bone metabolism in older women: a randomized controlled trial. *J Am Med Assoc* 2003; 290: 1042–8

20. Ettinger B, Ensrud KE, Wallace R, et al. Effects of ultralow-dose transdermal estradiol on bone mineral density: a randomized clinical trial. *Obstet Gynecol* 2004; 104: 443–51

21. Cummings SR, Yankov V, Ensrud K, et al. Ultralow estradiol increases BMD and decreases bone turnover in older women, particularly those with undetectable estradiol: the ULTRA Trial. *J Bone Miner Res* 2003; 18: S53 (abstr)

22. Prestwood KM, Kenny AM, Unson C, et al. The effect of low-dose micronized 17 beta-estradiol on bone turnover, sex hormone levels, and side effects in older women: a randomized, double blind, placebo-controlled study. *J Clin Endocrinol Metab* 2000; 85: 4462–9

23. Ettinger B, Black DM, Mitlak BH, et al. Reduction of vertebral fracture risk in postmenopausal women with osteoporosis treated with raloxifene: results from a 3-year randomized clinical trial. Multiple Outcomes of Raloxifene Evaluation (MORE) Investigators [Published erratum appears in *J Am Med Assoc* 1999; 282: 2124]. *J Am Med Assoc* 1999; 282: 637–45

24. Hersh AL, Stefanik ML, Stafford RS. National use of postmenopausal hormone therapy. *J Am Med Assoc* 2004; 291: 47–53

25. Ettinger B, Pressman A, Silver P. Effect of age on reasons for initiation and discontinuation of hormone replacement therapy. *Menopause* 1999; 6: 282–9

26. Speroff L, Whitcomb RW, Kempfert NJ, et al. Efficacy and local tolerance of a low-dose, 7-day matrix estradiol transdermal system in the treatment of menopausal vasomotor symptoms. *Obstet Gynecol* 1996; 88: 587–92

27. Utian WH, Burry KA, Archer DF, et al. Efficacy and safety of low, standard, and high dosages of an estradiol transdermal system (Esclim) compared with placebo on vasomotor symptoms in highly symptomatic menopausal patients. The Esclim Study Group. *Am J Obstet Gynecol* 1999; 181: 71–9

28. Utian WH, Shoupe D, Bachmann G, et al. Relief of vasomotor symptoms and vaginal atrophy with lower doses of conjugated equine estrogens and medroxyprogesterone acetate. *Fertil Steril* 2001; 75: 1065–79

29. Ettinger B. Pressman A, Van Gessel A. Low-dosage esterified estrogens opposed by progestin at 6-month intervals. *Obstet Gynecol* 2001; 98: 205–11

30. Grady D, Ettinger B, Tosteson ANA, et al. Predictors of difficulty when discontinuing postmenopausal hormone therapy. *Obstet Gynecol* 2003; 102: 1233–9

31. National Osteoporosis Foundation. *Physician's Guide to Prevention and Treatment of Osteoporosis*. Washington, DC: Excerpta Medica, 1998

32. Diagnostic Products Corporation. Immulite® Estradiol. Technical Bulletin PILKE2-5, 2003-08-12. Los Angeles: Diagnostic Products Corporation, 2003

33. Johnson SR, Ettinger B, Macer JL, et al. Uterine and vaginal effects of unopposed ultralow-dose transdermal estradiol. *Obstet Gynecol* 2005; in press

34. Glass TR, Ohmura N, Saiki H, Sackie SJ. A combination of labeled and unlabeled antibody enables self-calibration and reduction of sample matrix effects in immunoassay. *Anal Biochem* 2004; 331: 68–76

35. Key TJ, and Endogenous Hormones Breast Cancer Collaborative Group. Body mass index, serum sex hormones, and breast cancer risk in postmenopausal women. *J Natl Cancer Inst* 2003; 95: 1218–26

36. Rinaldi S, Dechaud H, Biessy C, et al. Reliability and validity of commercially available, direct radioimmunoassays for measurement of blood androgens and estrogens in postmenopausal women. *Cancer Epidemiol Biomark Prev* 2001; 10: 757–65

37. Falk RT, Dorgan JF, Kahle L, et al. Assay reproducibility of hormone measurements in postmenopausal women. *Cancer Epidemiol Biomark Prev* 1997; 6: 429–32

38. Hankinson SE, Manson JE, London SJ, et al. Laboratory reproducibility of endogenous hormone levels in postmenopausal women. *Cancer Epidemiol Biomark Prev* 1994; 3: 51–6

39. Stanczyk FZ, Cho MM, Endres DB, et al. Limitations of direct estradiol and testosterone immunoassay kits. *Steroids* 2003; 68: 1173–8

40. England BG, Parsons GH, Possley RM, et al. Ultrasensitive semiautomated chemiluminescent immunoassay for estradiol. *Clin Chem* 2002; 48: 1584–6

41. Dighe AS, Sluss PM. Improved detection of serum estradiol after sample extraction procedure. *Clin Chem* 2004; 50: 764–6

42. Nelson RE, Grebe SK, O'Kane DJ, Singh RJ. Liquid chromatography-tandem mass spectrometry assay for simultaneous measurement of estradiol and estrone in human plasma. *Clin Chem* 2004; 50: 373–84

Selective estrogen receptor modulators 22

A. Diez-Pérez

INTRODUCTION

Selective estrogen receptor modulators (SERMs) are a group of compounds characterized by binding to the estrogen receptor. Chemically, they are heterogeneous, and have been grouped into five categories[1]: triphenylethylenes (tamoxifen, droloxifene, idoxifene, clomiphene and toremiphene), benzothiophenes (raloxifene, arzoxifene), tetrahydronaphthylenes (lasofoxifene, nafoxidine), indoles (bazedoxifene) and benzopyrans (EM-800, levormeloxifene). Other compounds are currently in development. To date, few of them are approved for human use, and only raloxifene is indicated for patients with postmenopausal osteoporosis.

Their mechanism of action is mainly antiresorptive, by inhibiting the bone-resorbing cell, the osteoclast. However, the intimate process is largely unknown. SERMs are not hormones, but they act as ligands for the estrogen receptor (ER). After binding to the estrogen receptor, an intracellular factor called a response element combines with the ER–SERM complex, eliciting the genomic response. There are a number of other factors that regulate this response pathway.

The ER mainly comprises two categories, ERα and ERβ. These receptors map differently in different organs and tissues. Therefore, different SERMs (as well as the natural ligand, estradiol) can activate more predominantly one or the other. The conformational changes of the ER–ligand complex can vary for different ligands[2]. Furthermore, the various ligands can activate different intracellular pathways, combining with different response elements[3]. Considered together, the genomic responses for the various compounds differ among themselves and with respect to estradiol for the two receptor subtypes, and for different activating or repressing

genes expressed differently for the various SERMs[4].

EFFECTS OF SERMS ON BONE MINERAL DENSITY

A large number of animal models have been used for analyzing the effects of SERMs on bone mineral density (BMD). In general, investigators have worked with models of oophorectomy-induced bone loss in which SERMs are protective against the decline in BMD[3,5–9] and against the associated decline in bone strength[9,10].

Human data in postmenopausal women confirm this bone-sparing effect of the drugs. Data on tamoxifen show that the drug prevents bone loss in postmenopausal women. However, in premenopausal patients, tamoxifen use was followed by a decline of BMD in comparison with placebo[11]. The effects of raloxifene in the prevention of postmenopausal bone loss have been extensively tested[12]. The drug is able to prevent this loss for up to 7 years of continuous use[13]. Lasofoxifene also has reported efficacy in preventing postmenopausal bone loss[14].

SERMS AND FRACTURE PREVENTION

Results concerning fracture prevention are restricted to raloxifene, and mainly to the results of the Multiple Outcomes of Raloxifene Evaluation (MORE) study. This drug is the only one to date that has completed phase III trials with reduction in fracture risk as the primary outcome.

After 4 years of treatment, raloxifene reduces the risk of new vertebral fractures by 49% in women without pre-existing vertebral fractures (relative risk (RR) 0.51, 95% confidence interval (CI) 0.35–0.73). In cases with prevalent vertebral fractures at baseline, the risk reduction is 34% (RR 0.66, 95% CI 0.55–0.81)[15]. A meta-analysis of the efficacy of the drug for vertebral fracture prevention showed a RR value of 0.53 (95% CI 0.39–0.78), with no heterogeneity in the results and a robust sensitivity analysis[16]. The effect is apparent after 1 year of treatment; a 68% reduction in the risk of clinical vertebral fractures (RR 0.32, 95% CI 0.13–0.79) was observed in a *post hoc* analysis[17]. The antifracture efficacy for vertebrae is also sustained. In other words, the risk reduction achieved during the first 3 years of treatment is also apparent during the fourth year[15]. In another exploratory analysis of the MORE results, women with osteopenia, as defined by femoral neck BMD and the absence of prevalent vertebral fractures, also benefit from treatment, with a 45% reduction in the risk of radiological vertebral fracture (RR 0.55, 95% CI 0.32–0.95) and a 70% reduction in the risk of clinical vertebral fracture (RR 0.55, 95% CI 0.32–0.95)[18].

Vertebral fracture severity grade is a good predictor of risk of subsequent fracture, both vertebral and non-vertebral, and therefore constitutes a good marker of disease severity. In women with the most severe vertebral fractures at baseline, with a grade III fracture, raloxifene was able to reduce significantly the risk of both vertebral (27%) and non-vertebral (47%) fracture[19]. This reduction in the risk of non-vertebral fractures in a high-risk subset has been further confirmed in a *post hoc* analysis of the CORE population (Continuing Outcomes Relevant to Evista) after 8 years of treatment with the drug[20].

EFFECTS OF SERMS ON BONE QUALITY

An important observation was made in patients treated with raloxifene in the MORE study. The relationship between baseline BMD and fracture risk was different for placebo- and for raloxifene-treated patients. Likewise, the curves were different for the change in BMD and their associated

fracture risk[21]. Moreover, both curves and their respective confidence intervals were totally independent. In other words, bone behaved very differently when exposed to the drug, in the sense that only about 4% of the fracture risk reduction induced by raloxifene could be explained by BMD changes. Therefore, the vast majority of the effect needs to be explained by BMD-independent factors. These elements have been defined as bone quality[22], and this term encompasses material and structural properties of bone. Hip structural analysis has been used in patients treated with raloxifene. The drug induced significant improvement in femoral neck cross-sectional area and in section modulus.

In a short subgroup of cases of the MORE trial, volumetric quantitative computed tomography (vQCT) measurements were obtained at the lumbar spine. This technique permits isolated three-dimensional measurements of purely trabecular bone and predominantly cortical shell envelope of the vertebral body, among other regions of interest. After 2 years of treatment, raloxifene prevented trabecular bone loss with significant differences compared with placebo. Conventional BMD, although showing a similar trend, was not able to reach significant differences[23].

Biopsies of raloxifene-treated patients have been analyzed by microradiography. In the bone tissue exposed to raloxifene there was a shift toward a higher mineralization degree, although both this parameter and homogeneity of the bone were kept within the physiologic range[24].

Fatigue damage is measurable in bone tissue as the presence of microcracks. These elements are associated with aging and decreased toughness of bone. In animal experiments, treatment with raloxifene induces a decrease in the density of microcracks[25].

Osteocyte apoptosis is another relevant aspect of the quality of bone. Several drugs have shown a protective effect against this phenomenon. A raloxifene analog, LY 117018, inhibits the osteocytic apoptosis induced by oophorectomy in a rat model[26]. Moreover, in bone biopsies of patients treated with raloxifene for 2 years, no increase in the number of empty osteocyte lacunae was observed[27].

Relevant in favor of the physiologic effect of SERMs on bone are data supporting that patients treated with these drugs do not show an impaired or delayed response to anabolic agents[28], and even their association induces a better BMD increase than with the anabolic agent alone[29].

NON-SKELETAL EFFECTS

SERMs have shown in different trials and in preclinical studies positive effects on reproductive tissue. After 8 years of treatment, patients treated with raloxifene have a sustained reduction in the risk of ER-positive breast cancer[30].

Neutral effects on the endometrium, ovaries and pelvic structures have been demonstrated[31–34].

Post hoc and safety analysis also point toward positive effects on cardiovascular disease, both coronary heart disease and stroke, in patients at high risk for cardiovascular events[35]. Ongoing clinical trials will definitively clarify the actual role of SERMs in these other aspects of postmenopausal health.

We can conclude that SERMs are a first-line alternative for treatment of the postmenopausal woman with osteoporosis, given their positive effects on bone, with reduction in vertebral fractures, possible reduction in the risk of nonvertebral fractures in cases with severe disease and positive effects on the quality of bone.

References

1. Bryant H. Selective estrogen receptor modulators. *Rev Endocr Metab Disord* 2002; 3: 231–41
2. Katzenellenbogen BS. Defining the 'S' in SERMs. *Science* 2002; 295: 2380–1
3. Nuttall ME, Stroup GB, Fisher PW, et al. Distinct mechanisms of action of selective estrogen receptor modulators in breast and osteoblastic cells. *Am J Physiol Cell Physiol* 2000; 279: C1550–7
4. Kian Tee M, Rogatsky I, Tzagarakis-Foster C, et al. Estradiol and selective estrogen receptor modulators differentially regulate target genes with estrogen receptors alpha and beta. *Mol Biol Cell* 2004; 15: 1262–72
5. Sato M, Kim J, Short LL, et al. Longitudinal and cross-sectional analysis of raloxifene effects on tibiae from ovariectomized aged rats. *J Pharmacol Exp Ther* 1995; 272: 1252–9
6. Evans G, Bryant HU, Magee D, et al. The effects of raloxifene on tibia histomorphometry in ovariectomized rats. *Endocrinology* 1994; 134: 2283–8
7. Qu Q, Zheng H, Dahllund J, et al. Selective estrogenic effects of a novel triphenylethylene compound, FC1271a, on bone, cholesterol level, and reproductive tissues in intact and ovariectomized rats. *Endocrinology* 2000; 141: 809–20
8. Arshad M, Sengupta S, Sharma S, et al. In vitro anti-resorptive activity and prevention of ovariectomy-induced osteoporosis in female Sprague–Dawley rats by ormeloxifene, a selective estrogen receptor modulator. *J Steroid Biochem Mol Biol* 2004; 91: 67–78
9. Ammann P, Bourrin S, Brunner F, et al. A new selective estrogen receptor modulator HMR-3339 fully corrects bone alterations induced by ovariectomy in adult rats. *Bone* 2004; 35: 153–61
10. Turner CH, Sato M, Bryant HU. Raloxifene preserves bone strength and bone mass in ovariectomized rats. *Endocrinology* 1994; 135: 2001–5
11. Powles TJ, Hickish T, Kanis JA, et al. Effect of tamoxifen on bone mineral density measured by dual-energy X-ray absorptiometry in healthy premenopausal and postmenopausal women. *J Clin Oncol* 1996; 14: 78–84
12. Johnston CC Jr, Bjarnason NH, Cohen FJ, et al. Long-term effects of raloxifene on bone mineral density, bone turnover, and serum lipid levels in

early postmenopausal women: three-year data from 2 double-blind, randomized, placebo-controlled trials. *Arch Intern Med* 2000; 160: 3444–50

13. Harris ST, Siris ES, Stock JL, et al. Increases in bone mineral density are maintained after 7 years of raloxifene therapy: results from the Continuous Outcomes Relevant to Evista (CORE) study. *Bone* 2004; 35: 1164–8

14. McClung M, Omizo M, Weiss S, et al. Comparison of lasofoxifene and raloxifene for the prevention of bone loss in postmenopausal women. *J Bone Miner Res* 2004; 19 (Suppl 1): F424

15. Delmas PD, Ensrud KE, Adachi JD, et al. Multiple Outcomes of Raloxifene Evaluation Investigators. Efficacy of raloxifene on vertebral fracture risk reduction in postmenopausal women with osteoporosis: four-year results from a randomized clinical trial. *J Clin Endocrinol Metab* 2002; 87: 3609–17

16. Seeman E, Crans G, Diez-Perez A, et al. Meta-analysis of the efficacy of raloxifene on reduction of vertebral fracture risk. American Society of Bone and Mineral Research 25th Annual Meeting, Minneapolis, Minnesota, September 19–23 2003. *J Bone Miner Res* 2003; 18 (Suppl 2): SU164

17. Maricic M, Adachi JD, Sarkar S, et al. Early effects of raloxifene on clinical vertebral fractures at 12 months in postmenopausal women with osteoporosis. *Arch Intern Med* 2002; 162: 1140–3

18. Kanis JA, Johnell O, Black DM, et al. Effect of raloxifene on the risk of new vertebral fracture in postmenopausal women with osteopenia or osteoporosis: a reanalysis of the Multiple Outcomes of Raloxifene Evaluation trial. *Bone* 2003; 33: 293–300

19. Delmas PD, Genant HK, Crans GG, et al. Severity of prevalent vertebral fractures and the risk of subsequent vertebral and nonvertebral fractures: results from the MORE trial. *Bone* 2003; 33: 522–32

20. Siris ES, Harris ST, Eastell R, et al. Effects of raloxifene on the risk of nonvertebral fractures after 8 years: results from the Continuing Outcomes Relevant to Evista (CORE) study. *J Bone Miner Res* 2004; 19 (Suppl 1): SA428

21. Sarkar S, Mitlak BH, Wong M, et al. Relationships between bone mineral density and incident vertebral fracture risk with raloxifene therapy. *J Bone Miner Res* 2002; 17: 1–10

22. NIH Consensus Development Panel. Osteoporosis prevention, diagnosis, and therapy. *J Am Med Assoc* 2001; 285: 785–95

23. Genant HK, Lang T, Fuerst T, et al. Treatment with raloxifene for two years increases vertebral bone mineral density as measured by volumetric quantitative computed tomography. *Bone* 2004; 35: 1164–8

24. Boivin G, Lips P, Ott SM, et al. Contribution of raloxifene and calcium and vitamin D3 supplementation to the increase of the degree of mineralization of bone in postmenopausal women. *J Clin Endocrinol Metab* 2003; 88: 4199–205

25. Burr DB. Microdamage and bone strength. *Osteoporos Int* 2003; 14 (Suppl 5): 67–72

26. Colishaw S, Reeve J. Effects of SERM LY117018 on bone microdamage. *J Bone Miner Res* 2003; 18: S293

27. Ott SM, Oleksik A, Lu Y, et al. Bone histomorphometric and biochemical marker results of a 2-year placebo-controlled trial of raloxifene in postmenopausal women. *J Bone Miner Res* 2002; 17: 341–8

28. Ettinger B, San Martin J, Crans G, et al. Differential effects of teriparatide on BMD after treatment with raloxifene or alendronate. *J Bone Miner Res* 2004; 19: 745–51

29. Deal C, Omizo M, Schwartz EN, et al. Raloxifene in combination with teriparatide reduces teriparatide-induced stimulation of bone resorption but not formation in postmenopausal women with osteoporosis *J Bone Miner Res* 2004; 19 (Suppl 1): 1169

30. Martino S, Canley JA, Barret-Connor E, et al. Continuing outcomes relevant to Evista: breast cancer incidence in postmenopausal osteoporotic women in a randomized trail of raloxifene. *J Natl Cancer Inst* 2004; 96: 1751–61

31. Davies GC, Huster WJ, Shen W, et al. Endometrial response to raloxifene compared with placebo, cyclical hormone replacement therapy, and unopposed estrogen in postmenopausal women. *Menopause* 1999; 6: 188–95

32. Goldstein SR, Scheele WH, Rajagopalan SK, et al. A 12-month comparative study of raloxifene, estrogen, and placebo on the postmenopausal endometrium. *Obstet Gynecol* 2000; 95: 95–103

33. Cauley J, Norton L, Lippman ME, et al. Continued breast cancer risk reduction in post-menopausal women treated with raloxifene: 4-year results from the MORE trial. Multiple Outcomes of Raloxifene Evaluation. *Breast Cancer Res Treat* 2001; 65: 125–34

34. Goldstein SR, Neven P, Zhou L, et al. Raloxifene effect on frequency of surgery for pelvic floor relaxation. *Obstet Gynecol* 2001; 98: 91–6

35. Barrett-Connor E, Grady D, Sashegyi A, et al. Raloxifene and cardiovascular events in osteoporotic postmenopausal women: four-year results from the MORE (Multiple Outcomes of Raloxifene Evaluation) randomized trial. *J Am Med Assoc* 2002; 287: 847–57

Bisphosphonates in the management of osteoporosis

23

S. E. Papapoulos

INTRODUCTION

Bisphosphonates are synthetic compounds that have a high affinity for calcium-containing crystals, concentrate preferentially in the skeleton and affect bone surface-related processes. The first bisphosphonate was synthesized in the 19th century, but the relevance of these compounds to clinical medicine was recognized in the 1960s[1]. They were initially developed as inhibitors of growth and dissolution of calcium crystals, but were subsequently found to inhibit osteoclast-mediated bone resorption. Because of this action, bisphosphonates were used initially in the management of conditions characterized by excessive osteoclastic bone resorption, such as Paget's disease of bone and malignancy-associated hypercalcemia. Increasing understanding of bone physiology and pathology as well as of the pharmacological properties of bisphosphonates led to their application to the treatment of other skeletal disorders, including osteoporosis.

PHARMACOLOGY

Chemically, geminal bisphosphonates have a central carbon atom bound to two phosphonate groups to give a P–C–P structure, which is resistant to biological degradation, and two substitutions at the carbon atom, R_1 and R_2, respectively[2,3]. R_1 is usually short, and together with the phosphonate groups was previously thought to be solely responsible for the binding of bisphosphonate to bone mineral (bone hook). R_2 differs considerably among the various bisphosphonates, and was believed to be responsible for their cellular effects (bioactive moiety). Recent evidence, however, indicates that the whole molecule is essential for the action of bisphosphonates. According to the presence or not of a nitrogen atom in R_2, bisphosphonates are classified into nitrogen-containing and non-nitrogen-containing compounds. Nitrogen increases the potency and the specificity of bisphosphonates for bone resorption. Nitrogen-containing bisphosphonates include alendronate, ibandronate, incadronate, neridronate, olpadronate, pamidronate and risedronate. Non-nitrogen-containing bisphosphonates are clodronate, etidronate and tiludronate.

Bisphosphonates are taken up selectively by the skeleton at the bone surface, where they bind to hydroxyapatite crystals. They concentrate preferentially in bone resorption sites, are liberated from bone mineral by the decrease of local pH which occurs under osteoclasts during bone resorption, and are taken up by the osteoclasts[4]. Non-nitrogen-containing bisphosphonates are metabolized intracellularly to adenosine triphosphate analogs that induce osteoclast apoptosis. Nitrogen-containing bisphosphonates induce changes in the cytoskeleton of osteoclasts, such as loss of the ruffled border or disruption of the actin rings, leading to inactivation and subsequently apoptosis of osteoclasts[5]. The latter changes are due to inhibition of farnesylpyrophosphate synthase, an enzyme of the mevalonic acid metabolic pathway, leading to impaired synthesis of the isoprenoid geranylgeranyl pyrophosphate which is required for the isoprenylation of small guanosine triphosphate (GTP)-binding proteins such as ras, rho and rac. These proteins are essential for intracellular signal transduction and cytoskeletal integrity. There are considerable differences in antiresorptive potency among the various bisphosphonates. In general, the nitrogen-containing types are more potent, but the magnitude of the difference in potency depends on the experimental conditions used.

The intestinal absorption of orally administered bisphosphonates is poor, accounting for < 1% of the administered dose. It occurs across intestinal cells probably by the paracellular route (along the cells), rather than transcellularly (across the cells). This low absorption is attributed to the highly negative charge of phosphonates which inhibits their diffusion through lipophilic membranes. Bisphosphonates have a short plasma half-life. Plasma disappearance is multiexponential, and practically all bisphosphonate is cleared from the circulation within 6–10 h after administration. About half of the administered dose concentrates in the skeleton. The capacity of the skeleton to retain bisphosphonate is very large, and saturation of binding sites is impossible during treatment of osteoporosis even if this is given for decades[6]. The remaining bisphosphonate is excreted unaltered in urine. To date, no bisphosphonate metabolites have been identified *in vivo*. Bisphosphonates are embedded in the skeleton where they remain for long periods. Elimination from this compartment is extremely slow. The terminal half-life has been calculated for a number of them, and can be as long as 10 years in humans. There may be differences in the terminal half-life of bisphosphonates, the magnitude of which, however, can only be addressed in pharmacokinetics studies of similar design and length of observation period. Such studies are not yet available.

In early studies, Reitsma and colleagues[7] treated growing rats with daily subcutaneous injections of pamidronate, and followed the changes in bone resorption and calcium balance. Treatment suppressed bone resorption dose-dependently, and significantly increased calcium retention. More important, with all doses used, suppression of resorption reached a plateau that was also dose-dependent and did not decrease further, despite continuous administration of the drug. These results suggested for the first time that it might be possible to suppress bone resorption and to induce significant increases in calcium balance with low-dose bisphosphonate

given daily. Moreover, these authors demonstrated that the daily administration of bisphosphonate is not accompanied by progressive suppression of bone resorption, and thus accumulation of bisphosphonate in the skeleton is not associated with a cumulative effect on bone metabolism. This pattern of response has now been repeatedly shown in humans treated for up to 10 years with oral bisphosphonates given daily[8–10]. In addition, a recent report of bone biopsies from a small number of patients treated with oral alendronate for 10 years showed the presence of double tetracycline labels in all specimens examined, and values of activation frequency similar to those observed by these authors in premenopausal women[11]. Thus, from data currently available, there is no evidence of a cumulative effect or an adverse long-term effect of long-term treatment with bisphosphonates on bone metabolism.

EFFICACY

Bisphosphonates are very effective treatments of osteoporosis. When given daily for up to 5 years, they decrease the risk of fractures in postmenopausal women with osteoporosis[12–23]. In addition, the two worldwide-approved bisphosphonates, alendronate and risedronate, reduce the risk of non-vertebral fractures including those of the hip, as has been demonstrated by specifically designed randomized clinical trials. Systematic reviews with meta-analyses have further shown that the antifracture efficacy of the two bisphosphonates is consistent among trials and populations[24–26]. To improve patient convenience and long-term adherence to treatment, and to decrease potential gastrointestinal complications that may be associated with daily use, once-weekly regimens have been developed for both bisphosphonates. These regimens provide the sum of seven daily doses (alendronate 70 mg and risedronate 35 mg once a week) and are pharmacologically equivalent to the daily ones.

Consistent with the pharmacological properties of bisphosphonates and the principles of bone cell biology, once-weekly bisphosphonate administration should be considered 'continuous' treatment, distinct from administration at longer drug-free intervals, which are commonly referred to as 'intermittent' or 'cyclical' regimens[6].

Mechanism of antifracture efficacy

It is well established that bone mineral density (BMD) and increased rate of bone resorption are strong, independent risk factors for fractures. However, there has been disagreement regarding the relative contributions of changes in BMD to the antifracture efficacies of antiresorptive agents. This disagreement has stemmed from observations in clinical trials of antiresorptive agents showing reductions in the risk of vertebral fractures of a similar magnitude for agents with a smaller or a larger effect on BMD. Furthermore, reported estimates of the proportion of the reduction in fracture risk that can be explained by changes in BMD range between 4 and 50%, creating considerable confusion among physicians and raising questions about the validity of BMD measurements. These are only apparent discrepancies. In order to understand the action of a therapeutic agent on a clinical outcome, in this case fracture incidence, we need first to consider the mechanism of action of this agent in relation to the pathophysiology of the disease. In osteoporosis there is an imbalance between bone formation and bone resorption, resulting in bone loss with every remodeling cycle. When this imbalance is accompanied by an increase in the activation of new bone remodeling units, more bone will be lost within the same period. In addition, the latter will adversely affect structural and material properties of bone, increasing further the risk of fracture. This pathophysiological background provides the rationale for the use of agents that reduce bone resorption and bone turnover in the management of osteoporosis. The primary pharmacological action of bisphosphonates is the suppression of bone resorption. This occurs early after the initiation of treatment, and is followed by a slower decline in the rate of bone formation due to the coupling of the two processes until a new equilibrium between bone formation and resorption is achieved, at between 6 and 12 months, at a lower rate of bone turnover. Increases in BMD are secondary to this action. Thus, the demonstration that suppression of bone resorption early in the course of treatment with a bisphosphonate can explain a large part of its antifracture efficacy is consistent with the known pharmacological properties and mechanism of action of bisphosphonates. In addition, bisphosphonates have been shown to preserve bone microarchitecture in both preclinical and clinical studies. For example, Dufresne and colleagues[27] examined bone biopsies from early postmenopausal women (mean 3 years) who were marginally osteopenic (lumbar spine BMD T-score -1.3) before and after 1 year of treatment with risedronate or placebo, using microcomputed tomography (μCT). As expected, in the placebo-treated women, there was significant and rapid bone loss, shown by a decrease in bone volume (expressed as a percentage of tissue volume) of 20% and in BMD of 3.3% after 1 year. Risedronate reduced the rate of bone remodeling, as indicated by a reduction in activation frequency and in mineralizing surfaces, histomorphometrically assessed, and an increase in BMD of 2.02%, consistent with its primary pharmacological action. Importantly, risedronate induced substantial changes in a number of key architectural parameters, such as trabecular number and trabecular separation. In addition, bone biopsies from osteoporotic women treated with alendronate for 2 or 3 years showed significantly higher bone volume and lower trabecular spacing, compared with placebo-treated women[28]. Finally, a 46% significant decrease of cortical porosity, compared with placebo-treated patients, has been reported after alendronate treatment[29]. Information about the effects of bisphosphonates on bone material properties has been obtained from animal and human studies that assessed the degree of mineralization of bone. In all studies, either with alendronate or risedronate, a significant improvement was reported[30,31].

Thus, bisphosphonate treatment of patients with osteoporosis suppresses bone resorption, decreases the rate of bone remodeling, increases bone mineral density and affects favorably a number of bone structural and material properties leading to the desired clinical outcome, namely a reduction in fracture risk.

LONG-TERM EFFECTS ON SKELETAL FRAGILITY

Skeletal fragility on long-term bisphosphonate therapy has been examined in a series of extensions of three previously reported pivotal clinical trials (Vertebral Efficacy with Risedronate Therapy (VERT)-international, phase III, and Fracture Intervention Trial (FIT) with alendronate). It should be noted that none of these extension studies was specifically designed to assess antifracture efficacy, but rather safety and efficacy on surrogate end-points, as well as consistency of the effect of bisphosphonates over longer periods, were evaluated.

The first study consisted of two 2-year extensions of the VERT-international clinical trial[10]. During the first 5 years of the study, two groups of osteoporotic women received either placebo or risedronate 5 mg/day, while in the following 2 years all patients received active treatment. The rate of vertebral fractures during years 6 and 7 was similar in patients who received placebo previously and in those who continued on oral risedronate. In addition, the incidence of vertebral fractures in the risedronate group was similar to that observed in years 0–3 and years 4–5. Moreover, the number of women with non-vertebral fractures was not significantly different between the two groups during years 6–7 (7.4% vs. 6.0%).

The second study[9] was an extension of the clinical trial originally reported by Liberman and colleagues with alendronate[12]. In these extension studies, patients received alendronate either 5 mg/day or 10 mg/day continuously for 10 years or 20 mg/day for 2 years, followed by 5 mg/day for 3 years (providing a total dose equivalent to 10 mg/day for 5 years), followed by placebo for 5 years. The rate of non-vertebral fractures during years 6–10 in patients treated for 10 years with 10 mg/day was similar to that observed during the first 3 years of alendronate treatment, although patients were older and had a higher risk of fracture due to the increase in age.

The recently, in abstract form, reported results of the extension of the FIT trial (FLEX) support these conclusions[32]. In this study, 1099 patients who participated in the FIT and received alendronate for 5 years, on average, were randomized to placebo (PBO), alendronate (ALN) 5 mg/day or alendronate 10 mg/day and were followed for another 5 years. At the end of the 10-year observation period, the incidence of non-vertebral and hip fractures in the ALN/PBO group was similar to that of the ALN/ALN groups (20% vs. 19% and 3% vs. 3%, respectively). In addition, the incidence of clinical vertebral fractures was lower in the ALN/ALN groups compared with the ALN/PBO group (2% vs. 5%).

Taken together, these results are reassuring for clinicians, as they indicate that prolonged exposure of bone tissue to bisphosphonate is not associated with adverse effects on bone fragility and bone metabolism. In addition, the favorable effect of bisphosphonates on skeletal integrity appears to be sustained.

RESOLUTION OF THE EFFECT OF TREATMENT

In general, chronic diseases require chronic uninterrupted pharmacotherapy in order to maintain the desired clinical outcome. The nature of osteoporosis and the properties of bisphosphonates raise questions, however, about the general applicability of this approach to management of the disease. For many years, research in osteoporosis has focused on the development of effective and safe medications, and it is only recently that the issue of duration of treatment is systematically being investigated. In principle, the length of treatment with any antiosteoporotic medication will be determined by its pharmacological properties as well as by the risk for the individual patient. In practice, pharmacodynamic responses following discontinuation of treatment in different groups of women can be decisive.

Pharmacodynamic responses following cessation of bisphosphonate therapy given for prevention of bone loss were adequately investigated in the Early Postmenopausal Intervention Cohort (EPIC) study[33,34]. Early postmenopausal women were given alendronate for 2, 4 or 6 years, or placebo, and were followed for 6 years. Cessation of treatment after 2 or 4 years was associated with progressive increases of biochemical indices of bone resorption toward the levels of women treated with placebo, and BMD decreases at a rate similar to that of placebo-treated women. Thus, there was no rapid increase in the rate of bone resorption that may have consequences for trabecular architecture, and no 'catch-up' bone loss as observed in a parallel group that received hormone replacement therapy (HRT) for 4 years. Bagger and colleagues[35] analyzed all the results of studies of 203 women given different daily doses of alendronate or placebo for varying periods of up to 9 years for the prevention of postmenopausal bone loss. Women who received alendronate (2.5–10 mg/day) for 2 years had a 3.8% higher BMD than those receiving placebo, 7 years after withdrawal of treatment. The residual effect was proportionally larger in women who received treatment for 4 or 6 years (5.9% and 8.6%, respectively) but the largest residual effect was observed in women who received alendronate 20 mg/day for 2 years (9.7%). Similar to the EPIC study, the rate of bone loss following cessation of alendronate treatment was comparable to the bone loss observed in the placebo group. Bone turnover markers tended to reverse back to placebo levels. This study provides information additional to that obtained in EPIC. It shows that alendronate has a residual effect on bone metabolism that is proportional to the length of treatment with doses between 2.5 and 10 mg/day. The highest residual effect was obtained with the dose of 20 mg/day, although this was given for only 2 years, corresponding to 4 years of treatment with 10 mg/day or 8 years of treatment with 5 mg/day, the currently approved dose for prevention of postmenopausal bone loss. This residual response can be explained either by the larger initial suppression of bone resorption and consequently larger increase in BMD by the higher dose, or by liberation of higher concentrations of the bisphosphonate during follow-up. The data on bone markers support the first notion.

These results have important clinical implications, and can lead to recommendations about the use of alendronate for the prevention of osteoporosis. For example, the bisphosphonate can be given for a defined period of time (2–4 years) followed by a drug-free period, the length of which will be determined by the response of the individual woman. This is a remarkable pharmacological example in the management of chronic diseases, the medical rationale, risk/benefit ratio and cost-effectiveness of which need to be evaluated. However, for a number of reasons, discussion of which lies beyond the scope of this chapter, this is not a generally accepted indication in clinical practice. Moreover, these very interesting pharmacodynamic responses are specific for young postmenopausal women, and should not be extrapolated to the treatment of osteoporotic women with a different metabolic and fracture risk profile or to treatment with other bisphosphonates that may have a different pharmacological profile. There are, however, data available that help to define residual actions of bisphosphonates in older women with osteoporosis.

About 10 years ago, we reported in exploratory studies of women and men with osteoporosis treated with daily oral pamidronate that cessation of long-term treatment (6.5 years) was not associated with decreases in bone mineral density of the spine and the femoral neck, and that the rate of vertebral fractures remained stable during 2 years of follow-up without bisphosphonate[36]. These findings let us hypothesize that resumption of bone remodeling after stopping treatment led to the release of bisphosphonate previously embedded in bone. The concentration of the released bisphosphonate was sufficient to correct the imbalance between bone resorption and bone formation and to protect skeletal integrity, but insufficient to maintain the level of suppression of bone resorption achieved during treatment and further to increase BMD. The long-term responses of women with osteoporosis treated with alendronate are in agreement with these early conclusions. For example, cessation of alendronate treatment after 5 years was followed by modest increases in biochemical markers of bone turnover to levels clearly lower than those before any treatment was given[9]. The lack of a control group receiving placebo during the whole period of observation precludes any conclusions about the magnitude of this response. BMD at the spine remained stable during the 5 years off treatment, while it increased further on continuing treatment. Finally, the BMD of hip sites showed some decrease, but not back to baseline. Similarly, in the FLEX study, patients who received placebo after 5 years of alendronate therapy showed a 25% increase in urinary NTx (cross-linked N-telopeptides of type I collagen) that remained stable during the following 5 years without bisphosphonate[31]. Changes in BMD were similar to those in the extension of the phase III study, with the exception of total hip BMD, which reached pretreatment values after 5 years off treatment.

USE OF BISPHOSPHONATES AT INTERVALS LONGER THAN 1 WEEK

Intermittent administration of bisphosphonates to patients with osteoporosis has been used for many years, but studies have generally failed to show concrete evidence of antifracture efficacy. Interest in this form of treatment has recently been renewed with the development of more potent bisphosphonates that can be given at intervals longer than 1 week, either orally at safe doses or intravenously in convenient ways either by injection or by short-term infusion. Such regimens are thought to offer patient convenience, contributing to better long-term adherence to treatment. These administration regimens usually induce a fast decrease in the level of bone resorption, which reaches a nadir within a few days. The exact nadir reached depends on the sampling schedule, and it is greater than that of daily regimens since the dose size used in intermittent regimens is usually higher than that reached by daily treatments. Thereafter, bone resorption starts to increase again toward baseline until the administration of the next dose. The result is a fluctuating level of bone resorption. All such regimens can lead to some increases in BMD, but, until recently no clear-cut antifracture efficacy has been shown, suggesting that dose size or dosage interval may have been incorrect. A typical example of this is the intravenous injection of ibandronate 0.5 or 1.0 mg every 3 months to osteoporotic women. These doses increased BMD by about 3% after 3 years, but led to a non-significant reduction in the risk of new vertebral fractures[37]. The results suggested that a higher dose or a shorter dose interval might be needed for antifracture efficacy. In further phase II studies, intravenous ibandronate injections, 2 mg every 3 months, were associated with larger decreases in bone resorption and larger increases in BMD[38]. On the other hand, a single infusion of zolendronate 4 mg in patients with osteoporosis suppressed bone resorption during 1 year to a constant level, with a long-term pattern similar to that observed during daily oral administration of other bisphosphonates[39]. Similar data have previously been reported with intravenous alendronate (7.5 mg on four consecutive days) at a dose equivalent to about 430 days of treatment with 10 mg/day orally[40]. Of particular interest was a treatment regimen with oral ibandronate, given with a drug-free interval of longer than 2 months, that suppressed bone resorption significantly, with a response pattern similar to that induced by daily treatment. This was the first time that an intermittent bisphosphonate regimen was shown to have antifracture efficacy in a prospective, controlled trial[23]. These results opened the way to explore other treatment regimens with this bisphosphonate, such as once-monthly oral administration.

CONCLUSIONS

Bisphosphonates, because of their efficacy and safety, are generally accepted as first-line therapy for osteoporosis, and current research focuses on issues related to their optimal clinical use. Despite progress in our understanding of their action to reduce fracture risk and their long-term effects on bone, there are still questions regarding their long-term use that remain to be addressed. These focus mainly on the clinical question of length of treatment, and to potential differences among bisphosphonates. Will it be possible to offer to our patients 'drug holidays' with a bisphosphonate? Such a therapeutic approach can have substantial economic benefits, is more patient-friendly and may enhance adherence to treatment.

Can long-term results obtained with one bisphosphonate be extrapolated to the whole class? There are suggestions that this may not be the case. A number of ongoing studies are expected to provide more insight into these issues. When will efficacious regimens with intermittent administration of bisphosphonates either orally or parenterally become available? Current data indicate that this will be soon. Finally, how can we best use bisphosphonates in combination with other agents for the management of the rather small, but clinically very important, group of patients with severe disease? The first steps to answer this question have already been taken. Ongoing research is expected to provide more information that will help in the optimal management of the individual patient with osteoporosis with bisphosphonates.

References

1. Blomen LJMJ. History of bisphosphonates: discovery and history of non-medical uses of bisphosphonates. In Bijvoet OLM, Fleisch HA, Canfield RRE, Russell RGG, eds. *Bisphosphonates on Bones*. Amsterdam: Elsevier, 1995: 111–24

2. Fleisch H. Basic biology of bisphosphonates. In Marcus R, Feldman D, Kelsey J, eds. *Osteoporosis*, 2nd edn. San Diego: Academic Press, 2001: 449–70

3. Papapoulos SE. Bisphosphonates: pharmacology and use in the treatment of osteoporosis. In Marcus R, Feldman D, Kelsey J, eds. *Osteoporosis*. New York: Academic Press, 1996: 1209–33

4. Reszka AA, Rodan GA. Nitrogen-containing bisphosphonate mechanism of action. *Mini Rev Med Chem* 2004; 4: 711–19

5. Rogers MJ. From molds and macrophages to mevalonate: a decade of progress in understanding the molecular mode of action of bisphosphonates. *Calcif Tissue Int* 2004; 75: 451–61

6. Cremers CLM, Pillai G, Papapoulos SE. Pharmacokinetics/pharmacodynamics of bisphosphonates. *Clin Pharmacokinet* 2005; 44 (3): 551–70

7. Reitsma PH, Bijvoet OLM, Verlinden-Ooms H, Wee van der Plas LJA. Kinetic studies of bone and mineral metabolism during treatment with (3-amino-1-hydroxypropylidene)-1,1-bisphosphonate in rats. *Calcif Tissue Int* 1980; 32: 145–57

8. Papapoulos SE, Landman JO, Bijvoet OLM, et al. The use of bisphosphonates in the treatment of osteoporosis. *Bone* 1992; 13 (Suppl 1): S41–9

9. Bone HG, Hosking D, Devogelaer JP, et al. Alendronate Phase III Osteoporosis Treatment Group. Ten years' experience with alendronate for osteoporosis in postmenopausal women. *N Engl J Med* 2004; 350: 1189–99

10. Mellstrom DD, Sorensen OH, Goemaers S, et al. Seven years of treatment with risedronate in women with postmenopausal osteoporosis. *Calcif Tissue Int* 2004; 75: 462–8

11. Recker R, Ensrud K, Diem S, et al. Normal bone histomorphometry and 3D microarchitecture after 10 years alendronate treatment of postmenopausal women. *J Bone Miner Res* 2004; 19 (Suppl 2): S45

12. Liberman UA, Weiss SR, Broll J, et al. Effect of oral alendronate on bone mineral density and the incidence of fractures in postmenopausal osteoporosis. The Alendronate Phase III Osteoporosis Treatment Study Group. *N Engl J Med* 1995; 333: 1437–43

13. Black DM, Cummings SR, Karpf DB, et al. Randomised trial of effect of alendronate on risk of fracture in women with existing vertebral fractures. Fracture Intervention Trial Research Group. *Lancet* 1996; 348: 1535–41

14. Cummings SR, Black DM, Thompson DE, et al. Effect of alendronate on risk of fracture in women with low bone density but without vertebral fractures: results from the Fracture Intervention Trial. *J Am Med Assoc* 1998; 280: 2077–82

15. Pols HA, Felsenberg D, Hanley DA, et al. Multinational, placebo-controlled, randomized trial of the effects of alendronate on bone density and fracture risk in postmenopausal women with low bone mass: results of the FOSIT study. Fosamax

International Trial study group. *Osteoporos Int* 1999; 9: 461–8

16. Black DM, Thompson DE, Bauer DC, et al. Fracture risk reduction with alendronate in women with osteoporosis: the Fracture Intervention Trial. FIT Research Group. *J Clin Endocrinol Metab* 2000; 85: 4118–24

17. Harris ST, Watts NB, Genant HK, et al. Effects of risedronate treatment on vertebral and non-vertebral fractures in women with post-menopausal osteoporosis: a randomized controlled trial. Vertebral Efficacy with Risedronate Therapy (VERT) Study Group. *J Am Med Assoc* 1999; 282: 1344–52

18. Reginster JY, Minne HW, Sorensen OH, et al. Randomized trial of the effects of risedronate on vertebral fractures in women with established postmenopausal osteoporosis. Vertebral Efficacy with Risedronate Therapy (VERT) study group. *Osteoporos Int* 2000; 11: 83–91

19. McClung MR, Geusens P, Miller PD, et al. Hip Intervention Program Study Group. Effect of risedronate on the risk of hip fracture in elderly women. *N Engl J Med* 2001; 344: 333–40

20. Sorensen OH, Crawford GM, Mulder H, et al. Long-term efficacy of risedronate: a 5-year placebo-controlled clinical experience. *Bone* 2003; 32: 120–6

21. Brumsen C, Papapoulos SE, Lips P, et al. Daily oral pamidronate in women and men with osteoporosis: a 3-year randomized, placebo-controlled clinical trial with a 2-year open extension. *J Bone Miner Res* 2002; 17: 1057–64

22. McCloskey E, Selby P, Davies M, et al. Clodronate reduces vertebral fracture risk in women with postmenopausal osteoporosis: results of a double-blind, placebo-controlled 3-year study. *J Bone Miner Res* 2004; 19: 728–36

23. Chesnut Ch III, Skag A, Christiansen C, et al. Effects of oral ibandronate administered daily or intermittently on fracture risk in postmenopausal osteoporosis. *J Bone Miner Res* 2004; 19: 1241–9

24. Cranney A, Wells G, Willan A, et al. Meta-analysis of alendronate for the treatment of postmenopausal women. *Endocr Rev* 2002; 23: 508–16

25. Cranney A, Tugwell P, Adachi J, et al. Meta-analysis of risedronate for the treatment of postmenopausal osteoporosis. *Endocr Rev* 2002; 23: 517–23

26. Papapoulos SE, Quandt SA, Liberman UA, et al. Meta-analysis of the efficacy of alendronate for the prevention of hip fractures in postmenopausal women. *Osteoporos Int* 2005; 16: 468–74

27. Dufresne TE, Chmielewski PA, Manhart MD, et al. Risedronate preserves bone architecture in early postmenopausal women in 1 year as measured by three-dimensional microcomputed tomography. *Calcif Tissue Int* 2003; 73: 423–32

28. Recker R, Masarachia P, Santora A, et al. Trabecular bone microarchitecture after alendronate treatment of osteoporotic women. *Curr Med Res Opin* 2005; 21: 185–94

29. Roschger P, Rinnerthaler S, Yates J, et al. Alendronate increases degree and uniformity of mineralization in cancellous bone and decreases the porosity in cortical bone of osteoporotic women. *Bone* 2001; 29: 185–91

30. Boivin GY, Chavassieux PM, Santora AC, et al. Alendronate increases bone strength by increasing the mean degree of mineralization of bone tissue in osteoporotic women. *Bone* 2000; 27: 687–94

31. Borah B, Dufresne TE, Chmielewski PA, et al. Risedronate preserves bone architecture in postmenopausal women with osteoporosis as measured by three-dimensional microcomputed tomography. *Bone* 2004; 34: 736–46

32. Black D, Schwartz A, Ensrud K, et al. A 5 year randomized trial of the long-term efficacy and safety of alendronate: the FIT long-term extension (FLEX). *J Bone Miner Res* 2004; 19 (Suppl 2): S45

33. McClung MR, Wasnich RD, Hosking DJ, et al. Prevention of postmenopausal bone loss: six-year results from the Early Postmenopausal Intervention Cohort Study. *J Clin Endocrinol Metab* 2004; 89: 4879–85

34. Wasnich RD, Bagger YZ, Hosking DJ, et al. Early Postmenopausal Intervention Cohort Study Group. Changes in bone mineral density and turnover after alendronate or estrogen withdrawal. *Menopause* 2004; 11: 622–30

35. Bagger YZ, Tanko LB, Alexandersen P, et al. Alendronate has a residual effect on bone mass in postmenopausal Danish women up to 7 years after treatment withdrawal. *Bone* 2003; 33: 301–7

36. Landman JO, Hamdy NA, Pawels EK, Papapoulos SE. Skeletal metabolism in patients with

osteoporosis after discontinuation of long-term treatment with oral pamidronate. *J Clin Endocrinol Metab* 1995; 80: 3465–8

37. Recker R, Stakkestad JA, Chesnut CH III, et al. Insufficiently dosed intravenous ibandronate injections are associated with suboptimal antifracture efficacy in postmenopausal osteoporosis. *Bone* 2004; 34: 890–9

38. Adami S, Felsenberg D, Christiansen C, et al. Efficacy and safety of ibandronate given by intravenous injection once every 3 months. *Bone* 2004; 34: 881–9

39. Reid IR, Brown JP, Burckhardt P, et al. Intravenous zoledronic acid in postmenopausal women with low bone mineral density. *N Engl J Med* 2002; 346: 653–61

40. Khan SA, Kanis JA, Vasikaran S, et al. Elimination and biochemical responses to intravenous alendronate in postmenopausal osteoporosis. *J Bone Miner Res* 1997; 10: 1700–7

Phytoestrogens: food or drug? 24

L. Bacciottini, A. Falchetti, B. Pampaloni, E. Bartolini, A. M. Carossino and M. L. Brandi

INTRODUCTION

Within the past several years, the relationship between diet and health has been accepted by the mainstream nutrition community and, in this connection, interest in the physiological role of bioactive compounds present in plants has dramatically increased over the last decade. As a complex mixture of chemicals, foods provide essential nutrients, requisite calories and other physiologically active constituents that may be useful for life and health. A new paradigm for 'optimal nutrition' may be evolving that would identify physiologically active components that contribute to disease prevention. Thus, the functional foods concept unifies the medical, nutritional and food sciences (Figure 1). Collectively, plants contain several different families of natural bioactive products, among which are compounds with weak estrogenic or antiestrogenic activity toward mammals. Of particular interest in relation to human health are these plant-derived estrogens, or phytoestrogens, which embody several groups of non-steroidal estrogens widely distributed within the plant kingdom. Although *in vitro* and animal studies provide preliminary plausible mechanisms to explain how phytoestrogens act, the application of diets rich in such compounds and their consequent biological effects still need to be fully examined, tested and confirmed through traditional scientific experimental pathways (Table 1). Phytoestrogens are strikingly similar in chemical structure to the mammalian estrogen, estradiol, and bind to estrogen receptors (ERs) with a preference for ERβ[2]. This suggests that these compounds may exert tissue-specific effects, besides other non-receptor-mediated biological activities, such as antioxidant capacity and antiproliferative/antiangiogenic effects.

Natural estrogens are involved in a multiplicity of programmed events in target tissues such as the uterus, breast, pituitary gland and hormone-responsive tumors. The initiation of estrogen action by all of the estrogens is considered to be the same in each target tissue. Estrogen first binds to the nuclear ER, then an estrogenic ligand causes a conformational change that encourages dimerization and interaction with either specific DNA sequences or a protein–protein interaction with activator protein-1 (AP-1) or specificity protein 1 (SP1) sites in the promoter region of estrogen-responsive genes[3]. These events herald the biological effects of estrogen in the specific target tissue or tumor. A small percentage (2–3%) of ERs are located on the cell membrane and contribute to non-genomic

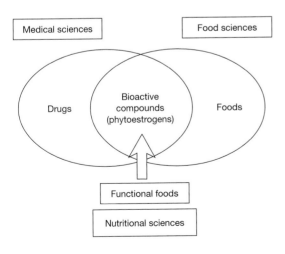

Figure 1 Phytoestrogens: scientific research areas

Table 1 Research needed to clarify possible roles of phytoestrogens in health. Modified from reference 1

Identify the specific types of phytoestrogens that provide health benefits
Characterize the sources, dietary or supplemental
Define the effective dose of phytoestrogens that provides protection against a specific symptom
Determine the concentration at which pharmacologic doses become a toxicologic problem
Identify new mechanisms by which the phytoestrogens produce protective effects
Identify specific binding proteins
Identify specific metabolites
Determine the effects of phytoestrogens on cell differentiation
Establish the pharmacokinetics of delivered doses
Identify the proportion of the population likely to respond positively to phytoestrogens
Examine more closely the dietary components relative to the diet as whole

---

effects of estrogen[4]. Two ERs are currently known, ERα and ERβ. Although the two ERs can be localized within the same cell, they vary in tissue distribution and can have different effects on mixed agonist and antagonist molecules.

Phytoestrogens include a wide variety of structurally diverse compounds such as isoflavones, mainly found in soy, lignans founds in grains and stilbenes found in the skins of grapes. Other less investigated compounds include flavones, flavans, isoflavanes and coumestans[5]. The estrogenic or antiestrogenic activity of any chemical depends on the ability of the compound to interact with the ERs (ERα, ERβ).

The aim of this chapter is to describe the substances that, up to date, have been validated from a pharmacological point of view for their estrogenicity or antiestrogenicity.

PHYTOESTROGEN-RICH FOODS

Phytoestrogens are present in many human foodstuffs including fruits (plums, pears, apples, grapes, berries, etc.), vegetables (beans, sprouts, cabbage, spinach, soybeans, grains, hops, garlic, onions, etc.), wines and teas, and have been identified in a number of botanical dietary supplements (Table 2). Plants vary both intra- and inter-species in the types and concentrations of phytoestrogens, due to variables in plant growth, soil, weather conditions and the age of the plant. Chemically, phytoestrogens are phenolic phytochemicals or polyphenols. These are the largest category of phytochemicals and the most widely distributed in the plant kingdom[7].

Polyphenols in plants show a multiple function: they act as antioxidants (protection against ultraviolet (UV) light), exert a protective action against insects, fungi, viruses and bacteria, and a visual attention–pollinator attraction (they are responsible for plant and flower colors), and they can also serve as feed-repellents and plant hormone controllers.

The study of phytoestrogens started in the 1950s when it was realized that some plant-derived substances could cause an estrogenic effect. Sheep that were grazing on pastures containing red clover had multiple fertility problems, and it was shown that the clover present in these pastures had high amounts of isoflavones[8], in particular formononetin and biochanin A.

The classification of phytoestrogens is controversial; however, currently we can subdivide the phytoestrogens into four main classes: flavonoids (flavonols and isoflavones), lignans, coumestans and stilbenes (Table 3).

Flavonoids

These are the largest group of plant phenols, including more than 4000 different compounds, which are the most studied phytochemicals. The basic flavonoid structure allows a multitude of variations in chemical structure, giving rise to flavonols (quercetin, kaempferol, myricetin), flavones (apigenin, luteolin), flavanones (catechin,

Table 2 Levels of isoflavones and lignans in various food sources. Values (in nanomoles per gram dry weight) were determined by isotope dilution gas chromatography–mass spectrometry with selected ion monitoring[6]

Plant species (common name)	Genistein	Daidzein	Secoisolariciresinol	Matairesinol
Soybean	993–3115	413–2205	< 1–8	< 1
Kidney bean	< 1–19	< 1–2	2–4	< 1
American groundnut	4–30	< 1	< 1–2	< 1
Chickpea	3–8	< 1–8	< 1	0
Pea	< 1	< 1	< 1	< 1
Lentil	< 1	< 1	< 1	< 1
Kudzu root	467	7283	< 1	< 1
Flaxseed	0	0	10–247	30
Sunflower seed	< 1	6	2	17
Peanut	2	1	8	< 1
Wheat bran	< 1	< 1	3	0
Barley	< 1	< 1	2	0
Rye bran	0	4	4	5
Strawberry	0	0	33	< 1
Cranberry	0	0	29	0
Blueberry	0	0	23	0
Raspberry	0	0	4	0
Red cabbage	< 1	< 1	4	< 1
Broccoli	< 1	< 1	11	< 1
Garlic	0	0	11	< 1
Zucchini	0	0	23	< 1
Carrot	0	0	10	< 1
Beetroot	0	0	3	< 1
Black tea	trace	trace	73	12
Green tea	trace	trace	75	5

Table 3 Main chemical categories of phytoestrogens

Lignans	Flavonols	Coumestans	Isoflavones	Stilbenes
Enterolactone Enterodiol	quercetin rutin	coumestrol	glycitein genistein daidzein	resveratrol

epicatechin), antocyanidins and isoflavonoids (genistein, daidzein)[9]. An important effect of flavonoids is the scavenging of oxygen-derived free radicals. The major source of isoflavonoids in the diet is from soy-based foods. The isoflavonoids from legumes, including genistein and daidzein, are the most studied phytoestrogens. They can exist as glycosides or as aglycones, the glucosides being readily hydrolyzed in the gut as their aglycones. The aglycones are easily transported across intestinal epithelial cells. Genistein has one-third the potency of estradiol when it interacts with ERβ, and one-thousandth the potency of estradiol when it interacts with ERα, as determined by the expression of luciferase reporter gene construct in kidney cells that have been cotransfected with ERα and ERβ[10]. Genistein may produce similar effects to estradiol in several different tissues such as breast, ovary, endometrium, prostate, vascular tissue, bone tissue and cell lines[11,12]. Furthermore, genistein also induces responses that are not associated with the ER, such as the inhibition of tyrosine kinase and DNA topoisomerase[13]. Such an effect is produced even in the presence of antiestrogen, revealing a non-genomic action that could explain a part of the difference between genistein and estradiol.

In vitro experimental systems have also shown that flavonoids possess anti-inflammatory, antiallergic, antiviral and anticarcinogenic properties[14], and various of these molecules, notably isoflavonoids, are identified as phytoestrogens being able to bind estrogen receptors, and possess estrogenic or antiestrogenic activities[15,16].

Lignans

These are constituents of higher plants, such as whole-grains, legumes, vegetables and seeds, with exceptionally high concentrations of lignans found in flaxseed. Although previously thought to be present only in higher plants, mammalian lignans have been detected in the biological fluids of humans and animals. The chemical structure of plant lignans is very different from that of mammalian lignans, and most of the changes occur in the colon, liver and small intestine. Enterolactone and enterodiol are metabolites of the plant lignans matairesinol and secoisolariciresinol, respectively[17]. A clinical study showed that excretion of the lignans enterodiol and enterolactone was significantly higher during a carotenoid (carrot and spinach) and cruciferous (broccoli and cauliflower) vegetable diet than during a vegetable-free diet[18].

Coumestans

Legumes are the main source of coumestrol, the coumestan showing the highest estrogenic activity, and low levels of coumestrol have also been found in brussels sprouts and spinach, while the highest concentrations are reported in clover and in soybean sprouts.

Stilbenes

Recently, the stilbene resveratrol has also been identified as a phytoestrogen. Resveratrol is a natural compound produced by some plants, such as grapevines, in response to injury. Peanuts are rich in resveratrol too. *Polygonium cuspidatum* roots, which have long been used in traditional oriental medicine, have been identified as the major active source of stilbene phytoalexins. Trans-resveratrol was first detected in grapevines in 1976 by Langcake and Pryce, who found that this compound was synthesized by leaf tissues in response to *Botrytis cinerea* fungal infection or exposure to UV light[19].

The biological activity of resveratrol was attested about 15 years ago by the health benefits obtained with orally administred resveratrol. An experimental study suggested that an average drinker of wine may, in the long term, absorb a quantity of resveratrol sufficient to explain the beneficial effect of red wine on human health[20]. Resveratrol possesses anticancer properties and antioxidant activity, and some observations have challenged the protective effects of resveratrol against atherosclerosis thus preventing cardiovascular disease. As a phytoestrogen it may favorably influence several physiological processes, and, given that resveratrol has a different structure, its mechanism of action might differ somewhat from that of other flavonoids[19,20].

HEALTH-BENEFICIAL EFFECTS OF PHYTOESTROGENS

In the past two decades, many clinical and epidemiological studies have been performed to test the health effects of foods and supplements rich in phytoestrogens. A recent review summarizes the main results from scientific studies[21]. The effects of phytoestrogen administration are evaluated on different clinical end-points as listed in Table 4.

Cardiovascular health

Estrogen may affect the vascular system both directly through the ERs located on vascular tissue, and indirectly through altering the

Table 4 Summary of phytoestrogen clinical studies. Modified from reference 21

Clinical end-points	Positive results (n)	Total (n)
Maintaining bone density	11	15
Relief of menopausal symptoms	4	17
Cardiovascular benefit	25	38
Cancer prevention	7	13
Hormone levels/ menstrual cycle	12	19
Effect of hormones in men	0	1
Immune system	1	1
Neurological	5	5
Total*	64	105

*Totals are less than the sum of the studies since some studies examined several clinical end-points

lipoprotein profile[22]. Initial epidemiologic studies showed that women taking hormone replace therapy (HRT) were 50% less likely to experience severe cardiovascular disease (CVD) than women not taking HRT[23]. Lately, a more comprehensive study performed by the Women's Health Initiative has demonstrated a significant increase in CVD in the first year of HRT use, which is still elevated after 5 years of continued use[24–26]. There are several clinical studies that have examined the effect of phytoestrogens on CVD. Isoflavonoids or soy/soy protein and flaxseed have the ability to lower total cholesterol[27,28] and low-density lipoprotein (LDL) cholesterol[27,29], and to raise high-density lipoprotein (HDL) cholesterol[30,31]. In contrast, other studies have shown no effect of isoflavonoids derived from soy or red clover on serum cholesterol levels or plasma lipids[32,33].

Although no clinical studies have shown that resveratrol improves cardiovascular function, the consumption of red wine has been linked to the 'French paradox', a phenomenon observed in French people who have a diet similar to the North American diet, with a significantly lower rate of CVD[34].

Cancer

There is a large body of evidence coming from epidemiologic studies showing that people who consume high amounts of isoflavonoids in their diets have lower rates of occurrence of several cancers, including breast, prostate and colon cancer[35].

The protective effect of phytoestrogens on cancer may be due to their role in lowering circulating levels of unconjugated sex hormones. Estrogens mainly circulate as inactive conjugates of sex hormone-binding globulin (SHBG) or albumin[36]. Dietary supplementation with soy isoflavonoids or lignans produced an increase of the levels of SHBG in postmenopausal women, lowering the serum levels of estradiol[37,38]. Furthermore, higher intakes of soya products and flaxseed produced a significant decrease of the urinary excretion of genotoxic estrogen metabolites[39]. Moreover, the role of phytoestrogens in preventing cancer in women may be related to changes in menstrual cycle length[40]. Increases in menstrual cycle length together with eating a diet rich in phytoestrogens correlate with a decreased rate of hormone-dependent cancer development, including endometrial, ovarian and breast cancers[41].

Menopausal symptoms

Epidemiological studies show that Asiatic women experience less severe, less frequent hot flushes than Western women, 20% vs. 80%, respectively.

Diet has been included among the various reasons proposed to explain such a proven difference. Indeed, the Asian diet is known to be rich in phytoestrogens, and, even though only a few clinical trials have been conducted to evaluate the role of these bioactive substances in regulating menopausal symptoms, most data from randomized studies indicate a significant drop in the severity and frequency of such symptoms. However, women given placebo also demonstrated a decline in menopausal symptoms[42,43]. The variability in frequency and severity of hot flushes and the high placebo-response rate make these clinical trials difficult to interpret, and, currently, they are not sufficient to demonstrate the effectiveness of phytoestrogens in reducing menopausal symptoms. However, considering the lower than expected effectiveness of HRT[24], it is not surprising that many new studies, planned to show a benefit by reduction of menopausal symptoms with phytoestrogen supplementation, are in progress.

Soy and cognitive function

There is clear evidence that treatment of postmenopausal women with mammalian estrogens improves memory, and may alleviate the decline of cognitive function and the risk of dementia[44]. A few studies have examined the effect of phytoestrogens on cognitive function. Data from a follow-up study of cognitive function showed an improvement in picture recall, sustained attention and ability to plan tasks, but on the other hand these women did not demonstrate any improvement in mood or sleepiness, suggesting a specific action on frontal lobe function[45]. In summary, there are too few studies to evaluate whether phytoestrogens may exert some effects on cognitive abilities resulting in a better quality of life in postmenopausal women.

A NUTRITIONAL MODEL: SOY FOODS AND BONE HEALTH

Soy intake is part of the regular diet of the Asian population. Observations that soy-consuming populations have lower hip fracture rates have given rise to the hypothesis that the intake of soy protein and/or soy-derived isoflavonoid phytoestrogens may be protective for bone health[46]. Researchers have long recognized that Asian women, consuming traditional diets, enjoy better cardiovascular and bone health than their counterparts in Western societies. Nutrition epidemiologists believe that this may partly be the result of the soya-rich diet. The scientific interest in isoflavones began with epidemiological studies of elderly women in Asian countries who consume high levels of isoflavones from soy products. The studies showed a positive correlation between a lower prevalence of hip fractures and the intake of soy food products[47]. However, this type of association is inconclusive, as Asian women have different hip geometry compared with Caucasian women[48]. Further epidemiological studies, conducted in Japan and in Hong Kong, to examine directly the linkage between dietary soy-food intake and lumbar spine bone mineral density (BMD) in Asian women, showed a significatively greater BMD in women consuming the highest level of dietary isoflavones compared with those who consumed the least[49]. These results do not demonstrate how this protective effect of soy and/or isoflavones is related to the length of exposure that, usually, for the majority of Asians, is over the entire life-span[50].

Various studies in animal models, using ovariectomized female rats fed with soy foods or soy derivatives, have shown comparable bone-sparing effects of 17β-estradiol and soy protein isolate[51], genistein[52] or daidzein[53].

Clinical trials of the effects of soy isoflavones on bone are too limited, and have shown mixed results[54,55]. Studies have used both soy protein isolate with isoflavones and isolated isoflavones, but the published clinical studies have been of short duration, with only one 12-month trial. The 6-month studies demonstrated promising effects of soy protein isolates containing isoflavones on spine BMD in peri- and postmenopausal women, but they were too short to evaluate adequately the impact of an intervention on BMD[54]. However, the 12-month trial provided confirmation of the positive effect of genistein on bone[55], although no consistent changes in biochemical markers of bone turnover have been reported.

None of the studies in either animals or humans have assessed the effects of soy isoflavones on calcium metabolism. Such information is essential in ascertaining the mode of action of isoflavones on the skeleton. In addition to the estrogenic role of isoflavones in bone health, it has also been demonstrated that many soy foods are a good source of calcium, and soy proteins are less calciuric than animal proteins. Although soybeans contain both oxalates and phytates, which are inhibitors of calcium absorption, calcium bioavailability from soybeans has been shown to be equivalent to that from milk[56]. An exception is represented by calcium-fortified soy beverage, from which calcium absorbtion was reported to be 75% of that from cows' milk[57]. In comparison with animal proteins, soy proteins incorporate fewer sulfur-containing amino acids. One study found that subjects consuming animal protein-based diets excreted 150 mg of urinary calcium per day, in comparison with about 100 mg in subjects consuming a soy protein-based diet[58].

In conclusion, the habitual intake of soy, as traditional Asian food, appears to be beneficial to bone health, though the effective or optimal dosage is still unclear. The soy–bone action could be mediated through its estrogenic or calcium-conserving effects. In addition, soy intake contributes to an increase in high-quality protein intake. Therefore, this traditional dietary practice should be encouraged and preserved in Asian populations.

Although European countries have no soy consumption tradition, another plant estrogen group, known as lignans, seems to have a positive impact on bone health in European countries, as well as in the vegetarian population. This is due to the relatively high levels of these compounds in certain grains, especially in rye, as well as in flaxseed, which are part of the daily diet in these populations. Interestingly, there is a striking similarity between the European vegetarian and Asian–Japanese populations, exhibiting a lower incidence of osteoporosis compared with the non-vegetarian populations[59].

A PHARMACOLOGICAL MODEL: PHYTOESTROGENS AND BONE HEALTH

Most studies suggest that phytoestrogens are somewhat effective in maintaining BMD in postmenopausal women[60–67]. Moreover, recent results from the Women's Health Initiative study, showing an unexpected lack of cardioprotective effects of HRT[24], pushed forward research into alternative and natural strategies for managing and preventing osteoporosis. The

most recent full review[68] concerning dietary phytoestrogens and their effect on bone justifies the bone-conserving properties of isoflavones by the following bodies of experimental evidence, showing close similarities to an experimental pharmacological model from in vitro studies of cultured bone cells, through animal models of osteoporosis to epidemiological and intervention studies in humans.

Most of the in vitro studies with human and animal osteoblasts and osteoblast-like cell lines have shown that daidzein and genistein have a stimulatory effect on protein synthesis and on alkaline phosphatase release[69,70]. This effect is blocked by the addition of actinomycin or cycloheximide, suggesting that these isoflavones influence transcriptional or translational events[68]. More recently, genistein has been found to stimulate the production of osteoprotegerin (OPG) by human osteoblasts, providing a further mechanism for the bone-sparing effects of soy isoflavones. Besides ER-dependent processes, genistein and daidzein both suppress osteoclast activity by several mechanisms, including apoptosis, activation of protein tyrosine phosphatase, inhibition of cytokines, changes in intracellular Ca^{2+}, membrane depolarization and antioxidant activity, much like many other polyphenols[71–73]. In some cases the antioxidant effect occurs in the nmol/l range. Furthermore, a positive synergy between phytoestrogens and other antioxidants has been described[74].

A number of observational and dietary intervention studies confirm the general findings of in vitro effects of phytoestrogens on human bone cells in culture. Thus far, observational or epidemiologic studies[75,76] and dietary intervention studies[77–82] have shown significant relationships between phytoestrogens and surrogate markers of bone turnover such as urinary calcium, magnesium and phosphorus, hydroxyproline and collagen cross-links and serum markers, including bone-specific alkaline phosphatase, osteocalcin, insulin-like growth factor I (IGF-I) and interleukin 6 (Tables 5 and 6). Most of the observational studies have been performed in women living in countries where the indigenous population have relatively high phytoestrogen intake, mostly related to soy protein foods.

Table 5 Intervention studies of phytoestrogen and bone health in women including findings on bone mineral density (BMD) and bone mineral content (BMC). Modified from reference 68

Reference	Subjects	Intervention (protein type and daily isoflavone level)	Study length	Findings (BMD or BMC end-point by DXA)
Dalais et al.[60], 1998	postmenopausal (n = 45)	soy grits 45 g wheat kibble 45 g flaxseed 45 g	3 months	all three groups had increase in BMC; soy group 5.2%, flax group 5.2% and control group 4.0%
Potter et al.[30], 1998	postmenopausal (n = 66)	casein 40 g/day soya 40 g/56 mg soya 40 g/90 mg Ca supplemented	6 months	+2.2% increase in lumbar spine BMD in soy 90 mg isoflavone group; 56 mg isoflavone group unchanged; no changes in other sites
Clifton-Bligh et al.[83], 2001	postmenopausal (n = 46)	clover-derived tablets: 28.5, 57 and 85.5 mg	6 months	BMD at proximal radius and ulna increased 4.1% with 57 mg/day and 3.0% with 85.5 mg/day; 28.5 mg remained unchanged; no increase in endometrial thickness was seen in any group
Anderson et al.[84], 2002	young healthy adult women (n = 27, age 21–25 years)	isoflavone-rich diet, 90 mg, compared with control diet	12 months	No effect of soy diet on BMD or BMC in healthy, menstruating women

DXA, dual-energy X-ray absorptiometry

CONCLUSIONS

Since it has now been established that life-style and particularly nutritional habits contribute significantly to the occurrence of different rates of degenerative disorders, such as cardiovascular disease, osteoporosis, cognitive disability and cancer, in recent years Eastern and Western governments and industries have started to invest in evaluation of the health effects of phytochemicals contained in the diet. This aspect is becoming a main feature of preventive medicine, since life expectancy is growing in the Western population.

To date, it is not still completely clear whether the foods rich in such compounds may really be protective for human health, and, if so, at which daily regimen they should be consumed to exert a real pharmacological action. Moreover, non-estrogenic compounds coexist with phyto-estrogens in the same plant-derived food, and the role that they may play in both activity and bioavailability of phytoestrogens themselves has not been elucidated. Since, at present, industries can produce extract compounds from these food-stuffs, researchers may take advantage to plan experimental studies and clinical trials in which these molecules can be tested in relation to bio-markers and other functional parameters connected with human pathophysiology. Consequently, the possibility of testing the purified phytochemical compounds, both in *in vitro* and *in vivo* experimental models, may offer the opportunity to corroborate data obtained from epidemiological studies.

Unfortunately, due to the great diversity of phytoestrogen compounds, including different bioavailabilities, pharmacokinetics, pharmacological properties and metabolic fates, it is quite complex to define, assess and understand their

Table 6 Intervention studies of phytoestrogen and bone health in women including findings on bone markers. Modified from reference 68

Reference	Subjects	Intervention (protein type and daily isoflavone level)	Study length	Findings (bone marker end-points)
Wong[82], 2000	postmenopausal ($n = 6$) open pilot study, mean age 55.4 years	soy isoflavones 160 mg/day	6 weeks	resorption markers: uDpy $-7 \pm 41\%$ urinary Ca concentration $-12 \pm 46\%$ sPTH $+3 \pm 60\%$ urinary Ca excretion $-5 \pm 29\%$ bone formation markers: sOC $9 \pm 15\%$, serum BAP $-16 \pm 23\%$, IGF-I $-8 \pm 27\%$, changes are of similar magnitude to those reported for ERT
Scheiber[85], 2001	postmenopausal ($n = 42$) open pilot study mean age 55.5 years	whole soy foods, 60 mg isoflavones/day, no Ca supplementation	3 months	Resorption markers: serum ALP unchanged, urinary NTx decreased 13.9%, formation markers: serum OC increased by 10.3%
Lu et al.[86], 2002	postmenopausal ($n = 12$) age range 49–66 years	soy milk 1.08 l/day ≈ 112 mg isoflavones	4 months	increase in uDpy 21% and serum BAP 18%, increase in OC 34%; values returned to pre-diet level 4 months after diet; no estrogenic effects on uterus; no changes in serum levels of PTH, follicle-stimulating hormone or estradiol

uDpy, urinary deoxypiridinoline; sPTH, serum parathyroid hormone; BAP, bone-specific alkaline phosphatase; IGF-I, insulin-like growth factor-I; ERT, estrogen replacement therapy; NTx, cross-linked N-telopeptides of type I collagen; OC osteocalcin; Ca, calcium; ALP, alkaline phosphatase

precise effects on human health, since large and long-term intervention studies are needed.

Osteoporosis represents one of the human disease models more widely studied for the potential therapeutic effects of phytoestrogens.

Currently, the results from the few studies on bone health are seductive but too few to draw definitive conclusions. Supporting data from *in vitro* and *in vivo* studies of models of osteoporosis strongly show bone-sparing effects of dietary phytoestrogens[87,88]. Such data may justify large-scale clinical dietary intervention studies of phytoestrogens in the near future.

Finally, the preliminary data in this field suggest that phytoestrogen-rich foods should be included in the health-food sector, and that scientists should push to isolate the active molecules to be used as potential new drugs.

References

1. Bidlack WR, Wang W. Designing functional foods. In Shils ME, Olson JA, Shike M, et al., eds. *Modern Nutrition in Health and Disease*. Lippincott, Williams & Wilkins, 1999: 1823–33

2. Cassidy A. Potential risks and benefits of phytoestrogen-rich diets. *Int J Vitam Nutr Res* 2003; 73: 120–6

3. Jordan VC, McGregor SJ, Levenson AS, et al. Molecular classification of estrogens. *Cancer Res* 2001; 61: 6619–23

4. Chen DB, Bird IM, Zheng J, et al. Membrane estrogen receptor-dependent extracellular signal-regulated kinase pathway mediates acute activation of endothelial nitric oxide synthase by estrogen in uterine artery endothelial cells. *Endocrinology* 2004; 145: 113–25

5. Mueller SO. Overview of in vitro tools to assess the estrogenic and antiestrogenic activity of phytoestrogens. *J Chromatogr B* 2002; 777: 155–65

6. Mazur W, Adelcreutz H. Naturally occurring oestrogens in food. *Pure Appl Chem* 1998; 70: 1759–76

7. UCLA Center for Human Nutrition. Phytoestrogens. http://www.cellinteractive.com/ucla/natural_remedies/phytoestrogens.html (26/04/2004)

8. Rossiter RC, Beck AB. Physiological and ecological studies on the estrogenic isoflavones in subterranean clover (*Tifolium subterraneum*) I. Effects of temperature. *Aust J Agric Res* 1996; 17: 29–37

9. UCLA Center for Human Nutrition. Flavonoids and Health. http://www.cellinteractive.com/ucla/natural_remedies/flavonoids.html (26/04/2004)

10. Kuiper GG, Lemmen JG, Carlsson B, et al. Interaction of estrogenic chemicals and phytoestrogens with estrogen receptor β. *Endocrinology* 1998; 139: 4252–63

11. Wang D, Gutkowska J, Marcinkiewicz M, et al. Genistein supplementation stimulates the oxytocin system in the aorta of ovariectomized rats. *Cardiovasc Res* 2003; 57: 186–94

12. Zhou S, Turgeman G, Harris SE, et al. Estrogens activate bone morphogenetic protein-2 gene transcription in mouse mesenchymal stem cells. *Mol Endocrinol* 2003; 17: 56–66

13. Jonas J, Plant T, Gilon P, et al. Multiple effects and stimulation of insulin secretion by the tyrosine kinase inhibitor genistein in normal mouse islets. *Br J Pharmacol* 1995; 114: 872–80

14. Nijveldt RJ, van Nood E, van Hoorn DEC, et al. Flavonoids: a review of probable mechanisms of action and potential applications. *Am J Clin Nutr* 2001; 74: 418–25

15. Van der Woude H, Gliszczynska-Swiglo A, Struijs K, et al. Biphasic modulation of cell proliferation by quercetin at concentrations physiologically relevant in humans. *Cancer Lett* 2003; 200: 41–7

16. Prouillet C, Mazière JC, Mazière C, et al. Stimulatory effect of naturally occurring flavonols quercetin and kaempferol on alkaline phosphatase activity in MG-63 human osteoblast through ERK and estrogen receptor pathway. *Biochem Pharmacol* 2004; 67: 1307–13

17. Tham DM, Gardner CD, Haskell WL. Potential health benefits of dietary phytoestrogens: a review of the clinical, epidemiological and mechanistic evidence. *J Clin Endocrinol Metab* 1998; 83: 2223–35

18. Kirkman LM, Lampe JW, Campbell DR, et al. Urinary lignan and isoflavonoid excretion in men and women consuming vegetable and soy diet. *Nutr Cancer* 1995; 24: 1–12

19. Frémont L. Biological effects of resveratrol. *Life Sci* 2000; 66: 663–73

20. Bertelli A, Bertelli AA, Gozzini A, et al. Plasma and tissue resveratrol concentrations and pharmacological activity. *Drugs Exp Clin Res* 1998; 24: 133–8

21. Cornwell T, Cohick W, Raskin I. Dietary phytoestrogens and health. *Phytochemistry* 2004; 65: 995–1016

22. Rubanyi GM, Johns A, Kaiser K. Effect of estrogen on endothelial function and angiogenesis. *Vasc Pharmacol* 2002; 38: 89–98

23. Lissin LW, Cook JP. Phytoestrogens and cardiovascular health. *J Am Coll Cardiol* 2000; 35: 1403–10

24. Writing Group for the Women's Health Initiative Investigators. Risks and benefits of estrogen plus progestin in healthy postmenopausal women: principal results from the Women's Health Initiative randomized controlled trial. *J Am Med Assoc* 2002; 288: 321–33

25. Hays J, Ockene JK, Brunner RL, et al. Women's Health Initiative Investigators. Effects of estrogen plus progestin on health related quality of life. *N Engl J Med* 2003; 348: 1835–7

26. Manson JE, Hsia J, Johnson KC, et al. The Women's Health Initiative Investigators. Estrogen plus progestin and the risk of coronary heart disease. *N Engl J Med* 2003; 349: 523–34

27. Lemay A, Dodin S, Kadri N, et al. Flaxseed dietary supplement versus hormone replacement therapy in hypercholesterolemic menopausal women. *Obstet Gynecol* 2002; 100: 495–504

28. Teede HJ, Dalais FS, Kotsopoulos D, et al. Dietary soy has both beneficial and potentially adverse cardiovascular effects: a placebo controlled study in men and postmenopausal women. *J Clin Endocrinol Metab* 2001; 86: 3053–60

29. Jayagopal V, Albertazzi P, Kilpatrick ES, et al. Beneficial effects of soy phytoestrogen intake in postmenopausal women with type 2 diabetes. *Diabetes Care* 2002; 25: 990–4

30. Potter S, Baum J, Teng H, et al. Soy protein and isoflavones: their effects on blood lipids and bone density in postmenopausal women. *Am J Clin Nutr* 1998; 68: 1375–9

31. Sanders TAB, Dean TS, Grainger D, et al. Moderate intakes of intact soy protein rich in isoflavones compared with ethanol-extracted soy protein increase HDL but do not influence transforming growth factor beta(1) concentrations and hemostatic risk factors for coronary heart disease in healthy subjects. *Am J Nutr* 2002; 76: 373–7

32. Howes JB, Sullivan D, Lai N, et al. The effect of dietary supplementation with isoflavones from red clover on the lipoprotein profiles of post menopausal women with mild to moderate hypercholesterolemia. *Atherosclerosis* 2000; 152: 143–7

33. Dewell A, Hollenbeck CB, Bruce B. The effects of the soy derived phytoestrogens on serum lipids and lipoproteins in moderately hypercholesterolemic postmenopausal women. *J Clin Endocrinol Metab* 2002; 87: 118–21

34. Asby J, Tinwell H, Pennie W, et al. Partial and weak estrogenicity of the red wine constituent resveratrol 4: consideration of its superagonist activity in MCF-7 cells and its suggested cardiovascular protective effects. *J Appl Toxicol* 1999; 19: 39–45

35. American Institute for Cancer Research. Food Nutrition and the Prevention of Cancer. A Global Perspective. Washington: World Cancer Research Fund, 1997

36. Dotsch J, Dorr HG, Wildt L. Exposure to endogenous estrogens during lifetime. In Metzler M, ed. *Endocrine Disruptors*, Part 1. Berlin: Springer-Verlag, 2001: 83–99

37. Hutchins AM, Martini MC, Olson BA, et al. Flaxseed compsumption influences endogenous hormone concentrations in postmenopausal women. *Nutr Cancer* 2001; 39: 58–65

38. Berrino F, Bellati C, Secreto G, et al. Reducing bioavailable sex hormones through a comprehensive change in diet: the diet and androgens (DIANA) randomized trial. *Cancer Epidemiol Biomarkers Prev* 2001; 10: 25–33

39. Xu X, Duncan AM, Merz BE, et al. Soy consumption alters endogenous estrogen metabolism in postmenopausal women. *Cancer Epidemiol Biomarkers Prev* 2000; 7: 1101–8

40. Nagata C, Takatsuka N, Inaba S, et al. Effect of soymilk consumption on serum estrogen concentrations in premenopausal Japanese women. *J Natl Cancer Inst* 1998; 90: 1830–5

41. Tsourounis C. Clinical effects of phytoestrogens. *Clin Obst Gynecol* 2004; 44: 836–42

42. Tice JA, Ettinger B, Ensrud K. Phytoestrogen supplements for the treatment of hot flashes: the isoflavone clover extract (ICE) study: a randomized controlled trial. *J Am Med Assoc* 2003; 290: 207–14

43. Nikander E, Kikkinen A, Metsa-Heikkila M, et al. A randomized placebo-controlled crossover trial with phytoestrogens in treatment of menopause in breast cancer patients. *Obstet Gynecol* 2003; 101: 1213–20

44. Yaffe K, Sawaya G, Lieberburg I, et al. Estrogen therapy in postmenopausal women: effects on cognitive function and dementia. *J Am Med Assoc* 1998; 279: 688–95

45. Duffy R, Wiseman H, File SE. Improved cognitive function in postmenopausal women after 12 weeks of consumption of a soya extract containing isoflavones. *Pharmacol Biochem Behav* 2003; 75: 721–9

46. Messina MJ. Legumes and soybeans: overview of their nutritional profiles and health effects. *Am J Clin Nutr* 1999; 70: 439S–50S

47. Lacey JM, Anderson JJB. Older women in Japan and the United States: physical and nutritional comparisons. In Takahashi HE, ed. *Bone Morphometry: Proceedings of the Fifth International Congress.* Nishimura, Japan, 1991; 562–5

48. Nakamura T, Turner CH, Yoshikawa T, et al. Do variations in hip geometry explain differences in hip fracture risk between Japanese and white Americans? *J Bone Miner Res* 1994; 9: 1071–6

49. Mei J, Yeung SS, Kung AW. High dietary phytoestrogen intake is associated with higher bone mineral density in postmenopausal but not premenopausal women. *J Clin Endocrinol Metab* 2001; 11: 5217–21

50. Cai DJ, Spence LA, Weaver CM. Soy isoflavones and bone health. In New SA, Bonjour JP, eds. *Nutritional Aspects of Bone Health.* Cambridge: The Royal Society of Chemistry, 2003: 421–38

51. Ajrmandi, BH, Alekel L, Hollis BW, et al. Dietary soybean protein prevents bone loss in an ovariectomized rat model of osteoporosis. *J Nutr* 1996; 126: 161–7

52. Fanti P, Monier-Faugere MC, Geng Z, et al. The phytoestrogen genistein reduces bone loss in short term ovariectomized rats. *Osteoporos Int* 1998; 8: 274–81

53. Ishida H, Uesugi T, Hirai K, et al. Preventive effects of the plants isoflavones, daidzeine and genisteine on bone loss in ovariectomized rats fed a calcium-deficient diet. *Biol Pharm Bull* 1998; 21: 62–6

54. Alekel L, St German A, Peterson CT, et al. Isoflavone-rich soy protein isolate exerts significant bone-sparing in the lumbar spine of perimenopausal women. *Am J Clin Nutr* 2000; 729: 844–52

55. Morabito N, Crisafulli A, Vergara C, et al. Effects of genistein and hormone-replacement therapy on bone loss in early postmenopausal women: a randomized double-blind placebo-controlled study. *J Bone Miner Res* 2002; 17: 1904–12

56. Poneros AG, Erdman JW Jr. Bioavailability of calcium from tofu, tortillas, nonfat dry milk and mozzarella cheese in rats, effect of supplemental ascorbic acid. *J Food Sci* 1993; 58: 382–4

57. Heaney RP, Dowell MS, Rafferty K, et al. Bioavailability of the calcium in fortified soy imitation milk: some observations on method. *Am J Clin Nutr* 2000; 71: 1166–9

58. .Breslau NA, Brinkley L, Hill KD, et al. Relationship of animal protein rich diet to kidney stone formation and calcium metabolism. *J Clin Endocrin Meter* 1988; 66: 140–6

59. Brouns F. Soy isoflavones: a new and promising ingredient for the health foods sector. *Food Res Int* 2002; 35: 187–93

60. Dalais FS, Rice GE, Wahlqvist ML, et al. Effects of dietary phytoestrogens in postmenopausal women. *Climateric* 1998; 1: 124–9

61. Kaardinal AFM, Morton MS, Bruggemann-Rotgans IEM, et al. Phytoestrogen excretion and rate of bone loss in postmenopausal women. *Eur J Clin Nutr* 1998; 52: 850–5

62. Alekel DL, Germain AS, Peterson CT, et al. Isoflavone rich soy protein isolate attenuates bone loss in the lumbar spine of perimenopausal women. *Am J Clin Nutr* 2000; 72: 844–52

63. Ho SC, Chan SG, Yi Q, et al. Soy intake and the maintenance of peak bone mass in Hong Kong Chinese women. *J Bone Miner Res* 2001; 16: 1363–9

64. Mei J, Yeung SS, Kung AW. High dietary phytoestrogen intake is associated with higher bone mineral density in postmenopausal but not premenopausal women. *J Clin Endocrinol Metab* 2001; 86: 5217–21

65. Chiechi LM, Secreto G, D'Amore M, et al. Efficacy of soy rich diet in preventing postmenopausal osteoporosis: the Menfis randomized trial. *Maturitas* 2002; 42: 295–300

66. Kim MK, Chung BC, Yu VY, et al. Relationships of urinary phyto-oestrogen excretion to BMD in postmenopausal women. *Clin Endocrinol* 2002; 56: 321–8

67. Morabito N, Crisafulli A, Vergara C, et al. Effects of genistein and hormone-replacement therapy on bone loss in early postmenopausal women: a randomized double-blind placebo-controlled study. *J Bone Miner Res* 2002; 17: 1904–12

68. Setchell KDR, Lydeking-Olsen E. Dietary phytoestrogens and their effect on bone: evince from in vitro and in vivo, human observational, and dietary intervention studies. *Am J Clin Nutr* 2003; 78: 593S–609S

69. Sugimoto E, Yamaguchi M. Anabolic effect of genistein in osteoblastic MC3T3-E1 cells. *Int J Mol Med* 2000; 5: 515–20

70. Yamaguchi M, Sugimoto E. Stimulatory effect of genistein and daidzein on protein synthesis in

osteoblastic MC3T3-E1 cells: activation of aminoacyl-tRNA synthetase. *Mol Cell Biochem* 2000; 214: 97–102

71. Blair HC, Jordan SE, Peterson TG, et al. Variable effects of tyrosine kinase inhibitors on avian osteoclastic activity and reduction of bone loss in ovariectomized rats. *J Cell Biochem* 1996; 61: 629–37

72. Williams JP, Jordan SE, Barnes S, et al. Tyrosine kinase inhibitor effects on avian osteoclastic acid transport. *Am J Clin Nutr* 1998; 68 (Suppl): 1369S–74S

73. Okamoto F, Okabe K, Kajiya H. Genistein, a soybean isoflavone, inhibits inward rectifier K+ channels in rat osteoclasts. *Jpn J Physiol* 2001; 51: 501–9

74. Gao YH, Yamaguchi M. Suppressive effects of genistein on rat bone osteoclasts: apoptosis is reduced through Ca++ signaling. *Biol Pharm Bull* 1999; 22: 805–9

75. Gao YH, Yamaguchi M. Suppressive effect of genistein on rat bone osteoclasts: involvement of protein kinase inhibition and protein tyrosine phosphatase activation. *Int J Mol Med* 2000; 5: 261–7

76. Chin-Dusting JP, Fisher LJ, Lewis TV, et al. The vascular activity of some isoflavone metabolites: implications for cardioprotective role. *Br J Pharmacol* 2001; 133: 595–605

77. Patel RP, Boersma B, Crawford JH, et al. Antioxidant mechanisms of isoflavones in lipid systems: paradoxical effects of peroxyl radical scavenging. *Free Rad Biol Med* 2001; 31: 1570–81

78. Horiuchi T, Onouchi T, Takahashi M, et al. Effect of soy protein on bone metabolism in postmenopausal women. *Osteoporosis* 2000; 11: 721–4

79. Somekawa Y, Chiguchi M, Ishibashi T, et al. Soy intake related to menopausal symptoms, serum lipids, and bone mineral density in postmenopausal Japanese women. *Obstet Gynecol* 2001; 97: 109–15

80. Pansini F, Bonaccorsi G, Albertazzi P, et al. Soy phytoestrogens and bone. Presented at the North American Menopause Society, 1997: 44

81. Wangen KE, Duncan AM, Merz-Demlow BE, et al. Effects of soy isoflavones on markers of bone turnover in premenopausal and postmenopausal women. *J Clin Endocrinol Metab* 2000; 85: 3043–9

82. Wong WW. Effects of soy isoflavones on blood lipids, blood pressure and biochemical markers of bone metabolism in postmenopausal women. *J Nutr* 2000; 130: 686S (abstr)

83. Clifton-Bligh PB, Baber RJ, Fulcher GR, et al. The effect of isoflavones extracted from red clover (Rimostil) on lipid and bone metabolism. *Menopause* 2001; 8: 259–65

84. Anderson JJ, Chen X, Boass A, et al. Soy isoflavones: no effects on bone mineral content and bone mineral density in healthy, menstruating young adult women after one year. *J Am Coll Nutr* 2002; 21: 388–93

85. Scheiber M, Liu J, Subbiah, et al. Dietary soy supplementation reduces LDL oxidation and bone turnover in healthy postmenopausal women. *Menopause* 2001; 8: 384–92

86. Lu L-JW, Anderson KE, Grady JJ, Nagamani M. Chronic soy consumption influences serum levels of steroid and peptide hormones without uterine effects in postmenopausal women. *J Nutr* 2002; 132: 615S (abstr)

87. Arjmandi BH, Khalil DA, Lucas EA, et al. Soy protein with its isoflavones improves bone markers in middle aged and elderly women. *FASEB J* 2001; 15: A728 (abstr)

88. Cook A, Pennington G. Phytoestrogen and multiple vitamin/mineral effects on bone mineral density in early postmenopausal women: a pilot study. *J Women's Health* 2002; 11: 53–60

Tibolone

25

M. R. McClung

INTRODUCTION

In response to estrogen deficiency at the menopause, an imbalance in bone remodeling occurs such that bone resorption exceeds bone formation. This results in a loss of bone mass, deterioration of bone architecture and trabecular structure and an increase in cortical porosity. All of these changes contribute to skeletal fragility and increased fracture risk that, in many older women, have significant clinical and social consequences. Estrogen therapy normalizes bone remodeling and effectively prevents bone loss in both younger and older postmenopausal women. Estrogen therapy with or without a progestin has been shown to reduce significantly the risk of both vertebral and non-vertebral fractures in large cohorts of low-risk women[1,2]. However, upon withdrawal from estrogen, relative rapid bone loss occurs, and the fracture protection effect gradually disappears[3,4]. Thus, long-term estrogen therapy is required to prevent osteoporosis and to reduce fracture risk effectively. Because concern exists about the safety of these agents, estrogen is no longer recommended for use long term to prevent bone loss in women who are not experiencing a symptomatic benefit of therapy[5]. Effective, safe and well-tolerated alternatives to estrogen are being sought for the prevention of bone loss in postmenopausal women.

Tibolone is a selective tissue estrogen activity regulator (STEAR) that has potent effects on the skeleton and may have important extraskeletal effects that would differentiate it from estrogen and other drugs used for the prevention of bone loss in postmenopausal women. This brief review summarizes and highlights some of the effects of tibolone.

MECHANISM OF ACTION

Tibolone is a synthetic steroid substance that has little if any inherent estrogenic effect[6]. However, it is converted to two 3-OH-metabolites that bind to and activate the estrogen receptor (ER). The metabolites preferentially interact with the ERα receptor, accounting for the estrogen-like activity of tibolone on bone metabolism. In breast tissue, metabolites of tibolone inhibit proliferation of and stimulate apoptosis of breast tissue cells[7]. In the uterus, the peripheral metabolite of tibolone (Δ^4-isomer) has progestational and possibly androgenic effects. This allows tibolone to be administered without concomitant progestin in women without an intact uterus. Studies with specific inhibitors of estrogenic, progestogenic and androgenic action have documented that the effects of tibolone on bone are mediated through the estrogen receptor[8].

EFFECTS ON THE SKELETON

Since the early study by Dr Lindsay and his colleagues of the effect of tibolone on bone density[9], several studies have evaluated the effects of tibolone in doses of 1.25 and 2.5 mg daily on bone mineral density (BMD) in placebo-controlled trials lasting 12–30 months[10–18]. Increases in spine BMD measured by dual-energy X-ray absorptiometry (DEXA) of 4.2–6.4%, compared with placebo, have been observed. The responses were similar in both older and younger postmenopausal women and in those with or without osteoporosis. In two identical studies, the BMD response over a broader range of doses of tibolone was evaluated[19]. Seven hundred and seventy postmenopausal women who were 1–4

233

years since the menopause and who had normal bone density values were randomly assigned to receive placebo or tibolone in doses of 0.3, 0.625, 1.25 or 2.5 mg daily. All received 500 mg calcium daily. Follow-up BMD studies were obtained in 656 subjects, and 519 women completed the entire 2-year study. Clear dose-related increases in bone density at both the spine and total hip regions were observed with tibolone, while density decreased modestly in the placebo group (Figure 1). Bone mass was preserved in the 0.3-mg group while the larger doses effected significant increases in bone density. Similarly, dose-related decreases in indices of bone resorption (urinary N-telopeptide) and bone formation (bone-specific alkaline phosphatase) were observed. The decrease in N-telopeptide was 40–50% with 1.25- and 2.5-mg doses. These effects on markers of bone turnover are similar to the results of previous studies[20,21].

The effect of tibolone on bone density has been followed for extended intervals in two small studies. In both, the initial increase in BMD was sustained over longer intervals. Women followed for 8 years while receiving 2.5 mg tibolone daily were noted to have increases in BMD of 4.1% in the lumbar spine and 1.6% in the hip region[22]. In a placebo-controlled, non-randomized study of women followed for 10 years, BMD in the lumbar spine and femoral neck increased by 4.8% and 3.7%, respectively, in 31 women receiving tibolone 2.5 mg daily, while, in the 26 subjects in the placebo group, decreases of 8.5% in the lumbar spine and 8.9% in the femoral neck were observed[23]. As with estrogen, spinal bone density decreased when tibolone therapy was withdrawn[7]. On the other hand, tibolone was effective in preventing bone loss in the radius in young women who had recently undergone ovarian resection[24].

Direct comparisons with estrogen of the effects of tibolone on BMD and bone metabolism have also been explored in several studies[16,17,25–29]. Bone density responses to 1.25 and 2.5 mg tibolone daily were generally similar to those with estrogen or estrogen–progestin. The similarity of BMD responses to tibolone and other estrogen therapies was confirmed in a meta-analysis of studies of at least 2 years'

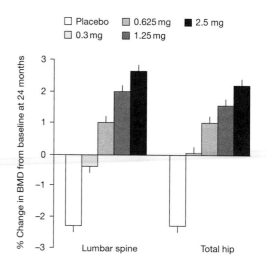

Figure 1 Bone mineral density (BMD) response (percentage change from baseline ± SE) at 24 months to tibolone or placebo. Data adapted from reference 19

duration[30]. In the largest direct comparison study to date, 866 women were randomly assigned to receive placebo, conjugated equine estrogen–medroxyprogesterone acetate (CEE–MPA) or tibolone 2.5 mg daily[31]. After 3 years, the women receiving tibolone experienced an increase of 4.2% in the lumbar spine compared with an increase of 4.6% with CEE–MPA. A decrease of 2% occurred in the placebo group. In the total hip region, BMD increased 3.6% and 3.0% in the tibolone and CEE–MPA treatment groups, respectively, while the value decreased by 1.0% in the placebo group. The responses to both tibolone and CEE–MPA were highly statistically significant when compared with the placebo group, but the responses to tibolone and CEE–MPA were not statistically different. Reductions in markers of bone turnover with tibolone have been similar to the effects observed with estrogen therapies[29,31].

No studies have yet prospectively evaluated the effect of tibolone therapy on fracture risk in patients with osteoporosis. None of the reported studies have been large enough to evaluate fractures as outcomes, and none have included fractures as formal end-points. Additionally, these bone density studies have generally evaluated relatively young postmenopausal women whose risk for fracture is low. In a large observational study performed in the United Kingdom involving 138 737 postmenopausal women aged 50–69 followed for an average of 2.8 years, the effect of estrogen-like drugs on the incidence of clinical fractures was evaluated[32]. Included in that study were 3037 women who had taken tibolone for an average of 4.8 years at baseline. Compared with non-estrogen users, the relative risk of experiencing a clinical fracture was 0.67 (95% confidence interval (CI) 0.54–0.83) in the women receiving tibolone, which was very similar to the effect observed with oral estrogen therapy (relative risk ((RR 0.65, 95% CI 0.58–0.71). A large prospective trial (Long-term Intervention on Fractures with Tibolone or LIFT) is now under way to evaluate the effect of tibolone on fracture risk in older women with low BMD.

NON-SKELETAL EFFECTS

Like estrogens and selective estrogen receptor modulators (SERMs), tibolone interacts with hormone receptors in many tissues. Its role in clinical practice will be shaped and defined by its extraskeletal effects and tolerability. In general, tibolone appears to be better tolerated than estrogen. Hot flushes and other menopausal symptoms are improved[19,27], and tibolone is approved for the management of menopausal symptoms in many countries. There is a suggestion that mood, libido and symptoms of vaginal atrophy improve with tibolone therapy[33,34]. Vaginal bleeding occurs in a small proportion of women receiving tibolone, but the frequency of bleeding is much less than with combined estrogen–progestin combinations[19,29,31,35,36]. Endometrial hyperplasia has not been described as a consequence of tibolone therapy, but larger or longer studies of endometrial monitoring are needed[37,38]. The incidence of breast tenderness is lower with tibolone than with estrogen therapy, but is generally higher than in subjects receiving placebo[19,28,30]. Unlike what occurs with estrogen, mammographic breast density does not increase in women who receive tibolone for as long as 10 years[39–41]. The incidence of breast

cancer assisted with tibolone therapy has not been adequately evaluated in randomized trials. In the Million Women Study, the risk of developing invasive breast cancer with current use of tibolone was 1.45 (95% CI 1.25–1.68) compared with non-estrogen users[42]. This risk was similar to that observed with users of preparations containing estrogen only, and was less than that observed with combined estrogen– progestin therapy. The significance of this observation is not known. The women evaluated in this large observational study were not randomly assigned to treatments. Because of the strong perception that tibolone might have less effect on the breast than estrogen, tibolone may have been preferentially prescribed to women at increased risk for breast cancer. A large prospective, randomized, placebo-controlled clinical trial is under way to address the effect of tibolone therapy on the risk of recurrence in women previously treated for, but without current evidence of, breast cancer.

Like other estrogens, tibolone therapy has been associated with a reduction in total and low density lipoprotein (LDL) cholesterol, and lipoprotein(a) (Lp(a)) and antithrombin III[43,44]. Unlike estrogen, however, serum levels of both high density lipoprotein (HDL) cholesterol and triglycerides also decrease significantly. Increases in C-reactive protein were similar with tibolone and estrogen–progestin[45]. Although lipid and antithrombin III levels are related to cardiovascular risk in untreated postmenopausal women, the relationships between treatment-induced changes in these markers with estrogen-like drugs and the effect on the risk of cardiovascular disease are uncertain. Thus, the effects of tibolone on the incidence of stroke, coronary heart disease and venous thrombotic episodes must await the results of the larger prospective studies now being conducted.

SUMMARY AND CONCLUSIONS

Tibolone is a unique medication that has important effects on the skeleton that are similar to those observed with conventional doses of estrogen. The responses to tibolone of bone mineral density and biochemical indices of bone metabolism are in the ranges that have been associated with significant fracture reduction in postmenopausal women with osteoporosis. The LIFT study will provide the information necessary to evaluate the effect of tibolone therapy on fracture incidence. Tibolone has other important extraskeletal actions. Its salutary effects on vasomotor symptoms, vaginal dryness and possibly on mood and libido offer potential benefits to women not available with bisphosphonates or SERMs. Important unanswered questions remain, however, about the effect of tibolone on the incidence of breast cancer, heart disease and stroke, venous thrombosis and long-term endometrial safety. Fortunately, large prospective trials are now in progress to address these issues. With those answers in hand, the role of tibolone as an alternative to estrogen for the prevention and treatment of osteoporosis, and the management of symptoms in postmenopausal women can be more clearly defined.

ACKNOWLEDGMENT

I thank Ms Philippa Jones for help in preparing the manuscript.

References

1. Writing Group for the Women's Health Initiative Investigators. Risks and benefits of estrogen plus progestin in healthy postmenopausal women: principal results from the Women's Health Initiative randomized controlled trial. *J Am Med Assoc* 2002; 288: 321–33

2. Anderson GL, Limacher M, Assaf AR, et al. Effects of conjugated equine estrogen in postmenopausal women with hysterectomy: the Women's Health Initiative randomized controlled trial. *J Am Med Assoc* 2004; 291: 1701–12

3. Greenspan SL, Emkey RD, Bone HG, et al. Significant differential effects of alendronate, estrogen, or combination therapy on the rate of bone loss after discontinuation of treatment of postmenopausal osteoporosis. A randomized, double-blind, placebo-controlled trial. *Ann Intern Med* 2002; 137: 875–83

4. Cauley JA, Zmuda JM, Ensrud KE, et al. Study of Osteoporotic Fractures Research Group. Timing of estrogen replacement therapy for optimal osteoporosis prevention. *J Clin Endocrinol Metab* 2001; 86: 5700–5

5. Burger H, Archer D, Barlow D, et al. Practical recommendations for hormone replacement therapy in the peri- and postmenopause. *Climacteric* 2004; 7: 210–16

6. Kloosterboer HJ. Tissue-selectivity: the mechanism of action of tibolone. *Maturitas* 2004; 48 (Suppl 1): S30–40

7. Berning B, van Kuijk C, Kuiper JW, et al. Increased loss of trabecular but not cortical bone density, 1 year after discontinuation of 2 years hormone replacement therapy with tibolone. *Maturitas* 1999; 31: 151–9

8. Ederveen AG, Spanjers CP, Quaijtaal JH, et al. Effect of 16 months of treatment with tibolone on bone mass, turnover, and biomechanical quality in mature ovariectomized rats. *J Bone Miner Res* 2001; 16: 1674–81

9. Lindsay R, Hart DM, Kraszewski A. Prospective double-blind trial of synthetic steroid (Org OD 14) for preventing postmenopausal osteoporosis. *Br Med J* 1980; 280: 1207–9

10. Geusens P, Dequeker J, Gielen J, et al. Non-linear increase in vertebral density induced by a synthetic steroid (Ord OD 14) in women with established osteoporosis. *Maturitas* 1991; 13: 155–62

11. Rymer J, Chapman MG, Fogelman I. Effect of tibolone on postmenopausal bone loss. *Osteoporos Int* 1994; 4: 314–19

12. Berning B, van Kuijk C, Kuiper JW, et al. Effects of two doses of tibolone on trabecular and cortical bone loss in early postmenopausal women: a

two-year randomized, placebo-controlled study. *Bone* 1996; 19: 395–9

13. Bjarnason NH, Bjarnason K, Haarbo J, et al. Tibolone – prevention of bone loss in late post-menopausal women. *J Clin Endocrinol Metab* 1996; 81: 2419–22

14. Studd J, Arnala I, Kicovic PM, et al. A random-ized study of tibolone on bone mineral density in osteoporotic postmenopausal women with previ-ous fractures. *Obstet Gynecol* 1998; 92: 574–9

15. Pavlov PW, Ginsburg J, Kicovic PM, et al. Dou-ble-blind, placebo-controlled study of the effects of tibolone on bone mineral density in post-menopausal osteoporotic women with and with-out previous fractures. *Gynecol Endocrinol* 1999; 13: 230–7

16. Milner M, Harrison RF, Gilligan E, et al. Bone density changes during two years treatment with tibolone or conjugated estrogens and norgestrel, compared with untreated controls in post-menopausal women. *Menopause* 2000; 7: 327–33

17. Castelo-Branco C, Vicente JJ, Figueras F, et al. Comparative effects of estrogen plus androgens and tibolone on bone, lipid pattern and sexuality in postmenopausal women. *Maturitas* 2000; 34: 161–8

18. Gambacciani M, Ciaponi M, Cappagli B, et al. A longitudinal evaluation of the effect of two doses of tibolone on bone density and metabolism in early postmenopausal women. *Gynecol Endocrinol* 2004; 18: 9–16

19. Gallagher JC, Baylink DJ, Freeman R, et al. Pre-vention of bone loss with tibolone in post-menopausal women: results of two randomized, double-blind, placebo-controlled, dose-finding studies. *J Clin Endocrinol Metab* 2001; 86: 4717–26

20. Bjarnason NH, Bjarnason K, Hassager C, et al. The response in spinal bone mass to tibolone treatment is related to bone turnover in elderly women. *Bone* 1997; 20: 151–5

21. Riera-Espinoza G, Ramos J, Carvajal R, et al. Changes in bone turnover during tibolone treat-ment. *Maturitas* 2004; 47: 83–90

22. Prevelic GM, Markou A, Arnold A, et al. The effect of tibolone on bone mineral density in post-menopausal women with osteopenia or osteo-porosis – 8 years follow-up. *Maturitas* 2004; 47: 229–4

23. Rymer J, Robinson J, Fogelman I. Ten years of treatment with tibolone 2.5 mg daily: effects on bone loss in postmenopausal women. *Climacteric* 2002; 5: 390–8

24. Lyritis GP, Karpathios S, Basdekis K, et al. Pre-vention of post-oophorectomy bone loss with tibolone. *Maturitas* 1995; 22: 247–53

25. Prevelic GM, Bartram C, Wood J, et al. Compar-ative effects on bone mineral density of tibolone, transdermal estrogen and oral estrogen/progesto-gen therapy in postmenopausal women. *Gynecol Endocrinol* 1996; 10: 413–20

26. Lippuner K, Haenggi W, Birkhaeuser MH, et al. Prevention of postmenopausal bone loss using tibolone or conventional per oral or transdermal hormone replacement therapy with 17 beta-estradiol and dydrogesterone. *J Bone Miner Res* 1997; 12: 806–12

27. Hammar M, Christau S, Nathorst-Boos J, et al. A double-blind, randomised trial comparing the effects of tibolone and continuous combined hor-mone replacement therapy in postmenopausal women with menopausal symptoms. *Br J Obstet Gynaecol* 1998; 105: 904–11

28. Thiebaud D, Bigler JM, Renteria S, et al. A 3-year study of prevention of postmenopausal bone loss: conjugated equine estrogens plus medroxy-progesterone acetate versus tibolone. *Climacteric* 1998; 1: 202–10

29. Roux C, Pelissier C, Fechtenbaum J, et al. Ran-domized, double-masked, 2-year comparison of tibolone with 17β-estradiol and norethindrone acetate in preventing postmenopausal bone loss. *Osteoporos Int* 2002; 13: 241–8

30. Doren M, Nilsson J-A, Johnell O. Effects of specific postmenopausal hormone therapies on bone mineral density in post-menopausal women: a meta-analysis. *Hum Reprod* 2003; 18: 1737–46

31. McClung MR, Omizo M, Langer RD, et al. The OPAL Study: BMD data from a three-year, dou-ble-blind, randomized study comparing the effects of tibolone, CEE/MPA and placebo in postmenopausal women. *J Bone Miner Res* 2003; 18 (Suppl 2): S381

32. Banks E, Beral V, Reeves G, et al; Million Women Study Collaborators. Fracture incidence in rela-tion to the pattern of use of hormone therapy in postmenopausal women. *J Am Med Assoc* 2004; 291: 2212–20

33. Rymer J, Chapman MG, Fogelman I, Wilson PO. A study of the effect of tibolone on the vagina in postmenopausal women. *Maturitas* 1994; 18: 127–33

34. Davis SR. The effects of tibolone on mood and libido. *Menopause* 2002; 9: 162–70

35. Doren M, Rubig A, Coelingh Bennink HJT, et al. Impact on uterine bleeding and endometrial thickness – tibolone compared with continuous combined estradiol and norethisterone acetate replacement therapy. *Menopause* 1999; 6: 299–306

36. Huber J, Palacios S, Berglund L, et al. Effects of tibolone and continuous combined hormone replacement therapy on bleeding rates, quality of life and tolerability in postmenopausal women. *Br J Obstet Gynaecol* 2002; 109: 886–93

37. Van Gorp T, Neven P. Endometrial safety of hormone replacement therapy: review of literature. *Maturitas* 2002; 42: 93–104

38. Volker W, Coelingh Bennink HJ, Helmond FA. Effects of tibolone on the endometrium. *Climacteric* 2001; 4: 203–8

39. Lundstrom E, Christow A, Kersemaekers W, et al. Effects of tibolone and continuous combined hormone replacement therapy on mammographic breast tissue. *Am J Obstet Gynecol* 2002; 186: 717–22

40. Valvidia I, Ortega D. Mammographic density in postmenopausal women treated with tibolone, estriol or conventional hormone replacement therapy. *Clin Drug Invest* 2000; 20: 101–7

41. Christodoulakos GE, Lambrinoudaki IV, Vourtsi AD, et al. Mammographic changes associated with raloxifene and tibolone therapy in postmenopausal women: a prospective study. *Menopause* 2002; 9: 110–16

42. Beral V. Million Women Study Collaborators. Breast cancer and hormone replacement therapy in the Million Women Study. *Lancet* 2003; 362: 419–27

43. Kalogeropoulos S, Petrogiannopoulos C, Gagos S, et al. The influence of 5-year therapy with tibolone on the lipid profile in postmenopausal women with mild hypercholesterolemia. *Gynecol Endocrinol* 2004; 18: 227–32

44. Farish E, Barnes JF, Fletcher CD, et al. Effects of tibolone on serum lipoprotein and apolipoprotein levels compared with a cyclical estrogen/ progestogen regimen. *Menopause* 1999; 6: 98–104

45. Garnero P, Jamin C, Benhamou CL, et al. Effects of tibolone and combined 17beta-estradiol and norethisterone acetate on serum C-reactive protein in healthy post-menopausal women: a randomized trial. *Hum Reprod* 2002; 17: 2748–53

Understanding the role of aromatizable androgens in bone-sparing

26

O. Tuncalp, V. Edusa, A. Fadiel and F. Naftolin

INTRODUCTION

Sex steroids decline in climacteric women, indicating sex steroid deficiency as a chief cause of osteoporosis. In this chapter, we focus on the possible role of androgens as prohormones for the ring A-reduced and aromatized metabolites that are thought to maintain bone mineral density (BMD) during the reproductive years and that may be useful in avoiding climacteric bone loss. Since maintenance of bone mass has tremendous importance for public health and quality of life, these considerations are particularly timely and appropriate as the length of the average post-reproductive life-span in the climacteric increases. After the end of reproduction there can be no natural selection for adaptive behavior during the climacteric, and women respond to low estrogen as they did during the reproductive years; bone resorbtion when estrogen falls is likely a replay of the adaptive furnishing of calcium for lactation during the postpartum period[1,2].

Osteoporosis is the most common metabolic bone disease, characterized by low bone mass and microarchitectural disruption that lead to increased bone fragility. Low bone mass is a major risk factor for fracture, leading to immense morbidity, mortality and expense. Osteoporosis annually affects more than 200 million individuals worldwide[3]. In the United States, the estimated cost of osteoporotic fractures in 1995 was $13.8 billion[4]. This number will continue to grow as more and older postmenopausal women appear on the scene. The burden of osteoporosis is borne disproportionately by women, although it is also a serious problem in men. For example, based on BMD measurements established by the World Health Organization, approximately 2

million men in the United States are currently affected[5]. In contradistinction to women, the precise mechanism of this loss in men has not been determined, although it is known that men begin to have decreased serum free testosterone levels with increasing age[6].

While osteoporosis may first be recognized by the presence of fragility fractures, diagnostic criteria for normal, osteopenic and osteoporotic bones based on BMD measurements by dual-energy X-ray absorptiometry (DXA) have been widely accepted[5], based on the well-documented inverse relationship between BMD and fracture risk[7]. At the cellular level, increased activity of individual osteoclasts (also termed high bone turnover) and/or an increase in the overall number of osteoclasts without compensation by osteoblasts result in bone-wasting[8]. In postmenopausal women, the major pathogenetic factor in the development of osteoporosis is estrogen deficiency. Since the estrogen deficiency reflects the lack of androgen production by the menopausal ovary, it is appropriate to consider the possible role of androgen therapy in women as an alternative means, preventing or even treating postmenopausal bone loss[9]. In addition, it is worth considering the possibility that treatment with androgens may act directly at the cellular level in bone.

To be sure, prevention and treatment of osteoporosis may include hormonal or/and non-hormonal therapy[10]: vitamin D, bisphosphonates, estrogen, selective estrogen receptor modulators, calcitonin, parathyroid hormone, and balance and exercise training programs[2]. Since androgens have not been approved for the prevention or treatment of osteoporosis in women, the provision of estrogen is most commonly by administration of various estrogenic compounds. However, the US Food and Drug Administration (FDA) has approved the use of the androgen methyl testosterone (MT) for menopausal symptoms[11]. Recently, the use of androgens has broadened from strict application in postsurgical menopausal women to include off-label use for hypoandrogenic sexual dysfunction and other menopausal complaints in normally menopausal women[12]. Therefore, increased numbers of women are receiving postmenopausal androgen treatment, and it is important to consider how this might impact upon bone health[13].

BONE METABOLISM

Bone has two main compartments: cortex and trabecular bone. But, in part because of the lack of information on cortical actions of sex steroids, we concentrate on information regarding the trabecular bone or marrow bone. Maintenance of trabecular bone is the result of an interaction between the three different bone cell types: osteoblasts, osteoclasts and osteocytes (Figure 1). Osteoblasts are derived from pluripotent mesenchymal stem cells and are responsible for bone formation and mineralization. The mesenchymal stem cells also give rise to chondrocytes, adipocytes, myoblasts and fibroblasts, as well as hematologic cells and immunocytes. After formation, the osteoblasts may undergo apoptosis, or become bone-lining cells or osteocytes, representing further stages of differentiation[9].

Osteocytes reside within the bone matrix, particularly in the cortical bone. They are believed to play a central role in response to physical stimuli, sensing mechanical strains and initiating an appropriate modeling or remodeling response via a number of chemical messengers. As the primary cells in the cortical bone, the osteocytes are of great importance in maintaining the tensile strength of long bones[9].

The *osteoclasts* patrol the trabecular bone surfaces and start the 'bone cycle' by inducing digestion of the bone matrix and the loss of bone mineral density. They derive from hematopoietic precursors of monocyte/macrophage lineage, and are considered to be terminally differentiated to

progress to apoptosis, the rate of which is influenced by many factors including estrogens and androgens. Thus, osteoclast apoptosis terminates the catabolic phase of the bone cycle[8].

SEX STEROIDS AND BONE REMODELING

In any given time, the bone turnover reflects the balance of resorption by osteoclasts and accretion of matrix and minerals via osteoblast action on the bone surfaces. In addition to sex steroid actions, the regulation of bone remodeling is influenced by diverse factors such as mechanical stress, locally produced factors (cytokines and growth factors)[14] and non-steroidal hormones[9]. However, sex steroids exert key effects on the bone cycle, acting directly on the bone cells themselves, or indirectly via regulation of local cytokines, growth factors and non-steroidal hormones. The mechanism of steroid action seems conventional, since both estrogen receptors (ERs) and androgen receptors (ARs) and aromatase have been identified in bone cells, and antihormones result in bone loss[15–19].

Earlier formulations of bone dynamics revolved around the effects of estrogen on osteoclast number and activity, and the androgens were considered mainly to stimulate the proliferation and possibly the differentiation of osteoblasts[20]. Such generalizations have been shown to be unduly restrictive of the understanding of bone remodeling and bone health. Therefore, we do not restrict discussion of the effects of specific sex steroids to individual bone cell types; rather, we start with the prohormonal androgens and follow them through bone metabolism. During the reproductive years, the main source of androgens and estrogens is the gonads, which furnish estradiol to the circulation and thereby to the bone cells. As the aging gonads furnish less testosterone and estradiol to the circulation, non-gonadal androgen formation, primarily androstenedione from the adrenal cortex, becomes the most important source of prohormonal androgen[11]. The oxido-reductase necessary to convert androstenedione to testosterone and estrone to estradiol is found in the

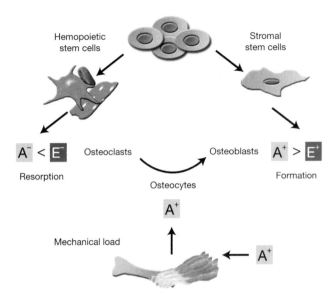

Figure 1 Representing the bone remodeling cycle in which three cell populations work in tandem under the influence of factors such as steroids and stress. As shown in this figure, the stem cells give rise to two cell populations (i.e. the osteoblasts and osteoclasts). Steroid hormones modulate the proliferation and/or apoptosis of both cells, thereby controlling the whole process of bone formation and resorption. A, androgen; E, estrogen

bone cells[21]. The bone cells also contain ring A-reductase to form the active androgenic metabolites[9], and aromatase to form estrogens locally[17,22]. However, just as the circulating estradiol is the main regulator of the bone cells during the reproductive period, it must be clear that the amount of prohormone androgen entering the bone from the circulation is a rate-limiting factor in bone maintenance during the climacteric[9]. We consider this metabolism more fully below.

THE SOURCE AND ROLE OF ANDROGENS IN THE BONES OF WOMEN

As mentioned, androgens may directly influence bone metabolism or undergo aromatization to estrogens, which then exert effects on bone cells. In either case, androgen effects include regulation of growth factors and cytokines that control bone cell kinetics and actions[8,9,23]. There are both genetic and epigenetic factors that interact

with the effects of the sex steroids, such as body mass, exercise and environmental exposure, but these effects are often general and apparently not specific to either androgens or estrogens[23].

There is a major difference in the origins and identity of androgens before and after the menopause

Prior to the menopause, androgen production in women takes place in three compartments: the ovary (testosterone and androstenedione), adrenal cortex (androstenedione) and peripheral tissues[24]. The androgens produced principally by the ovary and the adrenal are further metabolized in peripheral tissues. Although the largest quantity of androgen in the serum of cycling women is androstenedione[25], both the androgenic (ring A-reduced) and estrogenic (aromatized) metabolites of testosterone are by far more potent than those of androstenedione, and therefore are thought to furnish the main bone-sparing activity during the reproductive period. This is important, since pregnancy and lactation are, respectively, periods of functional and actual estrogen lack. The latter is due to the antiestrogenic action of progesterone during pregnancy. Between pregnancies, estrogen secreted by the ovarian follicles maintains bone mass. This is the main source of bone accretion that precedes the climacteric[11]. The net outcome of years of this interaction is the peak bone mass that is reached between ages 30 and 35. Thereafter, the fall of direct estrogen secretion is paralleled by a decrease in bone mass. While this is the picture that is seen, the precise factors that control the rate of postreproductive bone loss are not regularly active, i.e. both genetic and epigenetic factors are at work[26].

During the *natural menopause*, the ovarian (granulosa cell) production of estrogens stops completely. The production of androstenedione falls by 50%[27]. The fall is due to decreased ovarian production of the hormone, with the adrenal glands becoming the major site of androstenedione production. While testosterone secretion by the remaining ovarian tissue continues, it is considerably reduced. The reduction of circulating estradiol puts the burden for provision of estradiol from testosterone or reduced androstenedione on the non-gonadal tissues ('peripheral conversion'), including bone cells[17].

Following ovariectomy, the ovaries cease entirely to be a source of sex steroids, leaving adrenal androstenedione as the chief prohormone for ring A-reduced androgens and the aromatized androgens estrone and, to a much less extent, estradiol.

Androgens may be *administered* for medical indications, and then furnish metabolites.

METABOLISM OF ANDROGENS

Androgens undergo three types of metabolism (Figure 2):

(1) They are *interconverted* by oxidoreduction at C17, i.e. androstenedione to testosterone. This is a reversible reaction. The oxidoreductase is thus a bifunctional enzyme that regulates biological potency with tremendous leverage, since testosterone is manyfold potent compared with androstenedione. The 17β-oxidoreductase also reversibly metabolizes estrone to estradiol, with the same implications for biological efficacy. In the endometrium, this oxidoreductase is regulated by progesterone[28].

(2) Like other steroids, androgens are subject to *esterification*. This usually is a means of rendering them soluble for long-term storage in the body or rapid excretion. This is an important area about which little is known

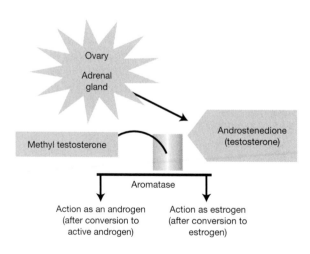

Figure 2   The metabolism and action of androgens

of physiological management, such as cleavage and release of free steroid[29].

(3) Androgens may be reduced by the addition of hydrogen to the A ring (ring A-reduction). This reaction is irreversible and furnishes the active metabolite dihydrotestosterone (DHT) or androstanediol from testosterone or androstenedione, respectively. Ring A-reduction accounts for most of the degradative metabolism of the androgens. DHT and androstanediol are anabolic steroids, meaning that they foster the accretion of muscle mass, etc.

(4) A minor portion of testosterone or androstenedione is degraded to estradiol or estrone, respectively. During this so-called aromatization, C19 is lost, irreversibly furnishing the cognate estrogen. It is of note that estrogens are generally two or three orders of magnitude more potent than their parent androgens. Thus, this small amount of aromatization has major consequences. The aromatase enzyme, a product of the CYP19 gene (cytochrome P450 enzyme complex), is responsible for the conversion[30]. A wide variety of tissue-specific regulators of aromatase expression and activity have been described[31]. The biological leverage arising from aromatization is dependent on the androgen substrate, i.e. androstenedione becomes estrone and testosterone becomes estradiol, with less or more estrogenic potency, respectively. For example, the loss of ovarian function shifts the onus to the weaker adrenal androgens.

PHARMACOLOGICALLY ADMINISTERED ANDROGENS

Androgen prohormones that can be aromatized or ring A-reduced are available on the market: testosterone and methyl testosterone (MT) (Figure 3). The former has not been approved for use in women. MT in oral form, as part of Estratest® (Solvay), is approved for use against menopausal symptoms. As well, one of the metabolites of tibolone (Livial®; Organon) is androgenic.

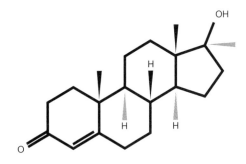

Figure 3　Methyl testosterone

Tibolone has been approved for use against menopausal symptoms in Europe and the UK. It is not clear that the androgenic metabolite of tibolone is aromatizable[32]. For simplicity, tibolone is not considered further, but it should be clear that a compound that furnishes androgenic, estrogenic and progestational metabolites could have cognate effects on bone[33]. Although *ring A-reduced androgens* have recently gained much notoriety because of their use as anabolic agents in sports, they are not discussed further except to note that their side-effects make anabolic steroids a poor choice for the treatment of women[34].

Aromatizable androgen, primarily MT, is increasingly employed in menopausal hormone treatment. Its use was originally limited to women who had their ovaries removed, and therefore were certain to undergo androgen deficiency. Recently, it has become clear that retained ovaries may cease function after hysterectomy or without previous surgery, in which case women may undergo androgen-deficiency syndromes, including hypoandrogenic sexual dysfunction[12]. This and recent formulations that furnish testosterone have reopened considerations regarding anabolic actions of androgen metabolites. Methyl testosterone and testosterone are aromatized to methyl estradiol and estradiol, respectively, and are also subject to ring A-reduction. These androgens furnish both potent estrogens and ring A-reduced anabolic steroids whose effects on women's bones have not been adequately investigated.

Methyl testosterone

17α-Methyl testosterone (MT) is a synthetic C19 androgen that is effectively absorbed from the intestine. Although it is now known to be aromatized[32], MT continues to be considered mainly as an anabolic–androgenic compound used in combination with estrogen to improve symptom relief and long-term effects of decreased sex steroids in menopausal women[35]. The US FDA first approved MT in the 1960s and allowed it to be added to esterified estrogen Estratest® (Solvay), for improvement of menopausal symptoms such as hot flushes. Although MT has been prescribed for nearly 50 years, usually to treat surgically menopausal, ostensibly androgen-deficient women for symptoms, little is known of MT's bone-sparing action. There are no published animal studies in this regard, and the data in humans are largely anecdotal. The emergence of hypogonadal sexual dysfunction as an entity in intact normal menopausal women will accelerate the use of MT and other androgens in this group of women at risk for osteoporosis and fracture[11,36].

Studies from our laboratory and others have shown that MT is a prohormone with both estrogenic and androgenic metabolites. Specifically, MT is a competitive aromatase inhibitor that preferentially blocks androstenedione aromatization to estrone and furnishes the more powerful estrogen, methyl estradiol (ME). In studies, we showed that the aromatization of MT furnishes ME even in the presence of testosterone[35].

Preliminary studies show MT is a powerful bone-sparing agent

As mentioned above, the recent emphasis on the use of androgens by naturally menopausal women has kindled interest in this form of treatment. Because of the dearth of studies, we examined the possibility that MT is a bone-sparing agent. We have performed preliminary studies of bone mineral density (BMD) in 1-week-castrated female mice who had received MT and other steroids and antihormones. These studies showed that, compared with androstenedione, MT is a more powerful bone-sparing agent that can forestall the loss of BMD by an order equivalent to

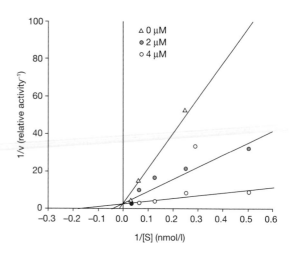

Figure 4 Lineweaver–Burke plot of methyl testosterone (MT) versus androstenedione showing MT's competitive inhibition of aromatase activity. From reference 34

that of testosterone or estradiol (Figure 4). These studies are ongoing, and will include bone histomorphometry as well as BMD studies (unpublished data). Since the experimental mice were ovariectomized, the main competitor for aromatase action was androstenedione from the adrenal cortex. We infer that the MT was aromatized and probably acted as both an estrogen and an androgen. Certainly, this is concordant with the reports of ER and AR expression by bone cells[9]. Although not designed for use as bone-sparing agents, it appears that the bone-sparing effects of MT and other aromatizable androgens may furnish added value to the treatment of climacteric women.

SUMMARY

In light of the public-health burden of osteoporosis in postmenopausal women, unraveling the mechanisms underlying the effects of sex steroids on bone is a high-priority research field. Different therapeutic agents and approaches to bone-sparing have been proposed and used over the years, but the need for new agents persists.

Aromatizable androgens are an important, currently available, form of menopausal hormone treatment that incidentally furnish the opportunity to avert bone loss. The evidence from preclinical and clinical studies suggests that such androgens may have an important positive effect on bone health. In preliminary studies, methyl testosterone (MT) has been found to be a powerful bone-sparing agent. MT apparently acts as a prohormone with both estrogenic and androgenic metabolites that affect bone cells. The cellular mechanisms underlying these actions are currently under investigation.

ACKNOWLEDGMENTS

This study was supported by an unrestricted educational grant from Solvay Pharmaceuticals and a grant from The Yale Center for Musculoskeletal Disorders. We appreciate the skilled technical assistance of Nancy Trioano.

References

1. Richman S, Naftolin F. *Climacteric Medicine: Where do we Go?* London: Taylor and Francis, 2005: 4–8
2. Lin JT, Lane JM. Osteoporosis: a review. *Clin Orthop Relat Res* 2004; 425: 126–34
3. Wolinsky FD, Fitzgerald JF, Stump TE. The effect of hip fracture on mortality, hospitalization, and functional status: a prospective study. *Am J Public Health* 1997; 87: 398–403
4. Ray NF, Chan JK, Thamer M, Melton LJ. Medical expenditures for the treatment of osteoporotic fractures in the United States in 1995: report from the National Osteoporosis Foundation. *J Bone Miner Res* 1997; 12: 24–35
5. World Health Organization Study Group. Assessment of fracture risk and its application to postmenopausal osteoporosis. Technical Report Series 843. Geneva: WHO, 1994
6. Deslypere JP, Vermeulen A. Leydig cell function in normal men: effect of age, life-style, residence, diet, and activity. *J Clin Endocrinol Metab* 1984; 59: 955–62
7. Cummings SR, Black DM, Nevitt MC, et al. Bone density at various sites for prediction of hip fractures. The Study of Osteoporotic Fractures Research Group. *Lancet* 1993; 341: 72–5
8. Teitelbaum SL, Ross FP. Genetic regulation of osteoclast development and function. *Nat Rev Genet* 2003; 4: 638–49
9. Compston JE. Sex steroids and bone. *Physiol Rev* 2001; 81: 419–47
10. NIH Consensus Development Panel. Osteoporosis prevention, diagnosis, and therapy. *J Am Med Assoc* 2001; 285: 785–95
11. Lobo RA. Androgens in postmenopausal women: production, possible role, and replacement options. *Obstet Gynecol Surv* 2001; 56: 361–76
12. Bachmann G, Bancroft J, Braunstein G, et al. Female androgen insufficiency: the Princeton consensus statement on definition, classification, and assessment. *Fertil Steril* 2002; 77: 660–5
13. Cameron DR, Braunstein GD. Androgen replacement therapy in women. *Fertil Steril* 2004; 82: 273–89
14. Pfeilschifter J. Changes in proinflammatory cytokine activity after menopause. *Endocr Rev* 2002; 23: 90–119
15. Pensler JM, Langman CB, Radosevich JA, et al. Sex steroid hormone receptors in normal and dysplastic bone disorders in children. *J Bone Miner Res* 1990; 5: 493–8
16. Lubahn DB, Joseph DR, Sar M, et al. The human androgen receptor: complementary deoxyribonucleic acid cloning, sequence analysis and gene expression in prostate. *Mol Endocrinol* 1988; 2: 1265–75
17. Roa-Pena L, Zreik T, Harada N, et al. Human osteoblast-like cells express aromatase immunoreactivity. *Menopause* 1994; 1: 73–8
18. Gennari L, Ranuccio N, Bilezikian JP. Aromatase activity and bone homeostasis in men. *J Clin Endocrinol Metab* 2004; 89: 5898–907

19. Ross RW, Small EJ. Osteoporosis in men treated with androgen deprivation therapy for prostate cancer. *J Urol* 2002; 167: 1952–6

20. Kasperk C, Wergedal JE, Farley JR, et al. Androgens directly stimulate proliferation of bone cells in vitro. *Endocrinology* 1989; 124: 1576–8

21. Czerwiec FS, Liaw JJ, Liu SB, et al. Absence of androgen-mediated transcriptional effects in osteoblastic cells despite presence of androgen receptors. *Bone* 1997; 21: 49–56

22. Jakob F, Siggelkow H, Homann D, et al. Local estradiol metabolism in osteoblast- and osteoclast-like cells. *J Steroid Biochem Mol Biol* 1997; 61: 167–74

23. Kearns AE, Khosla S. Potential anabolic effects of androgens on bone. *Mayo Clin Proc* 2004; 79 (Suppl): S14–18

24. Lobo RA. *The Treatment of Postmenopausal Women: Basic and Clinical Aspects*, 2nd edn. Philadelphia, PA: Lippincott Williams & Wilkins, 1999: 141–55

25. Judd HL, Fournet N. Changes of ovarian hormonal function with aging. *Exp Gerontol* 1994; 29: 285–98

26. Siris ES, Miller PD, Barrett-Connor E, et al. Identification and the fracture outcomes of undiagnosed low bone mineral density in postmenopausal women: results from the National Osteoporosis Risk Assessment. *J Am Med Assoc* 2001; 286: 2815–22

27. Judd HL, Judd GE, Lucas WE, Yen SSC. Endocrine function of the postmenopausal ovary: concentrations of androgens and estrogens in ovarian and peripheral vein blood. *J Clin Endocrinol Metab* 1974; 39: 1020–4

28. Markiewicz L, Hochberg RB, Gurpide E. Intrinsic estrogenicity of some progestagenic drugs. *J Steroid Biochem Mol Biol* 1992; 41: 53–8

29. Larner JM, Pahuja SL, Brown VM, Hochberg RB. Aromatase and testosterone fatty acid esters: the search for a cryptic biosynthetic pathway to estradiol esters. *Steroids* 1992; 57: 475–9

30. Conley A, Hinshelwood M. Mammalian aromatases. *Reproduction* 2001; 121: 685–95

31. Simpson ER, Mahendroo MS, Means GD, et al. Aromatase cytochrome P450, the enzyme responsible for estrogen biosynthesis. *Endocr Rev* 1994; 15: 342–55

32. de Gooyer ME, Oppers-Tiemissen HM, Leysen D, et al. Tibolone is not converted by human aromatase to 7alpha-methyl-17alpha-ethinylestradiol (7alpha-MEE): analyses with sensitive bioassay for estrogens and androgens with LC-MSMS. *Steroids* 2003; 68: 235–43

33. Hanifi-Moghaddam P, Gielen SC, Kloosterboer HJ, et al. Molecular portrait of the progestagenic and estrogenic actions of tibolone: behavior of cellular networks in response to tibolone. *J Clin Endocrinol Metab* 2005; 90: 973–83

34. Seeman A, Eisman JA. Treatment of osteoporosis: why, whom, and when and how to treat. *Med J Aust* 2004; 180: 298–303

35. Mor G, Eliza M, Song J, et al. 17a-Methyl testosterone is a competitive inhibitor of aromatase activity in JAR choriocarcinoma cells and macrophage-like THP-1 cells in culture. *J Steroid Biochem Mol Biol* 2001; 79: 239–46

36. Utian WH. Problems with desire and arousal in surgically menopausal women: advances in assessment, diagnosis and treatment. 2005; 14: 15–21

Strontium ranelate: a new first-line treatment for patients with postmenopausal osteoporosis

27

S. Ortolani

INTRODUCTION

The clinical challenge

Osteoporosis is a progressive systemic skeletal disorder characterized by low bone mass and a deterioration in the microarchitecture of bone tissue, leading to increased bone fragility and susceptibility to fracture. The most common sites of fragility fractures are in the vertebrae, hips and wrists. Many are associated with marked disability, pain and impaired quality of life. In the case of the hip, where fracture is typically associated with advanced age and concomitant disease, resulting complications are variously estimated to be fatal in 15–30% of cases, most of the excess deaths occurring within the first 6 months after the fracture. Hip fractures are associated with the highest morbidity and require hospitalization with a mean stay of 20–30 days, their major consequence being an inability to walk and consequently a loss of autonomy.

Although osteoporosis can occur in all age-groups and populations, its peak prevalence is in middle-aged and elderly women. One in two postmenopausal women will have an osteoporosis-related fracture in their lifetime. Not only does this in itself define an expanding at-risk population, but the situation is compounded by two further factors: the increasing incidence of osteoporosis within the elderly population[1,2], and the fact that fracture is an end stage in a disease for which it is often the presenting complaint. In other words, fracture is the tip of the osteoporosis iceberg. The clinical problem is thus vast, increasing and urgent.

Pathogenesis

Bone loss is a major determinant of the skeletal fragility in osteoporosis. It occurs postmenopausally due to a marked increase in osteoclast resorption, which is only partly offset by a moderate increase in the rate of bone formation by osteoblasts. Not only is there a cellular imbalance in bone remodeling, causing bone resorption to exceed bone formation, but the rate of tissue remodeling also increases[3]. The result is a decrease in bone tissue mass.

In addition to low bone mass, the increase in bone resorption reduces by itself the mechanical strength of bone.

Therapeutic options

A number of interventions preserve bone mass and prevent fracture. Compliance with recommended calcium and vitamin D intake is a *sine qua non* of any therapy, especially in the presence of demonstrated deficiency. But it is insufficient on its own. Worthwhile life-style changes include regular weight-bearing exercise, avoidance of smoking and moderation of alcohol intake. Yet, however great the general benefits of such changes, their specific impact on osteoporosis is relatively slight. In the elderly, fall-prevention measures, such as home modifications and anatomically designed hip protectors, have been advocated as reducing hip fractures, in some cases by more than 40%. However, the most recent evidence, from a randomized controlled trial in 561 Dutch elderly people living in sheltered accommodation, showed no significant difference in hip fracture rates between the hip-protector group and controls[4].

Most of the pharmaceutical interventions approved for the treatment of osteoporosis inhibit bone resorption and consequently reduce bone formation[5]. None of the agents so far available stimulate bone formation while inhibiting bone resorption, as strontium ranelate does.

Strontium ranelate

Strontium ranelate is composed of an organic moiety (ranelic acid) and two atoms of stable (non-radioactive) strontium. Its chemical name is 5-[bis(carboxymethyl)amino]-2-carboxy-4-cyano-3-thiophenacetic acid distrontium salt. Ranelic acid was chosen among 24 strontium salts and was the compound simultaneously presenting the best physicochemical characteristics (e.g. percentage of strontium with two atoms of strontium linked to the molecule, solubility, no chelating properties, chirality, stability, etc.), the best pharmacokinetic characteristics (e.g. bioavailability, exposure to strontium) and good safety. The purpose of this review is to examine the scientific rationale for its use in osteoporosis, and the results of the first major clinical studies.

PRECLINICAL RESULTS

In vitro studies

All *in vitro* studies have confirmed the osteotrophicity of strontium ranelate. They have provided extensive evidence of significant inhibition of bone resorption, e.g. the resorption induced by parathyroid hormone[6,7]. Other comparative investigations showed that, unlike calcium or sodium ranelate, strontium ranelate markedly inhibited ^{45}Ca release from prelabeled murine long-bone cultures[8], whether or not they were treated with vitamin D_3.

Strontium ranelate was also effective in the isolated rat osteoclast assay[9]: preincubation of bone slices with strontium ranelate at concentrations $\geq 10^{-4}$ mol/l dose-dependently inhibited bone resorption by untreated rat osteoclasts. At the highest test dose (10^{-3} mol/l), the effect reached −66%. Inhibition also increased after continuous incubation. To determine whether

this was caused by impairment of cell attachment and/or viability, the same study also evaluated the number of osteoclasts attached to bone slices at the end of the culture period under varying conditions. Neither preincubation nor continuous incubation with strontium ranelate at concentrations of 10^{-6}–10^{-3} mol/l significantly impaired osteoclast attachment or viability as determined by tartrate-resistant acid phosphatase (TRAP) activity staining. The effect of strontium ranelate was thus not a mere by-product of more general antiosteoclast activity.

Particularly striking were the *in vitro* studies in which sequential collagenase digestions were used to isolate bone cell populations enriched with fibroblasts and preosteoblasts, or in which mature osteoblasts were taken directly from fetal Sprague–Dawley rat calvaria[10]. Strontium ranelate (10^{-3} mol/l) increased DNA synthesis 3–4-fold in the fibroblast + preosteoblast population. In mature osteoblasts, collagen and non-collagen protein synthesis increased by 34%. Of particular interest was the effect on bone formation, determined in calvarial cultures using autoradiography and histomorphometry: strontium ranelate enhanced preosteoblast replication, producing a corresponding increase in bone formation ≤ 48 h later. Moreover, the activity appeared specific in that the related compounds, calcium ranelate and sodium ranelate, had no such effect at the same concentration. This study confirmed an earlier finding that strontium ranelate acted positively on bone formation[11].

The burden of the *in vitro* evidence was that strontium ranelate shared the characteristic profile of antiresorptive agents via direct and/or matrix-mediated inhibition of osteoclast activity and differentiation. At the same time, however, it stimulated bone formation by increasing the replication of preosteoblast cells. This was the novel profile informing the *in vivo* studies.

In vivo studies

Intact animal studies

In intact female rats, a 2-year period of exposure to strontium ranelate mixed in the diet (doses ranging from 225 to 900 mg/kg/day) induced a dose-dependent increase in bone mass at the level of the vertebral body containing a large proportion of trabecular bone, and of the mid-shaft femur containing a large proportion of cortical bone. This net gain in bone tissue was confirmed by histomorphometry as it showed an increase in trabecular bone volume, trabecular number and trabecular thickness as well as an increase in cortical thickness, measured at the proximal tibia and at the tibiofibular junction, respectively[12].

Subsequently, similar effects were found in primates. In a study from Yale, strontium ranelate dose-dependently decreased the histomorphometric indices of bone resorption in intact cynomolgus monkeys treated with 100, 275, 750 mg/kg/day, and vehicle for 6 months[13]. Osteoclast number and surface were significantly decreased, by 53% and 61%, respectively, at the 275-mg/kg/day dose. At the same time, bone-formation indices remained stable or increased, with borderline-significant increments in osteoid volume and osteoblast surface. A reassuring finding with respect to subsequent clinical applications was that no inhibition of mineralization was seen even at the highest dose, supporting earlier findings that chronic strontium ranelate does not impair crystallinity in the intact monkey[14].

Ovariectomy and immobilization models of bone loss

Strontium ranelate has been extensively tested in various ovariectomized rat models of estrogen deficiency, employing a battery of parameters: calcium balance and kinetics, histomorphometry and bone calcium levels.

In a comprehensive 1993 study[11], confirmed by subsequent studies[15], female rats were sham-operated or ovariectomized before receiving oral strontium ranelate 77, 154, 308 mg/kg/day, or vehicle, or subcutaneous 17β-estradiol (10 μg/kg/day) for 8 weeks. Bone loss in untreated animals was significant, along with high bone turnover (increases in both resorption and formation). In ovariectomized rats, strontium ranelate significantly increased femoral bone mineral content; it partially inhibited trabecular bone loss and totally inhibited the decrease in bone mineral content: bone volume was 30–36% higher in treated versus untreated

animals. Histological indices of bone resorption fell 13–24%, compared with untreated ovariectomized rats, and did not differ from those in sham-operated or estradiol-supplemented animals. Osteoclast surface and number were both reduced, suggesting an effect on osteoclast recruitment. Yet, unlike estradiol, strontium ranelate did not impair the bone formation response to ovariectomy. In contrast, osteoid surface, osteoblast surface, mineral apposition rate and bone formation rate all remained as high in strontium ranelate-treated rats as in untreated ovariectomized animals. In other words, under these conditions of careful strontium ranelate dosing, bone retained its vitality.

Strontium ranelate proved similarly effective in immobilization-induced osteoporosis[16]. Not only did it significantly increase trabecular bone volume versus controls (by 13% and 19% at 200 and 800 mg/kg/day, respectively), and significantly decrease bone resorption, but it did so without impairing the bone formation rate. Pre-treatment with 200 mg/kg/day had the same effect on bone histomorphometry as treatment for 10 days at the same dose.

Thus, the *in vivo* evidence confirmed that strontium ranelate consistently decreases bone resorption, but that in numerous models it also has a stimulatory effect on bone formation. Overall, the sum of these actions on bone formation and bone resorption means that strontium ranelate rebalances bone turnover in favor of formation.

In addition, strontium ranelate improves bone strength: in intact female rats, a 2-year period of exposure to strontium ranelate mixed in the diet dose-dependently increased bone mechanical properties of the vertebral body and of the mid-shaft femur. The increase in bone strength was related to a dose-dependent increase in bone mass and bone volume, along with normal bone mineralization[12].

CLINICAL RESULTS

The properties deduced from the preclinical studies have been, and are being, tested in a series of phase 2/3 trials, which, commensurate with expectations, are large-scale and multinational, and based exclusively on double-blind, placebo-controlled, randomized designs.

STRATOS trial

In a 2-year multicenter European phase-2 study of vertebral fractures (STrontium RAnelate for Treatment of Osteoporosis, STRATOS), 353 Caucasian women, mean age 66 years, received strontium ranelate (0.5, 1 or 2 g/day) or placebo. At inclusion, lumbar bone mineral density (BMD) by dual energy X-ray absorptiometry was 0.699 ± 0.098 g/cm^2, equivalent to a mean lumbar T-score of -3.9 ± 1.0. Mean prevalent vertebral fractures per patient were 2.7 ± 2.5, mean menopause duration was 18 ± 8 years and mean body mass index 25 ± 3 kg/m^2. All patients were supplemented with calcium 500 mg and vitamin D$_3$ 800 IU daily. In the 2-g treated group, lumbar BMD increased by 7.3% annually ($p < 0.001$ vs. placebo), combined with an increase in bone alkaline phosphatase ($p = 0.002$) over the 2 years, a decrease in N-telopeptide cross-links ($p < 0.004$) over 6 months and, in year 2, a significant 44% reduction in the number of patients with incident vertebral deformity. No defective mineralization was revealed by bone histomorphometry. Drop-outs due to adverse effects (10%) did not differ between strontium ranelate and placebo[17]. Moreover, the mean degree of bone mineralization was quantified by microradiography in transiliac biopsies together with strontium ranelate uptake and distribution. The drug was dose-dependently deposited in compact and trabecular bone, with significantly higher contents in new bone compared with old bone. New bone uptake was also dose-dependent. However, in confirmation of the animal data, the mean degree of bone mineralization in either compact or trabecular bone did not differ significantly from placebo[18].

Phase-3 program for the development of strontium ranelate in postmenopausal osteoporosis

A multinational phase-3 program is currently under way prefaced by a run-in study, from which patients were randomized into a 12-country, 75-center study comparing vertebral fracture risk (Spinal Osteoporosis Therapeutic Intervention, SOTI) or non-vertebral fracture risk in a second study between strontium ranelate 2 g/day and placebo. The purpose of the run-in was to begin normalizing calcium and vitamin D status. Patients remain supplemented throughout the studies, at doses determined by their degree of deficiency (calcium, 500 or 1000 mg; vitamin D$_3$, 400 or 800 IU)[19]. The studies extend over 5 years, with the main statistical analysis over 3 years in the intention-to-treat (ITT) group.

Over 9000 patients were enrolled in the run-in study, 1649 women (mean age 70 years) were included in the SOTI trial and 5091 (mean age 77 years) in the second treatment study[20]. The SOTI analysis, based on semiquantitative visual assessment of vertebral fracture[21], showed a decrease of 41% versus placebo in the number of patients experiencing a new vertebral fracture: 139 vs. 222 (relative risk (RR), 0.59, 95% confidence interval (CI) 0.48–0.73; $p < 0.001$) over 3 years (Figure 1). In practical terms, this means treating nine patients for 3 years to prevent one patient from having a vertebral fracture. In year 1, the RR of new vertebral fracture was reduced by 49% versus placebo (RR 0.51, 95% CI 0.36–0.74; Cox model $p < 0.001$). Similarly, the clinical vertebral fracture risk was reduced by 52% (RR 0.48, 95% CI 0.29–0.80; Cox model $p = 0.003$) and 38% (RR 0.62, 95% CI 0.47–0.83; Cox model $p < 0.001$) versus placebo at 1 and 3 years, respectively. Lumbar BMD increased progressively during the study, with no evidence of plateau formation versus placebo (+11.4% vs. -1.3%; $p < 0.001$), resulting in a difference of 14.4% between the two groups at 3 years. From month 3 to the end of year 3 in the treated group, serum bone-specific alkaline phosphatase levels were significantly higher, and serum type I collagen C-telopeptide cross-links levels significantly lower, than on placebo (Figure 2). These results for bone markers confirmed in a clinical setting the dual mode of action of strontium ranelate.

Treatment compliance over 3 years was similar on strontium ranelate (83%) and placebo (85%). Adverse events, serious adverse events

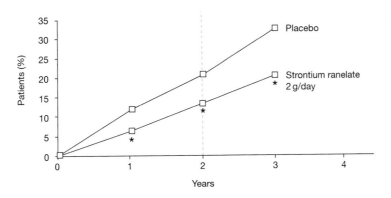

Figure 1 Relative risk (RR) of new vertebral fracture over 1 and 3 years, graded according to reference 21, using Kaplan–Meier analysis and the Cox model (Spinal Osteoporosis Therapeutic Intervention (SOTI) study). Over 1 year: RR 0.51, 95% confidence interval (CI) 0.36–0.74; $^*p < 0.001$. Over 3 years: RR 0.59, 95% CI 0.48–0.73; $^*p < 0.001$

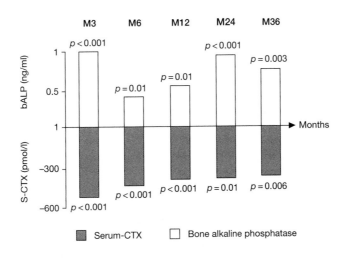

Figure 2 Differences over time in biochemical markers between the two groups (Spinal Osteoporosis Therapeutic Intervention (SOTI) study). Comparisons were performed with analysis of covariance in which baseline values were used as covariates. S-CTX, serum type I collagen C-telopeptide; bALP, bone alkaline phosphatase; M, month

and adverse event-related drop-outs were also similar in frequency in both groups. Diarrhea was initially the most frequent adverse event associated with active treatment (6.1% vs. 3.6%; $p = 0.02$), but it had resolved by month 3. Gastritis, as diagnosed clinically by the investigator, tended to be less frequent in the treated group (3.6% vs. 5.5%; $p = 0.07$)[22,23]. In addition, strontium ranelate was demonstrated to be safe at the bone-tissue level: all biopsy specimens analyzed consisted of lamellar bone normally mineralized.

Analysis over 3 years of the second treatment study revealed a significantly lower risk of peripheral fracture after strontium ranelate over 3 years versus placebo. In high-risk patients (aged 74 years or more and with femoral neck BMD < −3 standard deviations (SD)), hip fracture risk was significantly reduced[24]. The analysis also confirmed, as a secondary end-point, a significant reduction versus placebo in the RR of experiencing a first vertebral fracture[25].

DISCUSSION

Postmenopausal osteoporosis is a condition for which long-term treatment is required. Safety and tolerability are therefore particularly important for a candidate therapy, in particular to maintain high levels of compliance. Strontium ranelate satisfies these criteria. Evidence from animal studies is that its bone concentration halves within 10 weeks of treatment withdrawal[14]. It has shown no adverse effects to date on primary or secondary bone mineralization in laboratory animals or humans. In SOTI, the sole tolerability parameter in which it has differed significantly from placebo in the clinical trials – diarrhea – ceased to differ after the first 3 months.

At the same time, strontium ranelate is at least as effective as any conventional therapy for osteoporosis. Over the 3 years covered by the analyses of the phase-3 studies, efficacy against vertebral and hip fracture have been demonstrated and BMD increased continuously, without evidence of waning in effect over time. This too is an important credential for long-term therapy.

On the basis of the preclinical evidence, it can be assumed that strontium ranelate sustains this level of efficacy by stimulating bone formation as well as inhibiting bone resorption. This results in the rebalancing of bone turnover in favor of formation. The molecular basis for this dual mode of action is still under investigation. Current hypotheses include the regulation of cellular mechanisms governing bone cell differentiation and activity, since strontium ranelate has been shown *in vitro* to enhance osteoblastic cell replication and bone-forming activity and to decrease the differentiation and resorbing activity of osteoclasts[8–10]. Moreover, it may activate signaling pathways via the extracellular cation-sensing receptor expressed in bone cells[26], which is stimulated by divalent cations, including Sr^{2+}.

In view of its mode of action, its efficacy and its good long-term bone safety profile, strontium ranelate can thus be considered as a first-line therapy for postmenopausal women with osteoporosis.

References

1. Bengner U, Johnell O, Redlund-Johnell I. Change in incidence and prevalence of vertebral fractures during 30 years. *Calcif Tissue Int* 1988; 42: 293–6

2. The European Prospective Osteoporosis Study (EPOS) Group. Incidence of vertebral fracture in Europe: results from the European Prospective Osteoporosis Study. *J Bone Miner Res* 2002; 17: 716–24

3. Seeman E. Pathogenesis of bone fragility in women and men. *Lancet* 2002; 359: 1841–50

4. van Schoor NM, Smit JH, Twisk JW, et al. Prevention of hip fractures by external hip protectors: a randomized controlled trial. *J Am Med Assoc* 2003; 289: 1957–62

5. Eastell R. Treatment of postmenopausal osteoporosis. *N Engl J Med* 1998; 338: 736–46

6. Marie PJ, Ammann P, Boivin G, et al. Mechanisms of action and therapeutic potential of strontium in bone. *Calcif Tissue Int* 2001; 69: 121–9

7. Izumisawa T, Morohashi T, Amano H, et al. The effect of stable strontium on calcium metabolism. II. Effect of 1α-hydroxyvitamin D3 in strontium-fed rats and inhibitory effect of strontium on bone resorption in vitro. *J Bone Miner Metab* 1994; 12: 43–9

8. Takahashi N, Sasaki T, Tsouderos Y, et al. S12911-2 inhibits osteoclastic bone resorption in vitro. *J Bone Miner Res* 2003; 18: 1082–7

9. Baron R, Tsouderos Y. In vitro effects of S12911-2 on osteoclast function and bone marrow macrophage differentiation. *Eur J Pharmacol* 2002; 450: 11–17

10. Canalis E, Hott M, Deloffre P, et al. The divalent strontium salt S12911 enhances bone cell replication and bone formation in vitro. *Bone* 1996; 8: 517–23

11. Marie PJ, Hott M, Modrowski D, et al. An uncoupling agent containing strontium prevents bone loss by depressing bone resorption and maintaining bone formation in estrogen-deficient rats. *J Bone Miner Res* 1993; 8: 607–15

12. Ammann P, Shen V, Robin B, et al. Strontium ranelate improves bone resistance by increasing bone mass and improving architecture in intact female rats. *J Bone Miner Res* 2004; 12: 2012–20

13. Buehler J, Chappuis P, Saffar JL, et al. Strontium ranelate inhibits bone resorption while maintaining bone formation in alveolar bone in monkeys (*Macaca fascicularis*). *Bone* 2001; 29: 176–9

14. Boivin G, Deloffre P, Perrat B, et al. Strontium distribution and interactions with bone mineral density in monkey iliac bone after strontium salt (S12911) administration. *J Bone Miner Res* 1996; 11: 1302–11

15. Morohashi T, Sano T, Harai K, et al. Effects of strontium on calcium metabolism in rats. II. Strontium prevents the increased rate of bone turnover in ovariectomized rats. *Jpn J Pharmacol* 1995; 68: 153–9

16. Hott M, Deloffre P, Tsouderos Y, et al. S12911-2 reduces bone loss induced by short-term immobilization in rats. *Bone* 2003; 33: 115–23

17. Meunier PJ, Slosman D, Delmas P, et al. Strontium ranelate: dose-dependent effects in established postmenopausal vertebral osteoporosis: a 2-year randomized placebo controlled trial. *J Clin Endocrinol Metab* 2002; 87: 2060–6

18. Boivin G, Foos E, Tupinon-Mathieu I, et al. Strontium deposition in bone is dose dependent and does not alter the degree of mineralization of bone in osteoporotic patients treated with strontium ranelate. *J Bone Miner Res* 2000; 15 (Suppl 1): 305

19. Reginster JY, Diez-Perez A, Ortolani S, et al. Calcium-vitamin D supplementation in clinical trials of osteoporosis should be titrated on the basis of pre-study assessments. *Osteoporos Int* 2002; 13 (Suppl 1): S24

20. Reginster JY, Spector T, Badurski J, et al. A short-term run-in study can significantly contribute to increasing the quality of long-term osteoporosis trials. The strontium ranelate Phase III program. *Osteoporos Int* 2002; 13 (Suppl 1): S30

21. Genant HK, Wu CY, Van Kuijk C, et al. Vertebral semi-quantitative assessment using a semi-quantitative technique. *J Bone Miner Res* 1993; 8: 1137–48

22. Meunier PJ, Roux C, Ortolani S, et al. Strontium ranelate reduces the vertebral fracture risk in women with postmenopausal osteoporosis. *Osteoporos Int* 2002; 13 (Suppl 1): O45

23. Meunier PJ, Roux C, Seeman E, et al. The effect of strontium ranelate on the risk of vertebral fracture in women with postmenopausal osteoporosis. *N Engl J Med* 2004; 350: 459–68

24. Rizzoli R, Reginster JY, Diaz-Curiel M, et al. Patients at high risk of hip fracture benefit from treatment with strontium ranelate. *Osteoporos Int* 2004; 15 (Suppl 1): OC39

25. Reginster JY, Rizzoli R, Balogh A, et al. Strontium ranelate reduces the risk of vertebral fractures in osteoporotic post menopausal women without prevalent vertebral fracture. *Calcif Tissue Int* 2004; 74 (Suppl 1): P151

26. Quarles LD. Cation-sensing receptors in bone: a novel paradigm for regulating bone remodeling? *J Bone Miner Res* 1997; 12: 1971–4

Reconciling risks and benefits of hormone replacement therapy in a single outcome: the QALY approach

28

J. M. Alt, Y. Zöllner and J. Ryan

HISTORICAL PERSPECTIVE

Although hormone replacement therapy (HRT) is mainly prescribed for relief of vasomotor symptoms and urogenital atrophy, HRT has also been indicated for the prevention of postmenopausal osteoporosis. As shown by cohort studies and randomized controlled trials, HRT increases bone mineral density (BMD) and reduces the risk for fractures[1–4]. In addition, there is evidence that HRT reduces the risk for colorectal cancer[5,6]. HRT may also possibly reduce the risk of cognitive decline and dementia[7]. Until 2002, there was also fair evidence – mostly from large, prospective cohort studies – that HRT could protect women against cardiovascular disease[8–10]. However, the results from a secondary prevention trial (Heart and Estrogen/progestin Replacement Study (HERS) I and HERS II) did not demonstrate any benefit in terms of cardiovascular protection[11,12], and the results from the Women's Health Initiative (WHI)[1] study published in 2002 showed that HRT was also not effective for primary prevention of cardiovascular disease. This latter outcome has considerably changed the perceived balance of benefits and harms of HRT. For the Data and Safety Monitoring Board (DSMB), a 'global index' was devised for the WHI studies to estimate the risk/benefit ratio. The index included the two primary outcomes coronary heart disease and invasive breast cancer, plus stroke, pulmonary embolism, endometrial cancer, colorectal cancer, hip fracture and death due to other causes. It excluded menopausal symptoms and other osteoporotic fractures. Based on the 'global index', indicating

that risks were outweighing the benefits and that the design-specified weighted log-rank test statistic for breast cancer crossed the designated boundary, the independent DSMB decided to stop prematurely the combined estrogen– progestin (conjugated equine estrogens (CEE)–medroxyprogesterone acetate (MPA)) treatment arm of the WHI study.

The justification for stopping the WHI study, and the validity of a global index as a measure for the risk/benefit ratio, have been discussed ever since. The discussion was further fueled by publication of the Million Women Study, indicating an even larger risk of breast cancer in HRT users than reported in the WHI study[13]. The regulatory authorities and medical associations reacted promptly. The US Preventive Services Task Force (USPSTF) concluded that the harmful effects of combined estrogen-and-progestin HRT were likely to exceed the chronic disease prevention benefits in most women[14], and most organizations with guidelines on postmenopausal HRT have followed and revised their recommendations. Following the premature stop of the WHI study and the Million Women Study, HRT is now generally considered an acceptable treatment option for menopausal symptoms, but most organizations recommend against the long-term use of HRT for prevention. Also, the European Medicines Evaluation Agency (EMEA) no longer consider HRT as a first-line treatment for the long-term prevention of osteoporosis. HRT remains an option for postmenopausal women who are at high risk of future fractures, and who are intolerant of, or contraindicated for, other medicinal products approved for the prevention of osteoporosis[15].

In 2004, the results from the WHI estrogen-only treatment arm were published[16]. The data showed a different picture in that the women on unopposed CEE had no increased risk of breast cancer (hazard ratio (HR) 0.77; 95% confidence interval (CI) 0.59–1.01), even though the treatment duration in the estrogen-only treatment arm was longer than in the combined CEE–MPA treatment arm (6.8 and 5.2 years, respectively), whereas the protection against osteoporotic fractures was confirmed. The estimated excess risk for all monitored events was a non-significant two events per 10 000 person-years[16]. The conclusion to be drawn from these studies in respect to the overall risk–benefit profile of HRT depends not only on the incidence of an event but also on the weight that is placed on each of the different events: breast cancer, cardiovascular disease, osteoporotic fractures and cognition. Such a weight could be the impact of an event on the quality of life.

QUALITY OF LIFE WEIGHTS

Two of the most important outcome attributes when comparing health states are survival duration and quality of life. Indeed, recently, the American College of Obstetricians and Gynecologists (ACOG) has argued that any effort to determine the net health effect of any treatment is incomplete without an assessment of the effect of the treatment on the quality of life[17]. The 'global index' used in the WHI was not based upon women's own assessment of their quality of life, and it did not account for time in particular states of health. In addition, outcomes with significant impact on quality of life such as vertebral or other osteoporotic fractures were not included.

There are several disease-specific or generic instruments for individuals to assess quality of life, but, for the purpose of decision-making, it is often desirable to measure health outcomes in a single score that takes into account both quality of life and survival duration. In health economics, the concept of 'quality-adjusted life-years' (QALYs) is commonly used for assessing the rel-

ative cost-effectiveness of two treatment options. QALYs have several benefits. First, they assess the quality of life of a patient. Second, they also incorporate time in a particular health state. Third, they can be comparable across different therapeutic areas. Finally, they combine quality and quantity of life into one single figure.

The assessment of quality of life, as used in QALYs, is derived from the preferences of subjects for health states. There are three main methods for eliciting subjects' preferences, or utilities as they are often called. These methods are the time trade-off method, the standard gamble method and visual analog rating scales (VAS)[18]. Briefly, with the time trade-off method, a subject is given a choice between two alternatives, one being the certain event that a pre-existing chronic illness will continue for a specific period, and the other alternative consisting of undergoing a particular treatment that will result in perfect health but will shorten the subject's life-span. The time period of perfect health in the second alternative is then altered until a subject values both alternatives as the same. The utility of the first alternative is calculated from the ratio of the time during which health is perfect divided by the period during which health is poor. With the standard gamble method, a subject is asked to choose between two alternatives, one being a chronic illness that the subject is 100% certain to have for a specific number of years. For the second alternative, a treatment is introduced, which promises complete recovery at a certain probability, but on the other hand is associated with the risk that it will result in death. The probability for the two possible results of the second alternative are varied until the subject is indifferent to both alternatives. This probability is interpreted as the utility of the first alternative. When non-preference-based rating scales (such as VAS) are used to measure utilities, subjects are instructed to mark on such a scale where they feel a given health state ranks on a range from death to perfect health.

Despite methodological differences, each of the three methods results in a utility score for any particular health state. These utility values are then converted into a QALY by multiplying the number of years a subject is in a particular health state. For example, if someone values three different health states at a utility of 1, 0.8 and 0.4, respectively, and spends 10, 40 and 20 years in each health state, then their total QALYs would be 50. Their QALY value for each health state would be 10 (1×10), 32 (0.8×40) and 8 (0.4×20). A health state of death is usually assigned a utility value of 0.

Due to the general applicability and use across different health states, QALYs are the standard measure in cost–utility analyses. They are the primary outcome used in assessing the cost-effectiveness of health technology by the National Institute for Clinical Excellence (NICE) in England and Wales.

As demonstrated by the WHI, the effects of HRT are numerous, and impact on different health states. Therefore, a measure such as the QALY, which can incorporate the preference of the woman for each of these health states, as well as the time spent in each state, is an important tool for the decision-maker. In the following sections, an attempt is made to balance the outcomes 'breast cancer' and 'osteoporotic fractures' based on published data, and with a focus on scores that combine the quality of life with survival.

OSTEOPOROTIC FRACTURES

Osteoporotic fractures, particularly of the hip and spine, are common among postmenopausal women. These fractures are associated with significant mortality, and also have a significant and prolonged impact on quality of life, as hip fractures in particular often result in loss of independence. The event rates in postmenopausal women without prevalent vertebral fractures are 45.4 per 1000 patient-years for any fracture, 15.2 for vertebral fracture, 4.7 for clinical vertebral fracture and 0.9 for hip fracture. In women with prevalent vertebral fractures, the event rate per 1000 patient-years for any fracture is 117.4, and the event rates for vertebral fracture, clinical vertebral fracture and hip fracture are 77.1, 25.7 and 5.8, respectively[19]. The lifetime risk of hip fracture from age 50 onwards is estimated to be about 17% for white women, and the lifetime

risk of a clinically diagnosed vertebral fracture is about 16%[20]. The lifetime risk of suffering a vertebral fracture is 32% (including 'non-clinical' fractures)[21]. Excess mortality after a hip fracture ranges from 6 to 37%[22]. The risk of death is greatest immediately after the fracture, and then decreases over time. Nearly 8% of patients die within 180 days from the event, with having fractured femur mentioned on the death certificate, and this figure increases to nearly 25% when deaths of all causes are counted[23]. The age-adjusted relative risk to die within 3.8 years of observation from a hip fracture is 6.68 (95% CI 3.08–14.52), and the age-adjusted relative risk to die from a clinical vertebral fracture is 8.64 (95% CI 4.45–16.74)[22]. As clinical fractures constitute only approximately one-third of all vertebral fractures, the mortality from vertebral fractures is often underestimated. Morphometric vertebral fractures, which do not routinely come to medical attention, are associated with a modest excess morbidity and mortality (i.e. a relative risk of hospitalization of 1.18 (95% CI 1.06–1.31), and a relative risk of mortality of 1.60 (95% CI 1.10–2.32))[24,25].

The impact of vertebral and hip fractures on menopausal women's quality of life was investigated using the time trade-off method by Tosteson and co-workers in 2001[26]. This study found that 114 women with one or more vertebral fractures valued this health state with a utility of 0.82 (95% CI 0.76–0.87). For hip fractures, 67 women valued this health state at a utility of 0.63 (95% CI 0.52–0.74). These were compared with 199 women without fractures, who valued their health state at a utility value of 0.91 (95% CI 0.88–0.94). Estimated QALY differences (fracture minus non-fracture subjects) were equivalent to losses of 20–58 days and 23–65 days of perfect health per year for vertebral fracture and hip fracture subjects, respectively, depending on age[26]. Among older women, quality of life is profoundly threatened by hip fracture. A study in 195 older women showed that 80% would rather be dead than experience the loss of independence by a 'bad' hip fracture. On an interval scale between 0 and 1, a 'bad' hip fracture was valued at 0.05 and a 'good' hip fracture which permits maintaining independent living in the community at 0.31[27].

The burden that osteoporotic fractures place on women, their social supports and the health-care system is substantial, and the consequences of postmenopausal osteoporosis in terms of morbidity, mortality and costs have been quoted extensively as justification for preventive treatment[28,29]. HRT is among the most cost-effective treatments for prevention of osteoporosis and osteoporotic fractures[30,31]. It not only increases BMD, but also reduces the risk of fractures. Two systematic reviews of all randomized trials of HRT that reported or collected fracture data from women who had used HRT for at least 12 months showed an overall 33% reduction in vertebral fractures (95% CI 45–98), and an overall 27% reduction in non-vertebral fractures (95% CI 0.56–0.94). Women younger than 60 years had a larger reduction in non-vertebral fractures (i.e. a relative risk (RR) of 0.67, 95% CI 0.46–0.98), compared with women with a mean age of 60 years or older (RR 0.88, 95% CI 0.71–1.08). For hip and wrist fractures alone, the effectiveness of HRT appeared to be more marked (RR 0.60, 95% CI 0.40–0.91), particularly for women younger than 60 years (RR 0.45, 95% CI 0.26–0.79)[3,4]. A statistically significant beneficial effect of HRT on fracture incidence was also reported in the WHI study[2,16]. When considering all confirmed osteoporotic fracture events that occurred from enrollment to discontinuation of the CEE–MPA treatment arm of the trial in July 2002, 733 of 8506 women (8.6%) in the estrogen-plus-progestin group and 896 of 8102 women (11.1%) in the placebo group experienced a fracture (HR 0.76, 95% CI adjusted for multiple testing 0.63–0.92, nominal 95% CI 0.69–0.85)[2]. Reductions for hip and for vertebral fracture both amounted to 34% (nominal 95% CI 0.45–0.98 and 0.44–0.98, respectively)[2]. With estrogen-only treatment, an even further decreased risk for hip (HR 0.61, 95% CI 0.41–0.91), vertebral (HR 0.62, 95% CI 0.42–0.93) and total fractures (HR 0.70, 95% CI 0.63–0.79) was reported[16]. The annualized percentage of all fractures was 1.39% (503 out of 5310 patients) in the CEE treatment group, and 1.95% (724 out of 5429 patients) in the placebo group. Total hip bone mineral density (BMD), measured in a subset of 1024 women, increased

3.7% after 3 years of treatment with estrogen plus progestin, compared with 0.14% in the placebo group ($p < 0.001$)[2].

BREAST CANCER

Breast cancer is considered the most relevant adverse outcome from prolonged HRT use, and the greatest worry for the patient. Even though the mortality has been greatly reduced thanks to new therapies and earlier diagnosis, the risk of dying is still high. The lifetime risk of having breast cancer in the USA is 13%, and the risk of dying from it is approximately 23%. The lifetime risk of dying from breast cancer in the USA is 3%[32]. In Europe, the risk differs between countries. Overall, approximately 350 000 cases are diagnosed per year and approximately 130 000 women die per year of breast cancer, which corresponds to a death rate of approximately 37%[33]. The WHI estrogen-plus-progestogen study demonstrated a slightly increased risk of getting breast cancer compared with non-users, and the risk appears to increase with years of use. The WHI data indicated a 26% increased risk (95% CI 1.00–1.59) for invasive breast cancer in current HRT users after a mean treatment period of 5.2 years of combined HRT versus placebo[1], and the HERS indicated a similar (statistically not significant) 27% increased risk (95% CI 0.84–1.94)[34]. The relative risk in the Million Women Study was 1.66 (95% CI 1.58–1.75) in current users. Past users were not at an increased risk (1.01, 95% CI 0.94–1.09)[13]. The results of the WHI estrogen-alone study came as a surprise, as the hazard ratio of being diagnosed with breast cancer was 0.77 (95% CI 0.59–1.01) after a mean treatment duration of 6.8 years[16]. The rapid decline of the risk after stopping HRT reported in an earlier meta-analysis[35] has been confirmed by the Million Women Study[13]. This finding is quite puzzling, as cancer is considered to be an autonomous process.

Relatively few studies estimating utility values for different breast cancer stages have been conducted to date. Chie and colleagues[36] found that utility scores did not differ significantly between clinical phases of breast cancer. Another study estimated utility values based on 41 patients with early-stage breast cancer undergoing chemotherapy. Using the VAS, time trade-off and standard gambling techniques, they estimated utility values of 0.77 (standard deviation (SD) 0.15; $n = 41$), 0.90 (SD 0.12; $n = 41$) and 0.93 (SD 0.10; $n = 38$), respectively[18]. Two studies provided utility estimates for women with advanced breast cancer. One study used a VAS to assess quality of life during different treatments for advanced breast cancer. A total of 84 women were interviewed. The utility values for patients on hormonal therapies, mild chemotherapies and intensive chemotherapies were 0.628, 0.651 and 0.483, respectively. When not split by treatment, they rated their health at between 0.368 and 0.680[37]. The second study used a standard gamble approach in 129 oncology nurses across five countries. For partial response, stable disease, progressive disease and terminal disease, utility values of 0.81, 0.62, 0.41 and 0.16, respectively, were estimated[38]. Whether the mortality rate from breast cancer is increased in HRT users remains inconclusive[13,39]. Earlier studies indicated a better prognosis of breast cancer that had been diagnosed in HRT users, possibly because of less advanced tumor spread[40,41].

BALANCING OUTCOMES: BREAST CANCER AND OSTEOPOROTIC FRACTURES

Accepting an increased risk of breast cancer, the major question remains whether the beneficial effects on bone are outweighed by the negative effects on the breast. Only a few studies so far have used quantitative decision analysis to determine the net effect of HRT on women's health. Studies that were performed before the results from the WHI were published showed that HRT increased quality-adjusted life-years and was cost-effective relative to no therapy[42–45] but these analyses started from the assumption that HRT had a positive effect on coronary heart disease prevention. However, even when taking into account that HRT does not provide cardiovascular protection[46], or, as indicated by the WHI,

that HRT puts women at an increased risk of coronary heart disease, stroke, pulmonary embolism and breast cancer[1], and despite methodological differences, several studies have still indicated a net beneficial health effect of up to 20 years' treatment with HRT in symptomatic women[47–49]. Menopausal symptoms may affect as many as 75–80% of women at or around the time of the menopause, and almost one-third of postmenopausal women report symptoms that last up to 5 years after a natural menopause. Hot flushes can even persist for up to 15 years in 20% or more of women, and for the many women who experience hot flushes and other menopausal symptoms, these have a profound impact on the quality of life[50–52]. Utility values as low as 0.64 (95% CI 0.57–0.71) have been reported for severe menopausal symptoms and of 0.85 (95% CI 0.80–0.90) for mild symptoms, using the time trade-off method[53]. HRT effectively alleviates menopausal symptoms (i.e. a 77% reduction in frequency (95% CI 58.2–87.5) and an 87% reduction in symptom severity (95% CI 0.08–0.22) for HRT relative to placebo)[54]. The increase in the utility weight is 0.18 for women with mild symptoms, and 0.42 for women with severe symptoms[55]. The gain in quality-adjusted life-years with HRT thus depends on the severity of the women's symptoms and its impact on the quality of life, and probably also on the age at which HRT is started[39].

The outcomes of the quantitative decision analyses discussed above all indicated a net harmful effect of HRT for asymptomatic women[47–49], although the study by Kim and Kwok showed that the reduction in life expectancy would only be in the order of several days[49]. More important, however, is that these models only accounted for hip fractures, whereas the HRT-associated reduction in vertebral fractures and the impact thereof on the quality of life were not included. The lifetime risk for hip and vertebral fractures in the general population by far exceeds the lifetime risk of developing breast cancer, and the impact of hip and vertebral fractures on quality of life and survival is considerable, compared with breast cancer. When comparing the effect of HRT on both hip and vertebral fractures (five fewer hip fractures and approximately six fewer vertebral fractures per 10 000 person-years)[1] with the potential risk of breast cancer (i.e. eight more cases of breast cancer per 10 000 person-years)[1], it appears that the balance is clearly in favor of HRT, even in asymptomatic women.

References

1. Rossouw JE, Anderson GL, Prentice RL, et al. Writing Group for the Women's Health Initiative Investigators. Risks and benefits of estrogen plus progestin in healthy postmenopausal women. Principal results from the Women's Health Initiative randomized controlled trial. *J Am Med Assoc* 2002; 288: 321–33

2. Cauley JA, Robbins J, Chen Z, et al. Women's Health Initiative Investigators. Effects of estrogen plus progestin on risk of fracture and bone mineral density: the Women's Health Initiative randomized trial. *J Am Med Assoc* 2003; 290: 1729–38

3. Torgerson DJ, Bell-Syer SE. Hormone replacement therapy and prevention of nonvertebral fractures: a meta-analysis of randomized trials. *J Am Med Assoc* 2001; 285: 2891–7

4. Torgerson DJ, Bell-Syer SE. Hormone replacement therapy and prevention of vertebral fractures: a meta-analysis of randomised trials. *BMC Musculoskel Disord* 2001; 2: 7 and http://www.biomedcentral.com/1471-2474/2/7

5. Grodstein F, Newcomb PA, Stampfer MJ. Postmenopausal hormone therapy and the risk of colorectal cancer: a review and meta-analysis. *Am J Med* 1999; 106: 574–82

6. Nanda K, Bastian LA, Hasselblad V, et al. Hormone replacement therapy and the risk of colorectal cancer: a meta-analysis. *Obstet Gynecol* 1999; 93: 880–8

7. LeBlanc ES, Janowsky J, Chan BK, et al. Hormone replacement therapy and cognition: systematic review and meta-analysis. *J Am Med Assoc* 2001; 285: 1489–99

8. Wolf PH, Madans JH, Finucane FF, et al. Reduction of cardiovascular disease-related mortality among postmenopausal women who use hormones: evidence from a national cohort. *Am J Obstet Gynecol* 1991; 164: 489–94

9. Grodstein F, Stampfer MJ, Colditz GA, et al. Postmenopausal hormone therapy and mortality. *N Engl J Med* 1997; 336: 1769–75

10. Grodstein FG, Manson JE, Colditz GA, et al. A prospective, observational study of postmenopausal hormone therapy and primary prevention of cardiovascular disease. *Ann Intern Med* 2000; 133: 933–41

11. Hulley S, Grady D, Bush T, et al. Randomized trial of estrogen plus progestin for secondary prevention of coronary heart disease in postmenopausal women. Heart and Estrogen/progestin Replacement Study (HERS) Research Group. *J Am Med Assoc* 1998; 280: 605–13

12. Grady D, Herrington D, Bittner V, et al.; HERS Research Group. Cardiovascular disease outcomes during 6.8 years of hormone therapy: Heart and Estrogen/progestin Replacement Study follow-up (HERS II). *J Am Med Assoc* 2002; 288: 49–57

13. Beral V; Million Women Study Collaborators. Breast cancer and hormone-replacement therapy in the Million Women Study. *Lancet* 2003; 362: 419–27

14. US Preventive Services Task Force. Postmenopausal hormone replacement therapy for primary prevention of chronic conditions: recommendations and rationale. *Ann Intern Med* 2002; 137: 834–9

15. Core SPC for Hormone Replacement Therapy Revision 2: adopted revisions of the MRFG for the core SPC for HRT following the restriction of osteoporosis indication to second-line therapy, dated February 2004. http://heads.medagencies.org/index.html (5 November 2004)

16. Anderson GL, Limacher M, Assaf AR, et al. Women's Health Initiative Steering Committee. Effects of conjugated equine estrogen in postmenopausal women with hysterectomy: the

Women's Health Initiative randomized controlled trial. *J Am Med Assoc* 2004; 291: 1701–12

17. ACOG Task Force for Hormone Therapy, American College of Obstetricians and Gynecologists Women's Health Care Physicians. Summary of balancing risks and benefits. *Obstet Gynecol* 2004; 104 (Suppl 4): 128S–9S

18. Jansen SJT, Stiggelbout AM, Nooij MA, et al. The effect of individually assessed preference weights on the relationship between holistic utilities and non-preference-based assessment. *Qual Life Res* 2000; 9: 541–57

19. Silverman SL, Delmas PD, Kulkarni PM, et al. Comparison of fracture, cardiovascular event, and breast cancer rates at 3 years in postmenopausal women with osteoporosis. *J Am Geriatr Soc* 2004; 52: 1543–8

20. Cummings SR, Melton LJ. Epidemiology and outcomes of osteoporotic fractures. *Lancet* 2002; 359: 1761–7

21. Cummings SR, Black DM, Rubin SM. Lifetime risks of hip, Colles', or vertebral fracture and coronary heart disease among white postmenopausal women. *Arch Intern Med* 1989; 149: 2445–8

22. Cauley JA, Thompson DE, Ensrud KC, et al. Risk of mortality following clinical fractures. *Osteoporosis Int* 2000; 11: 556–61

23. Goldacre MJ, Roberts SE, Yeates D. Mortality after admission to hospital with fractured neck of femur: database study. *Br Med J* 2002; 325: 868–9

24. Ismail AA, O'Neill TW, Cooper C, et al. Mortality associated with vertebral deformity in men and women: results from the European Prospective Osteoporosis Study (EPOS). *Osteoporos Int* 1998; 8: 291–7

25. Ensrud KE, Thompson DE, Cauley JA, et al. Prevalent vertebral deformities predict mortality and hospitalization in older women with low bone mass. Fracture Intervention Trial Research Group. *J Am Geriatr* Soc 2000; 48: 241–9

26. Tosteson AN, Gabriel SE, Grove MR, et al. Impact of hip and vertebral fractures on quality-adjusted life years. *Osteoporos Int* 2001; 12: 1042–9

27. Salkeld G, Cameron ID, Cumming RG, et al. Quality of life related to fear of falling and hip fracture in older women: a time trade off study. *Br Med J* 2000; 320: 341–6

28. Chrischilles E, Shireman T, Wallace R. Costs and health effects of osteoporotic fractures. *Bone* 1994; 15: 377–86

29. Ethgen O, Tellier V, Sedrine WB, et al. Health-related quality of life and cost of ambulatory care in osteoporosis: how may such outcome measures be valuable information to health decision makers and payers? *Bone* 2003; 32: 718–24

30. Belchetz PE. Hormonal treatment of postmenopausal women. *N Engl J Med* 1994; 330: 1062–71

31. Francis RM, Anderson FH, Torgerson DJ. A comparison of the effectiveness and cost of treatment for vertebral fractures in women. *Br J Rheumatol* 1995; 34: 1167–71

32. SEERS Cancer Statistics Review 1975–2001. http://seer.cancer.gov/canques (5 November 2004)

33. Erbas B, Amos A, Fletcher A, et al. Incidence of invasive breast cancer and ductal carcinoma in situ in a screening program by age: should older women continue screening? *Cancer Epidemiol Biomarkers Prev* 2004; 13: 1569–73

34. Hulley S, Furberg C, Barrett-Connor E, et al. for the HERS Research Group. Noncardiovascular outcomes during 6.8 years of hormone therapy. Heart and Estrogen/progestin Replacement Study follow-up (HERS II). *J Am Med Assoc* 2002; 288: 58–66

35. Collaborative Group on Hormonal Factors in Breast Cancer. Breast cancer and hormone replacement therapy: colaborative reanalysis of data from 51 epidemiological studies of 52 705 women with breast cancer and 108 411 women without breast cancer. *Lancet* 1997; 350: 1047–59

36. Chie WC, Huang CS, Chen JH, et al. Measurement of the quality of life during different clinical phases of breast cancer. *J Formos Med Assoc* 1999; 98: 254–60

37. Hurny C, van Wegberg B, Bacchi M, et al. Subjective health estimations (SHE) in patients with advanced breast cancer: an adapted utility concept for clinical trials. *Br J Cancer* 1998; 77: 985–91

38. Hutton J, Brown R, Borowitz M, et al. A new decision model for cost–utility comparisons of chemotherapy in recurrent metastatic breast cancer. *Pharmacoeconomics* 1996; 9 (Suppl 2): 8–22

39. Salpeter SR, Walsh JM, Greyber E, et al. Mortality associated with hormone replacement therapy in younger and older women: a meta-analysis. *J Gen Intern Med* 2004; 19: 791–804

40. Willis DB, Calle EE, Miracle-McMahill HL, et al. Estrogen replacement therapy and risk of fatal breast cancer in a prospective cohort of postmenopausal women in the United States. *Cancer Causes Control* 1996; 7: 449–57

41. Schairer C, Byrne C, Keyl PM, et al. Menopausal estrogen and estrogen–progestin replacement therapy and risk of breast cancer (United States). *Cancer Causes Control* 1994; 5: 491–500

42. Weinstein MC, Schiff I. Cost-effectiveness of hormone replacement therapy in the menopause. *Obstet Gynecol Surv* 1983; 38: 445–55

43. Gorsky RD, Koplan JP, Peterson HB, et al. Relative risks and benefits of long-term estrogen replacement therapy: a decision analysis. *Obstet Gynecol* 1994; 83: 161–6

44. Kanis JA, Brazier JE, Stevenson M, et al. Treatment of established osteoporosis: a systematic review and cost–utility analysis. *Health Technol Assess* 2002; 6(29)

45. Armstrong K, Chen TM, Albert D, et al. Cost-effectiveness of raloxifene and hormone replacement therapy in postmenopausal women: impact of breast cancer risk. *Obstet Gynecol* 2001; 98: 996–1003

46. Beral V, Banks E, Reeves G. Evidence from randomised trials on the long-term effects of hormone replacement therapy. *Lancet* 2002; 360: 942–4

47. Minelli C, Abrams KR, Sutton AJ, et al. Benefits and harms associated with hormone replacement therapy: clinical decision analysis. *Br Med J* 2004; 328: 371–6

48. Col NF, Weber G, Stiggelbout A, et al. Short-term menopausal hormone therapy for symptom relief: an updated decision model. *Arch Intern Med* 2004; 164: 1634–40

49. Kim C, Kwok YS. Decision analysis of hormone replacement therapy after the Women's Health Initiative. *Am J Obstet Gynecol* 2003; 189: 1228–33

50. Kronenberg F. Hot flashes: phenomenology, quality of life and search for treatment options. *Exp Gerontol* 1994; 29: 319–36

51. Dennerstein L, Dudley E, Burger H. Well-being and the menopausal transition. *J Psychosom Obstet Gynecol* 1997; 18: 95–101

52. Hlatky MA, Boothroyd D, Vittinghoff E, et al. Heart and Estrogen/progestin Replacement Study (HERS) Research Group. Quality-of-life and depressive symptoms in postmenopausal women after receiving hormone therapy: results from the Heart and Estrogen/progestin Replacement Study (HERS) trial. *J Am Med Assoc* 2002; 287: 591–7

53. Daly E, Gray A, Barlow D, et al. Measuring the impact of menopausal symptoms on quality of life. *Br Med J* 1993; 307: 836–40

54. MacLennan A, Lester S, Moore V. Oral estrogen replacement therapy versus placebo for hot flushes: a systematic review. *Climacteric* 2001; 4: 58–74

55. Zethraeus N, Johannesson M, Henriksson P, et al. The impact of hormone replacement therapy on quality of life and willingness to pay. *Br J Obstet Gynaecol* 1997; 104: 1191–58

29

Prevent, treat and maintain: how to optimize the management of postmenopausal osteoporosis

D. Agnusdei

There is now a consensus that osteoporosis should be defined as a disease of decreased bone strength rather than a disease of decreased bone mass, and that all efficacious drugs should demonstrate increases in bone strength as evidenced by a decrease in fracture incidence. Bone strength primarily reflects the integration of bone density and bone quality[1]. From a skeletal metabolism standpoint, osteoporosis may be defined as a consequence of the imbalance of the physiological process of bone turnover (or coupling), i.e. a lack of equilibrium between the activity of osteoblasts (bone-forming cells) and osteoclasts (bone-resorbing cells), with a relative increase in the activity of the latter[2].

Osteoporosis is the most common metabolic bone disease among postmenopausal women, and it has a large impact on public health. All skeletal sites can be affected, with progressive bone mineral density (BMD) reduction and microarchitectural deterioration of bone tissue leading to an increase in fracture risk. Although bone mass is still the major determinant of bone strength, other determinants including bone geometry, bone material properties and bone microstructure play an important role as well[3].

Although pharmacological interventions to prevent bone loss are necessary in patients at the greatest risk of fracture, the first priority in osteoporosis secondary prevention should be to avoid falls, the major determinant of fractures in the elderly. A therapeutic choice must include treatments that are effective in reducing the risk and incidence of fractures, demonstrated in controlled clinical trials.

In postmenopausal women, using currently available treatment options, we should be able to implement a new strategy emerging from the following concept: prevent, treat and maintain (PTM). The need to clarify this matter is critical. As has already been evidenced for other clinical conditions, it would be ideal to achieve a rationale regarding the use of available treatment options, in order to optimize the balance between the efficacy of a drug and its potential side-effects. According to current knowledge, the priorities that should be considered for the satisfactory management of osteoporosis are: first, prevention of postmenopausal bone loss with preservation and/or restoration of normal bone structure and skeletal health; and second, prevention of first and/or subsequent fractures with a decrease of fracture risk that should be both statistically significant and clinically relevant. Furthermore, considering that this treatment should probably be continued long-term, pharmacological choices should take into account – primary end-point, cost/effectiveness issues and side-effects according to the mechanism of action.

In addition, patients with low bone mass and osteoporosis have several different clinical profiles. In our daily clinical practice, we see patients with different expectations: early-postmenopausal women, with and without menopausal symptoms, for whom the aim is to relieve symptoms, prevent bone loss and maintain bone density level; patients with osteoporosis, for whom it is essential to prevent the first vertebral fracture; and patients with prevalent vertebral fractures, for whom it is important to prevent subsequent fractures including hip fractures, and the associated well-known burden of increased morbidity and mortality. These scenarios are not necessarily linked to a particular age range or to a chronological sequence of events.

It is well known that, in the early-postmenopausal period, the main pathogenetic factor for osteoporosis is the cessation of ovarian activity that causes a disruption of bone homeostasis, leading to bone loss and deterioration of bone structure. In postmenopausal women with normal or low bone density, and with menopausal symptoms, the first treatment goal should be to maintain bone health, thus preventing occurrence of the first fracture, but also to prevent and/or treat vasomotor symptoms to maintain the patient's compliance. The first-choice treatment option for these women, in the absence of specific contraindications, should be hormone therapy (HT) or estrogen therapy (ET) in women without a uterus[4]. Estrogens of different types, dosages and delivery forms have been shown to prevent bone loss and to decrease fracture risk in many retrospective studies and in one randomized placebo-controlled clinical trial[4,5]. In particular, the results of the recent Women's Health Initiative (WHI) study, performed in 16 608 postmenopausal women of mean age 63.3 years, randomized to daily placebo or continuous combined conjugated equine estrogens 0.625 mg plus medroxyprogesterone acetate 2.5 mg, has demonstrated the efficacy of HT in decreasing the risk of osteoporotic fractures[5,6] (hazard ratio (HR) for hip fractures 0.66, HR for vertebral fractures 0.66). The population of the WHI study was not selected according to bone density or fracture risk status. The study, planned for 8 years, was stopped after 5.2 years because of the presence of a slight, but significant, increase in the incidence of breast cancer[7] (HR 1.26). This effect was evident only in the HT arm of the study. Moreover, the study failed to show any protection by HT against coronary heart disease (HR 1.24), the primary end-point in WHI[8]. Whether these results can be applied to other types and delivery forms of HT, and to different populations, such as younger postmenopausal women, or women with a lower body mass index, is still under debate.

After the publication of these results, scientific societies and regulatory authorities released recommendations to physicians that can be summarized as follows: the duration of HT should be maintained for the shortest possible time and with the lowest effective dosage; and, more important, the treatment should always be individualized to the patient's need[9–12].

Looking through the clinical continuum of osteoporosis, the next patient profile that clinicians should consider is the postmenopausal woman with normal or low BMD, but without vasomotor symptoms. For this woman, a selective estrogen receptor modulator (SERM) such as raloxifene (RLX) would be the most appropriate treatment option. In a recently published study, 5 years of RLX treatment in healthy postmenopausal women was shown to preserve BMD and significantly reduce the likelihood of development of osteoporosis, and was not associated with an increased rate of vaginal bleeding, endometrial hyperplasia or endometrial carcinoma, compared with women receiving calcium supplements[13]. These results confirmed the excellent uterine safety profile of RLX treatment shown in a large number of postmenopausal women with osteoporosis enrolled in the Multiple Outcomes of Raloxifene Evaluation (MORE) study[14]. Another important objective of the PTM strategy should be to prevent the first fracture in women with low bone mass, or osteopenia. A large cohort study, National Osteoporosis Risk Assessment (NORA), performed in the USA, has recently shown that low bone mass is largely undetected in the general population, and that more than half of these women are at risk for fractures to the same extent as in those with osteoporosis diagnosed by peripheral dual-energy X-ray absorptiometry (DXA)[15]. Indeed, occurrence of the first fracture is already a signal of bone qualitative and quantitative changes. A *post hoc* analysis of the MORE study has recently shown that 3 years of treatment with RLX significantly decreases the risk of all new radiographic vertebral fractures and new clinical vertebral fractures, irrespective of baseline total hip BMD, in postmenopausal women with low BMD but without prevalent vertebral fractures. Raloxifene is the first antiresorptive therapy able to reduce the risk of vertebral fractures among women with osteopenia defined by total hip BMD. Therefore, in this clinical situation, RLX should be considered the first-line treatment.

As the mean age of the general population increases, the incidence of osteoporotic fracture is expected to rise dramatically during the next few decades. Older patients are more susceptible to fracture at any given BMD than are younger patients. Many factors are responsible for this phenomenon, including an age-related deterioration of bone quality, which involves more than BMD. Therefore, in these women, the main objective should be to stop bone loss, thus decreasing the risk of first and subsequent fractures. Suppression of increased bone turnover by antiresorptive therapies, even if this produces only small changes in BMD, can significantly reduce fracture risk, particularly at the spine. All the antiresorptives currently available for clinical use, including raloxifene, bisphosphonates and calcitonin, have been shown in randomized controlled trials to reduce significantly, between 30 and 50%, vertebral fractures over 3 years[16–20]. Moreover, bisphosphonates and raloxifene in prospective and *post hoc* analyses have been shown to reduce consistently and significantly, from 50 to 65%, the risk of new morphometric and clinical vertebral fractures after 12 months of treatment in postmenopausal osteoporotic women, with and without prevalent vertebral fractures[17,19,21]. These results are clinically relevant, since these fractures are associated with significant pain and disability, and, more important, are predictive of future fragility fractures, including hip fractures[22].

In addition, in two different studies, alendronate and risedronate have been shown to reduce significantly the risk of hip fractures in elderly osteoporotic women with prevalent vertebral fractures[16,23]. A reduction in the incidence of hip fractures has not been shown after raloxifene treatment[17], although, in a *post hoc* analysis of the MORE study, a significant reduction of non-vertebral fracture incidence has been shown in osteoporotic women with severe prevalent vertebral fractures[24]. On the other hand, raloxifene, due to its SERM profile, has recently been associated with a consistent reduction of the risk of invasive breast cancer, by 66%, in postmenopausal women with osteoporosis over 8 years of treatment[25].

Since osteoporosis is a chronic degenerative disease, it requires long-term treatment. To this end, it is important to evaluate the overall pharmacological profile, efficacy and safety presented by the different bone-active agents used in management of the disease. Recently, important results concerning the safety profile of antiresorptive drugs have been published. Ten years' treatment with alendronate in postmenopausal women with osteoporosis has demonstrated sufficient skeletal safety of this compound[26]. Risedronate has been given for 7 years, and bone biopsies have shown preservation of bone architecture, without defects of mineralization[27]. However, there is still significant debate on the optimal duration of therapy with these potent inhibitors of bone turnover. For long-term therapies designed to prevent osteoporosis, over-suppression of bone turnover could determine, via the coupling phenomenon, an oversuppression of bone formation that in turn could impair the ability to repair microdamage, which is the physiological role of bone turnover. In osteoporotic patients treated with antiresorptives, the optimal level of bone formation rate remains uncertain. An ideal outcome of this osteoporosis management program would be to maintain bone formation within values found in premenopausal women. Results from the MORE and Continuing Outcome, Relevant to Evista (CORE) studies have shown that for 8 years RLX treatment was safe and did not elicit additional side-effects, compared with shorter treatment[25]. Thus, in postmenopausal patients with low BMD and in older patients with osteoporosis and osteopenia, raloxifene should be considered a valid treatment, with an excellent balance between long-term efficacy and safety. In elderly patients at highest risk for hip fractures, the treatment of choice should be with aminobisphosphonates.

Despite different changes of BMD observed in studies performed using antiresorptive agents, the decrease in relative risk of fracture was almost identical. Recent meta-analysis demonstrated that only 4–28% of the decrease of fracture risk could be explained by an increase of bone density. The recent introduction of the bone quality paradigm might explain these apparent contradictory results[28]. It appears that modulation of the increased postmenopausal bone turnover induced by antiresorptive therapies, even with only small changes in BMD, could play a pivotal role in the reduction of fracture risk, by preserving bone architecture[29].

A different approach to the PTM concept could consider, particularly for elderly patients with very low bone mass and prevalent fractures, the use of combined therapies. Although there is no theoretical rationale, combinations of different antiresorptives (HT–bisphosphonates, RLX–bisphosphonates) have been used in clinical practice, mainly to stop the fracture cascade in patients with severe osteoporosis and fractures. The effects of combined treatment have been investigated in several clinical trials. Recent clinical data have shown that combination therapy with HT and alendronate was efficacious and well tolerated, with significant additional increase in BMD, and preserving their tolerability profiles. In these studies, alendronate was superior to HT, and combination therapy was superior to either therapy alone. Therefore, combination therapy may represent an option for women with very high bone turnover, and with an urgent need to increase BMD, or for those who have failed to achieve an adequate response to monotherapy[30–32].

In patients with severe osteoporosis, the main goal of the PTM strategy would be to prevent further fractures, rebuild lost bone, restore structure and architecture of the bone tissue and manage frailty. Until recently, bisphosphonates were the agents of choice for most patients with severe osteoporosis. Treatment with these agents determined significant increase of BMD at different skeletal sites, and significantly reduced the risk of osteoporotic fractures, including hip fractures.

Although antiresorptive therapies prevent further bone loss and reduce fracture incidence by 50% in patients with osteoporosis, they do not restore bone mass or lost bone microarchitecture. The recent introduction of bone-forming agents such as parathyroid hormone peptides, in particular teriparatide (recombinant human parathyroid hormone 1–34 (rhPTH 1–34)) significantly modified the therapeutic approach to severe osteoporosis with fractures. Teriparatide directly stimulates new bone formation and bone turnover to increase bone mass and improve lost bone microarchitecture[33–42].

Teriparatide 20 µg/day (Forteo) has been available in the United States since November 2002, and received regulatory approval across all 15 member states of the European Union in June 2003. In Europe, teriparatide 20 µg/day is marketed under the trade name Forsteo. Successful regulatory approvals of Forsteo/Forteo are based on the Fracture Prevention Trial, in which 1637 postmenopausal women with osteoporosis and a history of at least one prior vertebral fracture received daily injections of teriparatide (20 or 40 µg/day) or placebo for an average of 19 months. Patients treated with teriparatide 20 µg experienced a 65% reduction in the risk for vertebral fracture, and a 53% reduction in the risk for non-vertebral fracture, versus placebo. Treatment with teriparatide 20 µg increased lumbar spine BMD by 9.7% and femoral neck BMD by 2.8%, compared with placebo. New or worsening back pain was reported less frequently in teriparatide 20 µg-treated patients versus placebo-treated patients. Teriparatide treatment was well tolerated; the only significant adverse event occurring in the teriparatide 20-µg group was a slight increase in leg cramps[43].

Following termination of the active treatment phase of the Fracture Prevention Trial, 77% (1262) of the women entered a 30-month post-treatment observational follow-up study. During follow-up, women previously treated with teriparatide continued to have a lower incidence of both vertebral and non-vertebral fractures compared with those who were originally randomized to placebo during the treatment study. The lower risk of fracture was apparent after adjusting for the use of other osteoporosis treatments that were used in the observational study[44].

Based on these results, teriparatide represents an important new advance in the therapy of this skeletal disorder. As the first bone-forming agent, its potential might be substantially greater than that of antiresorptive agents. Clear evidence in clinical trials now documents the ability of teriparatide to stimulate cancellous bone formation and to reduce fractures in postmenopausal women and men with osteoporosis[45,46].

In conclusion, metabolic bone disease is a rapidly advancing field of clinical investigation. The management of these diseases has been quite challenging in the past, and the 'prevent, treat and maintain' (PTM) concept represents an innovative approach. However, it is possible that further knowledge and availability of new treatment options may enrich and modify this strategy in the near future. There is clear evidence today that, with the recent advent of true anabolic agents, the evaluation of bone quality will probably become more important in the management of postmenopausal osteoporosis.

References

1. Consensus Conference. Osteoporosis prevention, diagnosis and treatment. NIH Consensus Development Panel on Osteoporosis. *J Am Med Assoc* 2001; 285: 785

2. Del Puente A, Migliaccio S, Esposito A, et al. A reappraisal of osteoporosis therapeutic approach. *Aging Clin Exp Res* 2004; 16: 42–6

3. Bouxsein ML. Biomechanics of age-related fractures. In Marcus R, Feldman D, Kelsey J, eds. *Osteoporosis*, 2nd edn. San Diego, CA: Academic Press, 2001: 509–31

4. Lindsay R, Gallagher JC, Kleerekoper M, Pickar JH. Effect of lower doses of conjugated equine estrogens with and without medroxyprogesterone acetate on bone in early postmenopausal women. *J Am Med Assoc* 2002; 287: 2668–76

5. Writing Group for the Women's Health Initiative Investigators. Risks and benefits of estrogen plus progestin in healthy postmenopausal women. *J Am Med Assoc* 2002; 288: 321–33

6. Cauley JA, Robbins J, Chen Z, et al. Effects of estrogen plus progestin on risk of fracture and bone mineral density. The Women's Health Initiative Randomized Trial. *J Am Med Assoc* 2003; 290: 1729–38

7. Chlebowski RT, Hendrix SL, Langer RD, et al. Influence of estrogen plus progestin on breast cancer and mammography in healthy postmenopausal women. *J Am Med Assoc* 2003; 289: 3243–53

8. Manson JA, Hsia J, Johnson KC, et al. Estrogen plus progestin and the risk of coronary heart disease. *N Engl J Med* 2003; 349: 523–34

9. Neves-e-Castro M, Samsioe G, Doren M, Skouby S. On behalf of the European Menopause & Andropause Society (EMAS). Results from WHI and HERS II – Implication for women and the prescriber of HRT. *Maturitas* 2002; 42: 255–8

10. Schneider HPG. The view of the International Menopause Society on the Women's Health Initiative. *Climacteric* 2002; 5: 211–161

11. Consensus Paper. The European Consensus Development Conference 2002: Sex Steroids and Cardiovascular Diseases. On the route to combined evidence from OC and HRT/ERT. *Maturitas* 2003; 44: 69–82

12. Prestwood KM, Kenny AM, Kleppinger A, Kulldorff M. Ultralow-dose micronized 17β-estradiol and bone density and bone metabolism in older women. A randomized controlled trial. *J Am Med Assoc* 2003; 290: 1042–8

13. Jolly EE, Bjarnason NH, Neven P, et al. Prevention of osteoporosis and uterine effects in postmenopausal women taking raloxifene for 5 years. *Menopause* 2003; 2: 35–40

14. Cummings SR, Eckert S, Krueger KA, et al. The effect of raloxifene on risk of breast cancer in postmenopausal women: results from the MORE randomized trial. Multiple Outcomes of Raloxifene Evaluation. *J Am Med Assoc* 1999; 281: 2189–97

15. Miller PD, Siris ES, Barrett-Connor E, et al. Prediction of fracture risk in postmenopausal white women with peripheral bone densitometry: evidence from the National Osteoporosis Risk Assessment. *J Bone Miner Res* 2002; 17: 2222–30

16. Black DM, Thompson DE, Bauer DC, et al. Fracture risk reduction with alendronate in women with osteoporosis: the fracture intervention trial. *J Clin Endocrinol Metab* 2000; 85: 4118–24

17. Ettinger B, Black DM, Mitlak BH, et al. Reduction of vertebral fracture risk in postmenopausal women with osteoporosis treated with raloxifene: results from a 3-year randomized clinical trial. *J Am Med Assoc* 1999; 282: 637–45

18. Harris ST, Watts NB, Genant HK, et al. Effects of risedronate treatment on vertebral and nonvertebral fractures in women with postmenopausal osteoporosis: a randomized controlled trial. Vertebral Efficacy with Risedronate Therapy (VERT) Study Group. *J Am Med Assoc* 1999; 282: 1344–52

19. Cummings S, Black D, Thompson DE, et al. Effect of alendronate on risk of fracture in women with low bone density but without vertebral fractures. *J Am Med Assoc* 1998; 280: 2077–84

20. Reginster J, Minne HW, Sorensen OH, et al. Randomized trial of the effects of risedronate on vertebral fractures in women with established postmenopausal osteoporosis. *Osteoporos Int* 2000; 11: 83–91

21. Maricic M, Adachi JD, Sarkar S, et al. Early effects of raloxifene on clinical vertebral fractures at 12 months in postmenopausal women with osteoporosis. *Arch Intern Med* 2002; 162: 1140–3

22. Lindsay R, Silverman SL, Cooper C, et al. Risk of new vertebral fracture in the year following a fracture. *J Am Med Assoc* 2001; 285: 320–3

23. McClung M, Geusens P, Miller PD, et al. Effect of risedronate on the risk of hip fracture in elderly women. *N Engl J Med* 2001; 344: 333–40

24. Delmas PD, Genant HK, Crans GG, et al. Severity of prevalent vertebral fractures and the risk of subsequent vertebral and nonvertebral fractures: results from the MORE trial. *Bone* 2003; 33: 522–32

25. Martino S, Cauley J, Barrett-Conner E, et al. Continuing Outcomes Relevant to Evista: a randomized trial of raloxifene in postmenopausal women with osteoporosis. *J Natl Cancer Inst* 2004; 96: 1751–61

26. Bone HG, Hosking D, Devogelaer JP, et al. Ten years' experience with alendronate for osteoporosis in postmenopausal women. *N Engl J Med* 2004; 350: 1189–99

27. Watts R. Bisphosphonate treatment of osteoporosis. *Clin Geriatr Med* 2003; 19: 395–414

28. Seeman E. Bone quality. *Osteoporos Int* 2003; 14 (Suppl 5): S3–7

29. Sarkar S, Mitlak BH, Wong M, et al. Relationships between bone mineral density and incident vertebral fracture risk with raloxifene therapy. *J Bone Miner Res* 2002; 17: 1–10

30. Davas I, Altintas A, Yoldemir T, et al. Effect of daily hormone therapy and alendronate use on bone mineral density in postmenopausal women. *Fertil Steril* 2003; 80: 536–40

31. Bone HG, Greenspan SL, McKeever C, et al. Alendronate and estrogen effects in postmenopausal women with low bone mineral density. *J Clin Endocrinol Metab* 2000; 85: 720–6

32. Johnell O, Scheele WH, Lu Y, et al. Additive effects of raloxifene and alendronate on bone density and biochemical markers of bone remodeling in postmenopausal women with osteoporosis. *J Clin Endocrinol Metab* 2002; 87: 983–4

33. Cosman Nieves J, Woelfert L, Gordon S, et al. Parathyroid responsivity in postmenopausal women with osteoporosis during treatment with parathyroid hormone. *J Clin Endocrinol Metab* 1998; 83: 788–90

34. Cosman Nieves J, Woelfert L, Formica C, et al. Parathyroid hormone added to established hormone therapy: effects on vertebral fracture and maintenance of bone mass after parathyroid hormone withdrawal. *J Bone Miner Res* 2001; 16: 925–31

35. Lane NE, Sanchez S, Modin GW, et al. Parathyroid hormone treatment can reverse corticosteroid-induced osteoporosis. Results of a randomized controlled clinical trial. *J Clin Invest* 1998; 102: 1627–33

36. Lane NE, Sanchez S, Genant HK, et al. Short-term increases in bone turnover markers predict parathyroid hormone-induced spinal bone mineral density gains in postmenopausal women with glucocorticoid-induced osteoporosis. *Osteoporos Int* 2000; 11: 434–42

37. Lane NE, Sanchez S, Modin GW, et al. Bone mass continues to increase at the hip after parathyroid hormone treatment is discontinued in glucocorticoid-induced osteoporosis: results of a randomized controlled clinical trial. *J Bone Miner Res* 2000; 15: 944–51

38. Rittmaster RS, Bolognese M, Ettinger MP, et al. Enhancement of bone mass in osteoporotic women with parathyroid hormone followed by alendronate. *J Clin Endocrinol Metab* 2000; 85: 2129–34

39. Lindsay R, Nieves J, Formica C, et al. Randomised controlled study of effect of parathyroid hormone on vertebral-bone mass and fracture incidence among postmenopausal women on oestrogen with osteoporosis. *Lancet* 1997; 350: 550–5

40. Finkelstein JS, Hayes A, Hunzelman JL, et al. The effects of parathyroid hormone, alendronate, or both in men with osteoporosis. *N Engl J Med* 2003; 349: 1216–26

41. Reeve J, Mitchell A, Tellez M, et al. Treatment with parathyroid peptides and estrogen replacement for severe postmenopausal vertebral osteoporosis: prediction of long-term responses in spine and femur. *J Bone Miner Metab* 2001; 19: 102–14

42. Neer M, Slovik DM, Daly M, et al. Treatment of postmenopausal osteoporosis with daily parathy-roid hormone plus calcitriol. *Osteoporos Int* 1993; 3 (Suppl 1): 204–5

43. Neer RM, Arnaud CD, Zanchetta JR, et al. Effect of parathyroid hormone (1-34) on fractures and bone mineral density in postmenopausal women with osteoporosis. *N Engl J Med* 2001; 344: 1434–41

44. Lindsay R, Scheele WH, Neer R, et al. Sustained vertebral fracture risk reduction after withdrawal of teriparatide in postmenopausal women with osteoporosis. *Arch Intern Med* 2004; 164: 2024–30

45. Rubin MR, Cosman F, Lindsay R, Bilezikian JP. The anabolic effects of parathyroid hormone. *Osteoporos Int* 2002; 13: 267–77

46. Dempster DW, Cosman F, Kurland ES, et al. Effects of daily treatment with parathyroid hor-mone on bone microarchitecture and turnover in patients with osteoporosis: a paired biopsy study. *J Bone Miner Res* 2001; 16: 1846–53

Transdermal hormone therapy: effects on bone   30

R. E. Nappi, F. Albani, F. Ferdeghini, S. Detaddei, A. Sommacal, A. Verza, A. Ornati and F. Polatti

INTRODUCTION

Estrogen deficiency plays a major role in the pathogenesis of bone loss and contributes to the impairment of quality of life in a large number of postmenopausal women. On the other hand, the positive effect of hormone therapy (HT) on bone density and fractures is well established, as is the beneficial action of HT on several aspects of well-being throughout the menopause and beyond[1,2].

There are many options available for conventional HT, differing mainly in terms of biochemical properties, route of administration, dosage and metabolism. The route of HT delivery may induce specific actions on target tissues, as may the combination of different types of estrogens with different types of progestins. As a net result, biological effects may differ according to the nature of HT combination, which needs to be tailored to women's needs and preferences[3].

The transdermal (transdermal therapeutic system, TTS) route of administration (patch or gel) replicates premenopausal physiology by replacing estradiol at a fairly constant rate, and by closely matching the estradiol/estrone ratio as a consequence of no first-pass effect in the liver[4]. Even some progestins (norethisterone acetate and levonorgestrel) may be delivered transdermally (patch or gel), and are essential to endometrial protection in postmenopausal women[5]. Being aware of the potential advantages of the transdermal route of estradiol administration on some specific symptoms that are very common during postmenopausal years, such as, for example, depression[6], headache[7] and androgen-insufficiency syndrome[8], herein we briefly summarize the effects of TTS HT on bone density and fractures.

TRANSDERMAL HORMONE THERAPY AND BONE

Randomized trials provide evidence that, among osteoporosis therapies, HT has a positive, strong impact on bone density at both trabecular and cortical sites[9]. Such an effect is not dependent on the route of HT administration, since both transdermal and oral HT improved bone density significantly in the vertebrae and proximal femur as well as biochemical measurements indicating a significant reduction in bone turnover, in comparison with untreated women, after 18 months[10]. Combining the results of all prevention and treatment trials for both opposed and unopposed estrogen[5], the pooled percentage change in bone density was statistically significantly in favor of HT at all measurement sites. After 1 year of HT, bone density increased at the lumbar spine (5.4%) and at the forearm and femoral neck (3.0% and 2.5%, respectively). After 2 years of treatment, the percentage change in favor of HT increased by about 1.5% at all sites, with differences of 6.8%, 4.5% and 4.1% for the lumbar spine, forearm and femoral neck, respectively[1]. As far as studies of the effect of HT on fractures are concerned, the resulting pooled estimate indicates a 34% reduction in relative risk (RR) of vertebral fractures. Lufkin and colleagues[11] evaluated the tolerance to and effectiveness of transdermal estrogen for women with established postmenopausal osteoporosis and vertebral fractures. In comparison with placebo, the median annual percentage change in bone mineral density in the estrogen group reflected increased or steady-state bone mineral density at the lumbar spine, femoral trochanter and mid-radius, but showed no significant difference at the femoral neck. Estrogen treatment uniformly decreased bone turnover as assessed by several methods, including serum osteocalcin concentration. Histomorphometric evaluation of iliac biopsy samples confirmed the effect of estrogen on bone formation rate per unit of bone volume. Finally, eight new fractures occurred in seven women in the estrogen group, whereas 20 occurred in 12 women in the placebo group, yielding a lower vertebral fracture rate in the estrogen group (RR 0.39, 95% confidence interval (CI) 0.16–0.95). Concerning non-vertebral fractures, the pooling of study results indicates a reduction in RR of 13%[1]. Michaelsson and colleagues, in a population-based case–control study conducted in six counties in Sweden[12], concluded that HT should be continued for long periods for optimal protection against hip fracture, and that no overall substantial hip fracture protection remains after 5 years without HT. In addition, therapy can be initiated several years after the menopause without loss of fracture protection, and the observed interactions with weight and physical activity suggest that HT has the best protective effect against hip fracture among high-risk women[13]. Oral or transdermal therapy was equally effective in reducing the risk of hip fracture, and the addition of progestins permitted lower doses of estrogens[12]. Indeed, in the meta-analysis by Wells and colleagues[1], for the lumbar spine, the difference between HT and control in percentage change in bone density for different types of estrogen preparations was 5.45 for transdermal, 5.36 for oral estradiol and 5.62 for oral conjugated equine estrogens (CEE)–Premarin®. It is interesting to note that the protective effect of estrogens is dose-related, and is significant for any regimen. Indeed, there was a significant difference in bone density at 2 years between low and high doses of estrogen for the lumbar spine and femoral neck[1].

After 2 years, transdermal estradiol was well tolerated and highly effective at doses of between 50 and 100 µg/day in preventing bone loss and reducing bone turnover in early postmenopausal women. The dose of 50 µg/day, the lowest dose tested, appears to be a suitable dose, because there is little clinical benefit of increasing the dosage from 75 to 100 µg/day in both the lumbar spine and the femoral neck[14]. Even the lower dose of a matrix transdermal 17β-estradiol system is efficacious in preventing bone loss, and 25 mg/day offers an effective option for those women who cannot tolerate higher doses[15]. After 2 years, there was a significant gain (increase greater than 2.08%) in lumbar spine bone mass, compared with placebo, and significant increases in femoral neck, trochanter and total hip BMD with all doses of estradiol, compared with placebo. Patients who received estradiol also experienced clinically significant and dose-related decreases in total serum osteocalcin, serum bone alkaline phosphatase and urinary C-telopeptides, with all three markers of bone turnover returning to premenopausal levels[15]. Similar data were reported by Weiss and colleagues[16], indicating that transdermal estradiol at doses of 0.025, 0.05, 0.06 and 0.1 mg/day effectively prevented bone loss at lumbar vertebrae L2–L4, radius, proximal femur and total hip in hysterectomized postmenopausal women. In addition, consistent and significant improvements in biochemical markers of bone turnover (serum osteocalcin and urinary pyridinoline and deoxypyridinoline) were also noted at various intervals in all treatment groups[16]. The lowest effective transdermal estradiol dose in improving lumbar bone mineral density in healthy, post-menopausal women was 0.025 mg/day, with a responder rate (defined as no change or increase in BMD at end-point) of 59.6%[17]. Recently, Ettinger and associates[18] reported that even very-low-dose (0.014 mg/day) unopposed trans-dermal estradiol increased bone mineral density and decreased markers of bone turnover without causing endometrial hyperplasia in post-menopausal women over 60 years.

From the data available, there are no indications that the various progestins used in clinical practice add or subtract much of the protective action of estrogens on bone[19]. As far as the efficacy and safety of the transdermal route of administration, with the addition of norethisterone acetate, is concerned, it is interesting to note that such an HT regimen decreased the turnover rate of mineralized bone matrix even in liver transplant patients, just as in healthy postmenopausal women[20].

Even at low doses in a continuous combined regimen, estradiol and norethisterone acetate were more effective than placebo in reducing the activation frequency of bone remodeling and in preventing bone loss at the spine and hip after 2 years. Effects on the hip were similar to those observed for higher doses of estrogen[21].

CONCLUSIONS

All doses of transdermal estradiol, even the lowest, increased bone mineral density in the lumbar spine and total hip from baseline to study end. No differences in bone density were found following spontaneous or surgical menopause with different estrogen preparations, and the positive effect was irrespective of age and menopausal age.

References

1. Wells G, Tugwell P, Shea B, et al. Meta-analysis of the efficacy of hormone replacement therapy in treating and preventing osteoporosis in postmenopausal women. *Endocrine Rev* 2002; 23: 529–39

2. Genazzani AR, Gambacciani M, Simoncini T, Schneider HP. Hormone replacement therapy in climacteric and aging brain. International Menopause Society Expert Workshop, 15–18 March 2003, Pisa, Italy. *Climacteric* 2003; 6: 188–203

3. Gambacciani M, Genazzani AR. Hormone replacement therapy: the benefits in tailoring the regimen and dose. *Maturitas* 2001; 40: 195–201

4. Ansbacher R. The pharmacokinetics and efficacy of different estrogens are not equivalent. *Am J Obstet Gynecol* 2001; 184: 255–63

5. Van Gorp T, Neven P. Endometrial safety of hormone replacement therapy: review of literature. *Maturitas* 2002; 42: 93–104

6. Schmidt PJ, Nieman L, Danaceau MA, et al. Estrogen replacement in perimenopause-related depression: a preliminary report. *Am J Obstet Gynecol* 2000; 183: 414–20

7. Nappi RE, Cagnacci A, Granella F, et al. Course of primary headaches during hormone replacement therapy. *Maturitas* 2001; 38: 157–63

8. Kraemer GR, Kraemer RR, Ogden BW, et al. Variability of serum estrogens among postmenopausal women treated with the same transdermal estrogen therapy and the effect on androgens and sex hormone binding globulin. *Fertil Steril* 2003; 79: 534–42

9. Cranney A, Guyatt G, Griffith L, et al. Meta-analyses of therapies for postmenopausal osteoporosis. IX. Summary of meta-analyses of therapies for postmenopausal osteoporosis. *Endocr Rev* 2000; 23: 570–8

10. Stevenson JC, Cust MP, Gangar KF, et al. Effects of transdermal versus oral hormone replacement therapy on bone density in spine and proximal femur in postmenopausal women. *Lancet* 1990; 336: 265–9

11. Lufkin EG, Wahner HW, O'Fallon WM, et al. Treatment of postmenopausal osteoporosis with transdermal estrogen. *Ann Intern Med* 1992; 117: 1–9

12. Michaelsson K, Baron JA, Farahmand BY, et al. Hormone replacement therapy and risk of hip fracture: population based case–control study. The Swedish Hip Fracture Study Group. *Br Med J* 1998; 316: 1858–63

13. Michaelsson K, Baron JA, Johnell O, et al. Variation in the efficacy of hormone replacement therapy in the prevention of hip fracture. Swedish Hip Fracture Study Group. *Osteoporos Int* 1998; 8: 540–6

14. Delmas PD, Pornel B, Felsenberg D, et al. A dose-ranging trial of a matrix transdermal 17beta-estradiol for the prevention of bone loss in

early postmenopausal women. International Study Group. *Bone* 1999; 24: 517–23

15. Cooper C, Stakkestad JA, Radowicki S, et al. Matrix delivery transdermal 17beta-estradiol for the prevention of bone loss in postmenopausal women. The International Study Group. *Osteoporos Int* 1999; 9: 358–66

16. Weiss SR, Ellman H, Dolker M. A randomized controlled trial of four doses of transdermal estradiol for preventing postmenopausal bone loss. Transdermal Estradiol Investigator Group. *Obstet Gynecol* 1999; 94: 330–6

17. Notelovitz M, John VA, Good WR. Effectiveness of Alora estradiol matrix transdermal delivery system in improving lumbar bone mineral density in healthy, postmenopausal women. *Menopause* 2002; 9: 343–53

18. Ettinger B, Ensrud KE, Wallace R. Effects of ultralow-dose transdermal estradiol on bone mineral density: a randomized clinical trial. *Obstet Gynecol* 2004; 104: 443–51

19. Thijssen JH. Overview on the effects of progestins on bone. *Maturitas* 2003; 46: S77–87

20. Isoniemi H, Appelberg J, Nilsson CG, et al. Transdermal oestrogen therapy protects postmenopausal liver transplant women from osteoporosis. A 2-year follow-up study. *J Hepatol* 2001; 34: 299–305

21. Rubinacci A, Peruzzi E, Modena AB, et al. Effect of low-dose transdermal E2/NETA on the reduction of postmenopausal bone loss in women. *Menopause* 2003; 10: 241–9

Progestogens and bone

31

D. W. Sturdee

INTRODUCTION

In considering the many factors which influence bone remodeling, it is inevitable that most discussions will concentrate on the influence of estrogen, and the recent developments in non-hormonal therapies such as bisphosphonates and strontium-containing products. However, the hormonal influence on bone is not limited to estrogens alone. Other steroids such as androgens and corticosteroids are important, as well as hormones such as growth hormone, thyroid hormones, parathyroid hormone, calcitonin and 1,25-dihydroxyvitamin D[1]. In addition, there is an increasing body of evidence that progesterone and progestogens can influence bone metabolism.

PROGESTERONE RECEPTORS AND BONE

The expression of both estrogen receptors (ERs) and progesterone receptors (PRs) in normal human osteoblast-like cells has been well documented[1–3], and several lines of evidence support a role for steroid hormones in regulating the expression and function of matrix proteins and metalloproteinases involved in bone remodeling and resorption[4].

Progesterone may also influence bone remodeling by acting as a ligand for the glucocorticoid receptor. Glucocorticoids have been implicated in the process of bone loss through their ability to block $1,25(OH)_2$-vitamin D-induced osteocalcin synthesis[5] and to prevent the attachment of osteoblasts to matrix proteins. Progesterone may antagonize these effects, resulting in a reduction of the glucocorticoid-induced bone loss[6].

There are two progesterone receptors, a and b, both of which are promoted by estradiol. PRb is a strong activator of target genes, but PRa acts as a dominant repressor of PRb. Therefore, the response of individual cells depends on the ratio of PRa/PRb. Estrogen receptor α is the predominant inducer of PRa[7,8].

CLINICAL EVIDENCE

The clinical evidence of the effect of progestogens on bone is found in fertile women taking contraception, premenopausal women receiving gonadotropin-releasing hormone (GnRH) therapy with additional progestogen or combinations of estrogen and progestogen, and postmenopausal women taking hormone therapy.

Progestogen-only contraception

Breast-feeding mothers experience a reversible reduction in bone mineral density (BMD) due to lowered estrogen levels associated with ovulation suppression. In a study of 31 women followed for 1 year postpartum, breast-feeding together with barrier methods of contraception resulted in a mean reduction in spinal BMD of $4.9 \pm 1.5\%$ by 6 months, whereas those who were breast-feeding and using oral progestogen-only contraception had a spinal BMD at 1 year that was $2.95 \pm 0.75\%$ higher than immediately postpartum[9]. This study concluded that the small amount of progestogen in the progesterone-only pill would appear to protect against the loss of bone resulting from breast-feeding.

Levonorgestrel subdermal implants (Norplant®) are used widely, and especially in China, for contraception. In a prospective randomized clinical trial involving 61 women of childbearing age studied over 1 year in China, a small but significant increase in lumbar spine (2.4%)

and proximal femur (3.34%) BMD ($p < 0.01$) was reported[10]. Similar findings were reported by Naessen and colleagues[11] in a study comparing the differential effects of depot medroxyprogesterone acetate (DMPA) and subdermal levonorgestrel implants over 6 months. While there was a significant increase in forearm BMD of 2.94% ($p = 0.006$) in women who were prescribed levonorgestrel, there was no effect on bone density during treatment with DMPA at standard clinical doses for contraception. Other recent studies with DMPA have raised concern about bone loss due to the suppression of ovulation. A 2-year study of 38 premenopausal women using DMPA, and randomized to receive in addition either conjugated equine estrogens (CEE) 0.625 mg daily or a matching placebo, showed a significant decline in lumbar spine BMD in the placebo group, but no change in those receiving CEE[12] (Figure 1). A further study of adolescent females using DMPA compared with combined oral contraception and a control group has also reported a significant loss of bone, compared with controls, which was not seen in those on combined oral contraceptive pills[13] (Table 1) . Such data have prompted the Committee on Safety of Medicines (CSM) in the UK to send advice to prescribers that the prolonged use of DMPA in adolescents may impair the attainment of peak bone mass. Although BMD starts to recover when DMPA is stopped in adult women, and at the menopause the bone density of users may be no different from that of women who have never used DMPA[14,15], the extent of recovery in adolescents is not known. In women with significant life-style and/or medical risk factors for osteoporosis, the CSM has advised that other methods of contraception should be considered[16]. When DMPA was used together with GnRH therapy for women with symptomatic fibroids prior to surgery, DMPA had no effect on the bone loss associated with GnRH[17]. However, when norethisterone is used in conjunction with GnRH, the bone loss is prevented[18] (Figure 2).

Postmenopausal hormone therapy

In symptomatic postmenopausal women, progestogens such as norethisterone[19] and megestrol[20] have been shown to give some relief from vasomotor symptoms. In addition, several studies have also demonstrated that norethisterone will prevent bone loss in postmenopausal women. A study of 43 symptomatic postmenopausal women in Glasgow, of whom 20 received norethisterone 5 mg twice daily for 2

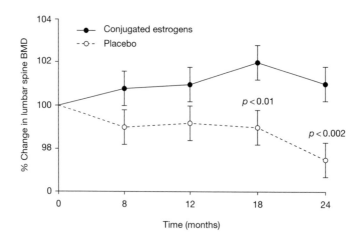

Figure 1 Lumbar spine bone mineral density (BMD) in 38 premenopausal women using depot medroxyprogesterone acetate (MPA) and randomized also to receive either conjugated equine estrogens 0.625 mg daily or matching placebo. Difference between the groups was 3.2% at 18 months and 3.5% at 24 months. Reproduced from reference 12, with permission

Table 1 Lumbar vertebral bone mineral density in adolescent females using depot medroxyprogesterone acetate (DMPA) or combined oral contraception (COC) compared with controls[13]

	6 months		12 months		18 months	
	n	*Change (%)*	*n*	*Change (%)*	*n*	*Change (%)*
DMPA	36	−0.249[*]	27	−1.59[**]	24	−2.91[***]
COC	27	1.170	16	2.35	11	3.82
Control	14	2.768	10	2.45	5	0.73

*$p < 0.014$; **$p = 0.001$; ***$p < 0.001$

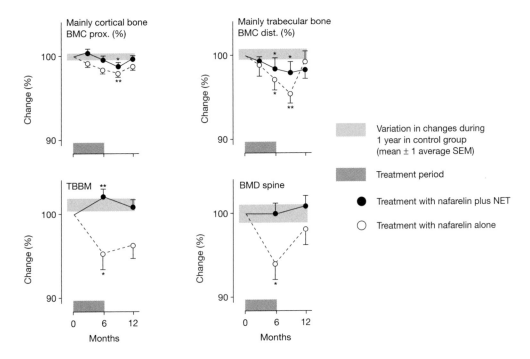

Figure 2 Changes in bone mass during treatment and after withdrawal of treatment with nafarelin plus norethisterone (NET) 1.2 mg daily and nafarelin alone. BMC, bone mineral content; TBBM, total body bone mineral; BMD, bone mineral density. *$p < 0.05$; **$p < 0.01$ (vs. baseline). Reproduced from reference 18, with permission

years and the others had placebo, showed a marked difference in the metacarpal bone mineral content ($p < 0.001$)[21] (Figure 3). Horowitz and colleagues[22] also demonstrated that norethisterone 5 mg per day in women with postmenopausal osteoporosis prevents further bone loss by decreasing bone turnover, increasing serum parathyroid hormone and having an independent effect on vitamin D and calcium absorption. However, progestogens are not commonly given alone to postmenopausal women, but are included in combination therapy predominantly for protection of the endometrium. Combinations of norethisterone with ethinylestradiol have produced a dose-related significant increase in BMD that was not present with

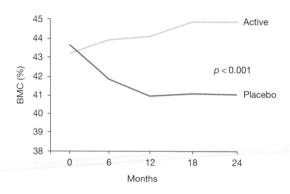

Figure 3 Metacarpal bone mineral content (BMC) in women receiving norethisterone 5 mg twice daily compared with placebo over 2 years. Reproduced from reference 21, with permission

unopposed ethinylestradiol[23]. A similar effect has been demonstrated when norethisterone is combined with estradiol, showing a positive effect on postmenopausal bone metabolism and an increase in bone mass more than expected and more than with treatment with alendronate[24] (Figure 4). Conversely, the addition of oral medroxyprogesterone acetate or oral micronized progesterone to CEE does not appear to give any additional benefit to the bone-sparing effects of CEE alone[25]. Other progestogens, such as dydrogesterone[26], that have been studied either alone or in combination with estrogen have not shown any obvious additive effect on bone loss. The new progestogen trimegestone, when given alone or in combination with 17β-estradiol, also does not inhibit the effect of estrogen in maintaining bone mass, while at the same time completely blocking its proliferative effect on the endometrium[27].

Progesterone cream has been advocated as a natural replacement for postmenopausal women who are lacking progesterone, but the claims for an effect on osteoporosis[28] have not been substantiated. Several studies have failed to demonstrate any clinically significant increase in serum progesterone following the application of progesterone cream, and, in a 12-week study of women using transdermal progesterone cream 32 mg daily, there were no detectable changes in clinical symptoms or bone mineral activity markers[29–31].

Thus, in postmenopausal women, the combination of norethisterone with estrogen does seem to have an additive effect on preventing bone loss, whereas such an effect has not been demonstrated with any other progestogen. Norethisterone is one of the few progestogens to demonstrate some estrogenic activity, with bioconversion to estrogenic compounds that activate both ERα and ERβ[32,33] in addition to other progesterone-like activities. This may be the main reason why it has a different effect on bone metabolism compared with the other progestogens.

In a review on the apparent lack of effect of progestogens on bone, Lindsay[34] stated that 'evidence so far suggests that when used alone at normally prescribed dosages, progestogens have neither direct effect on osteoporosis nor an additive effect when used as a component of HRT. Positive effects of HRT on bone seen in postmenopausal women are more likely a direct result of the estrogen component'. Furthermore, although progesterone receptors are evident in bone tissue and on osteoblasts in particular, it is not clear whether the currently available progestogens are able to bind specifically to the PR isoforms PRa and PRb[35]. None of the data presented above have demonstrated any effects on bone remodeling from a progestogenic action mediated through PR.

CONCLUSIONS

Progestogens may have more relevance to bone metabolism in premenopausal than in postmenopausal women. DMPA is associated with loss of bone, especially in adolescent girls, due to suppression of ovarian function. In addition, the bone loss associated with breast-feeding may be prevented by progestogen-only oral contraceptive preparations. In the postmenopausal woman, micronized progesterone, medroxyprogesterone acetate, megestrol, dydrogesterone and trimegestone do not prevent postmenopausal bone loss. Norethisterone acetate, however, may have an independent positive effect as well as additional benefits when combined with estrogen in postmenopausal women, although this may be due more to some estrogenic activity rather than a pure progestogenic action.

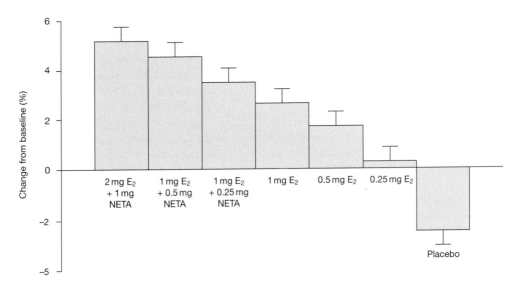

Figure 4 Effects of oral estradiol ± norethisterone acetate (E$_2$ ± NETA) at different doses on spinal bone mineral density after 26 months. Reproduced from reference 24, with permission

References

1. Thijssen JHH, Druckmann R. Effects of progestins on bone: an update. *Gynecol Endocrinol* 1999; 13 (Suppl 4): 25–39

2. Wei LL, Leech MW, Miner RS, Demers LM. Evidence for progesterone receptors in human osteoblast-like cells. *Biochem Biophys Res Commun* 1993; 195: 525–32

3. Eriksen EF, Colvard DS, Berg NJ, et al. Evidence of estrogen receptors in normal human osteoblast-like cells. *Science* 1998; 241: 84–6

4. Graham JD, Clarke CL. Physiological action of progesterone in target tissues. *Endocr Rev* 1997; 18: 502–19

5. Beresford JN, Gallagher JA, Poser JW, Russell RGG. Production of osteocalcin by human bone cells in vitro. Effects of 1,25(OH)$_2$D$_3$, parathyroid hormone, and glucocorticoids. *Metab Bone Dis Relat Res* 1984; 5: 229–34

6. Prior JC. Progesterone as a bone-trophic hormone. *Endocr Rev* 1990; 11: 386–98

7. Rickard DJ, Waters KM, Ruesink TJ, et al. Estrogen receptor isoform-specific indication of progesterone receptors in human osteoblasts. *J Bone Miner Res* 2002; 17: 580–92

8. MacNamara P, Loughrey HC. Progesterone receptor a and b isoform expression in human osteoblasts. *Calcif Tissue Int* 1998; 63: 39–46

9. Caird L, Reid-Thomas V, Hannan W, et al. Oral progestogen-only contraception may protect against loss of bone mass in breast-feeding women. *Clin Endocrinol* 1994; 41: 739–45

10. Di X, Li Y, Zhang C, et al. Effects of levonorgestrel-releasing subdermal contraceptive implants on bone density and bone metabolism. *Contraception* 1999; 60: 161–6

11. Naessen T, Olsson SE, Gudmundson J. Differential effects on bone density of progestogen-only methods for contraception in pre-menopausal women. *Contraception* 1995; 52: 35–9

12. Cundy T, Ames R, Horne A, et al. A randomised controlled trial of estrogen replacement in long-term users of depot medroxyprogesterone acetate. *J Clin Endocrinol Metab* 2003; 88: 78–81

13. Lara-Torre E, Edwards CP, Perlman S, Hertweck SB. Bone mineral density in adolescent females using depot medroxyprogesterone acetate. *J Pediatr Adolesc Gynecol* 2004; 17: 17–21

14. Cundy T, Cornish J, Evans MC, et al. Recovery of bone density in women who stop using medroxyprogesterone acetate. *Br Med J* 1994; 308: 247–8

15. Cundy T, Cornish J, Roberts H, Reid IR. Menopausal bone loss in long-term users of depot medroxyprogesterone acetate contraception. *Am J Obstet Gynecol* 2002; 186: 978–83

16. Medicines and Healthcare products Regulatory Agency/Committee on Safety of Medicines. http://www.mca.gov.uk/csmhome, 2004

17. Caird LE, West CP, Lumsden MA, et al. Medroxyprogesterone acetate with Zoladex™ for long-term treatment of fibroids: effects on bone density and patient acceptability. *Hum Reprod* 1997; 12: 436–40

18. Riis BJ, Christiansen C, Johansen JS, Jacobson J. Is it possible to prevent bone loss in young women treated with luteinising hormone-releasing hormone agonists? *J Clin Endocrinol Metab* 1990; 70: 920–4

19. Paterson MEL. A randomised double-blind crossover trial into the effect of norethisterone on climacteric symptoms and biochemical profiles. *Br J Obstet Gynaecol* 1982; 89: 464–72

20. Farish E, Barnes JF, O'Donoghue F, et al. The role of megestrol acetate as an alternative to conventional hormone replacement therapy. *Climacteric* 2000; 3: 125–34

21. Abdalla HI, Hart DM, Lindsay R, et al. Prevention of bone mineral loss in postmenopausal women by norethisterone. *Obstet Gynecol* 1985; 66: 789–92

22. Horowitz M, Wishart JM, Need AG, et al. Effects of norethisterone on bone-related biochemical variables and forearm bone mineral in post-menopausal osteoporosis. *Clin Endocrinol* 1993; 39: 649–55

23. Speroff L, Rowan J, Symons J, et al. The comparative effect on bone density, endometrium, and lipids of continuous hormones as replacement therapy (CHART Study). A randomised controlled trial. *J Am Med Assoc* 1996; 276: 1397–403

24. Riis BJ, Lehmann HJ, Christiansen C. Norethisterone acetate in combination with estrogen: effects on the skeleton and other organs. A review. *Am J Obstet Gynecol* 2002; 187: 1101–16

25. The Writing Group for the PEPI Study. Effects of hormone therapy on bone mineral density: results from the Postmenopausal Estrogen/Progestin Interventions (PEPI) Trial. *J Am Med Assoc* 1996; 276: 1389–96

26. de Valk-de Roo GW, Netelenbos JC, Peters-Muller IR, et al. Continuously combined hormone replacement therapy and bone turnover: the influence of dydrogesterone dose, smoking and initial degree of bone turnover. *Maturitas* 1997; 28: 153–62

27. Lepescheux L, Secchi J, Gaillard-Kelly M, Miller P. Effects of 17β-estradiol and trimegestone alone, and in combination, on the bone and uterus of oophorectomised rats. *Gynecol Endocrinol* 2001; 15: 312–20

28. Lee JR. Osteoporosis reversal: the role of progesterone. *Int Clin Nutr Rev* 1990; 10: 384–9

29. Wren BG, Champion S, Manga R, Eden JA. Transdermal progesterone and its effect on vasomotor symptoms, blood lipid levels, bone metabolic markers, moods, and quality of life for postmenopausal women. *Menopause* 2003; 10: 13–18

30. Wren BG. Progesterone creams: do they work? *Climacteric* 2003; 6: 184–7

31. Leonetti H, Longa S, Anasti J. Transdermal progesterone cream for vasomotor symptoms and postmenopausal bone loss. *Obstet Gynecol* 1999; 94: 225–8

32. Pasapera AM, Gutierrez-Sagal R, Herrera J, et al. Norethisterone is bioconverted to oestrogenic compounds that activate both the oestrogen receptor alpha and oestrogen receptor beta in vitro. *Eur J Pharmacol* 2002; 452: 347–55

33. Schindler AE. Role of progestins in the premenopausal climacteric. *Gynecol Endocrinol* 1999; 13 (Suppl 6): 35–40

34. Lindsay R. The lack of effect of progestogen on bone. *J Reprod Med* 1999; 44: 215–20

35. Sitruk-Ware R. New progestogens; a review of their effects in peri-menopausal and postmenopausal women. *Drugs Ageing* 2004; 21: 865–83

Effect of different dose options of continuous combined hormone therapy on bone and bone marker N-terminal propeptide of type I procollagen: results from a long-term study in Finnish postmenopausal women

J. Heikkinen and J. Haapalahti

32

INTRODUCTION

Estrogen–progestogen therapy has long been the treatment of choice for the prevention of osteoporosis, and the Women's Health Initiative study results confirmed its efficacy in preventing fractures in a randomized setting[1]. However, the results of the same study raised concern about the safety of long-term hormone replacement therapies in postmenopausal women, and turned the focus toward shorter-term therapies[2].

In 2000, we published the 4-year bone mineral density (BMD) results from an ongoing clinical trial involving 419 women randomized to four different estradiol valerate (E_2V) and medroxyprogesterone acetate (MPA) dose options in six treatment regimens, as in two treatment groups the E_2V component was doubled after the initial 6 months while, in the remaining four groups, the dose combinations remained the same throughout the study[3]. The four dose combinations were: 1 mg E_2V + 2.5 mg MPA (1 + 2.5); 1 mg E_2V + 5 mg MPA (1 + 5); 2 mg E_2V + 2.5 mg MPA (2 + 2.5) and 2 mg E_2V + 5 mg MPA (2 + 5).

After 7 treatment years, the long-term safety results were reported[4]. When all women had completed the 8th year, the focus was turned toward the lowest dose regimen for the rest of the period, with switching all women still in the study ($n = 232$) to this dose option for the last 6 months of the total active study period of 9 years. The main interest was to see whether lowering the dose before stopping hormone replacement therapy (HRT) would have any effects on the parameters studied, e.g. bone. This phase was completed in early 2004. There will still be one follow-up visit, with BMD and other measurements, approximately 1 year after discontinuation of study treatments.

The aim of bone marker determinations was to elucidate whether a single baseline measurement of serum intact N-terminal propeptide of type I procollagen (PINP) can reliably predict short-term skeletal treatment response 12 months after treatment start, using lumbar spine BMD as reference.

DESIGN AND METHODS

The study, starting in 1994 as a parallel-group, double-blind, dose-finding trial with 419 women randomized to six HRT regimens, containing 1 or 2 mg of E_2V combined with 2.5 or 5 mg of MPA (Indivina®; Orion Pharma, Finland), was continued after the 2-year double-blind period, first as a single-blind and later as an open study, in order to gather more efficacy – especially regarding bone – and safety information.

Three of the dose options were registered for marketing in 1999. The unregistered dose combination of 2 mg E_2V with 2.5 mg MPA was no longer manufactured, and therefore women receiving this dose option had to discontinue the study after the completion of 7 years. Results for this dose option are not reported here.

Bone mineral density measurements

BMD was measured at the lumbar spine (L2–L4) and the hip (femoral neck, Ward's triangle, trochanter) by dual-energy X-ray absorptiometry at baseline, 6 months, 12 months and annually thereafter. The final measurement will be made when the women have been without study treatment for approximately 1 year.

Bone marker (PINP) determinations

For PINP determination, serum samples from a subgroup of 44 women on the lowest dose option of $1 + 2.5$ were taken at baseline and at 12 months. Further PINP determinations were performed at the end of the active study period (9 years). The last PINP determination will be made 1 year after treatment stop. PINP is measured using commercially available reagents (Orion Diagnostica UniQ® PINP radioimmunoassay).

In order to assess the power of the initial PINP level to predict treatment response at the 12-month time-point on bone metabolism, the baseline PINP results from 44 patients were divided into quartiles and, after combining quartile 1 with 2 and 3 with 4, two groups were formed: group A (low bone turnover) with baseline PINP $< 40\,\mu g/l$ ($n = 22$), and group B (high bone turnover) with basal PINP $> 40\,\mu g/l$ ($n = 22$).

RESULTS

The main baseline characteristics of the study population at baseline are given in Table 1.

Bone mineral density

After 4 years of treatment, with 296 women completing this period, the mean increases from baseline in femoral and lumbar BMD were similar in the 1-mg and 2-mg E_2V groups, but at all sites the increase was most pronounced in the groups where the estrogen dose had been doubled 6 months after treatment start. The increases were more pronounced in women with

Table 1 Baseline characteristics of women in study

	Group			
	1–2 + 5 (n = 70)	*2 + 5* (n = 70)	*1 + 2.5* (n = 69)	*1 + 5* (n = 70)
Age (years, mean ± SD)	56.2 ± 1.8	56.1 ± 2.0	56.0 ± 2.0	56.3 ± 2.1
Age at menopause (years, mean ± SD)	48.9 ± 2.6	49.0 ± 3.2	49.4 ± 2.2	48.8 ± 3.0
Body mass index (BMI) (kg/m^2, mean ± SD)	25.6 ± 3.16	25.4 ± 2.9	25.2 ± 2.8	25.4 ± 2.8
Previous HRT (n (%))	38 (54.3%)	32 (45.7%)	38 (55.1%)	36 (51.4%)
Smokers (%)	12.9	7.1	14.5	14.3
Women (%) with	lumbar spine (L2–L4)		femoral neck	
normal BMD	43		57	
osteopenia	45		40	
osteoporosis	12		3	

SD, standard deviation; HRT, hormone replacement therapy; BMD, bone mineral density low bone mass at baseline. The MPA dose did not seem to have any effect on bone (Figures 1 and 2).

In all groups, BMD increased more rapidly during the first 3–4 years, with mean annual increases of 1–2%. Then the increases began to level out, but still a slightly increasing trend could be seen at the lumbar spine (Figure 3).

At the femoral neck, BMD values started to decrease slightly around 72–84 months from the peak increases of 3.5–4% (Figure 4).

At the end of the active study period, the mean increases from baseline at the lumbar spine ranged between 8% (group 1 + 5) and 10% (2 + 5), and at the femoral neck between 1% (1 + 5) and 2% (2 + 5) (Figure 5). Based on preliminary analyses, no effect of the dose reduction for the last 6 months could yet be established.

Using the cut-off point of ± 2%, over 85% of women who completed the 9-year period had gained BMD of more than 2% during the study, and in approximately 5% no relevant change in BMD was observed. In less than 5% of women, a decrease of more than 2% could be seen at the end of the study. By the end of the active 9-year study period, the proportion of women with low bone mass (osteopenia or osteoporosis) had decreased, compared with baseline (Table 1), with the majority of women now having normal BMD values (Figure 6).

Bone marker PINP

By the 6th treatment month, the PINP values determined from 44 women receiving the lowest dose option showed a significant decrease from

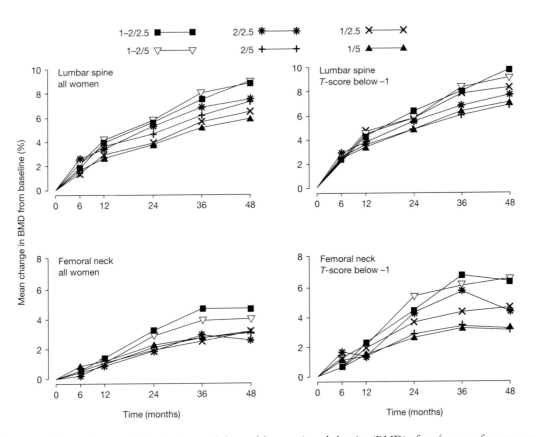

Figure 1 Mean changes (%) in lumbar and femoral bone mineral density (BMD) after 4 years of treatment. All women and women with low bone mass at baseline (BMD *T*-score below -1). Figure reproduced with permission from *Osteoporosis International*[3]

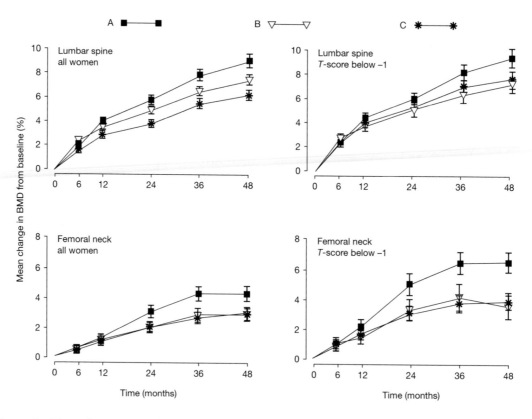

Figure 2 Mean changes (%) in lumbar and femoral bone mineral density (BMD) after 4 years of treatment. All women and women with low bone mass at baseline (BMD *T*-score below -1). Groups pooled according to the estrogen dose regimen. Group A, 1–2 mg E_2V (dose increased from 1 mg to 2 mg after 6 months); Group B, 2 mg E_2V; Group C, 1 mg E_2V. MPA dose in all groups either 2.5 mg or 5 mg. Figure reproduced with permission from *Osteoporosis International*[3]

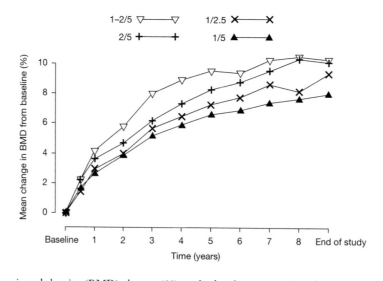

Figure 3 Bone mineral density (BMD) change (%) at the lumbar spine (L2–L4) from baseline until 9 years

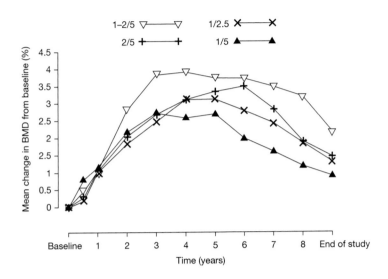

Figure 4 Bone mineral density (BMD) change (%) at the femoral neck from baseline to 9 years

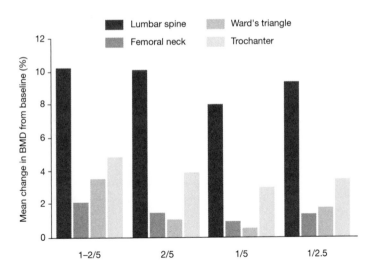

Figure 5 Increases in bone mineral density (BMD) (%) after 9 treatment years in lumbar spine, femoral neck, Ward's triangle and trochanter

baseline values, and the changes remained significant at the 12-month and end-of-study measuring points (Figure 7).

In group A (low turnover), no statistically significant responses to treatment at 12 months (PINP, $p = 0.626$; lumbar spine BMD, $p = 0.117$) were found. PINP changed $+ 4.7\%$, from 29.7 to 31.1 µg/l (Figure 8) and lumbar BMD changed $+ 0.7\%$, from 1.171 to 1.180 g/cm^2 (Figure 9).

In women with high turnover (group B), statistically highly significant responses to treatment at 12 months were found (PINP, $p < 0.0001$; lumbar spine BMD, $p < 0.0001$).

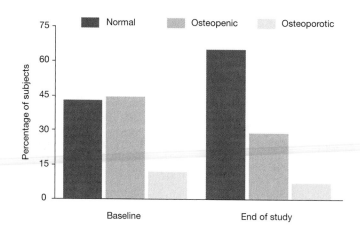

Figure 6 Proportion of women with normal bone mineral density (BMD), osteopenia or osteoporosis at baseline and at 9 years

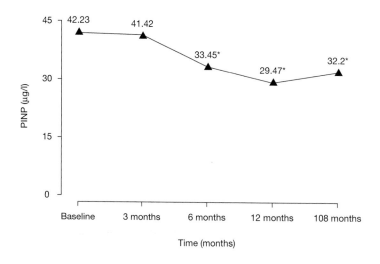

Figure 7 Serum N-terminal propeptide of type I procollagen (PINP) levels for subgroup receiving 1 + 2.5 regimen ($n = 44$) at baseline, 3 months, 6 months, 12 months and 9 years. $^*p < 0.001$

PINP changed –49.1%, from 54.8 to 27.9 µg/l (Figure 8), and lumbar spine BMD increased 5.1%, from 0.996 to 1.047 g/cm² (Figure 9).

When an increase of 2% in lumbar spine BMD was considered a reliable sign of response, 18 of 22 in group A and only four of 22 in group B exceeded this limit, leading to 81.8% sensitivity and 81.8% specificity at the cut-off of 40 µg/l of baseline PINP.

Occurrence of fractures and overall safety

The occurrence of fractures was very low in this study: five foot or leg fractures, four radial and two vertebral fractures. No hip fractures occurred. All fractures occurred following an accident, such as falling on an icy street, or car accident. None of the women with fractures had osteopenic or osteoporotic BMD.

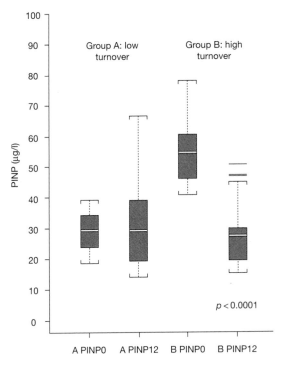

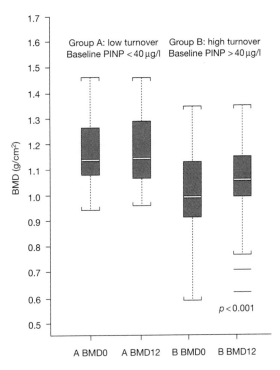

Figure 8 Serum N-terminal propeptide of type I procollagen (PINP) at baseline and after 12 months of treatment. Subgroups divided into women with low (A) or high (B) bone turnover

Figure 9 Lumbar bone mineral density (BMD) at baseline and at 12 months in N-terminal propeptide of type I procollagen (PINP) subgroups A and B

Overall, all treatments had a favorable safety profile with a low frequency of adverse drug reactions or serious clinical outcomes, as reported in the published article on 7-year results of this study[4].

CONCLUSIONS

Our results suggest that starting postmenopausal hormone therapy with a lower estrogen dose and then increasing the dose after a few months can be beneficial, especially for women with low BMD. However, for most women, 1 mg E_2V dose level seems to be adequately effective in the long-term prevention of postmenopausal bone loss.

The baseline level of serum PINP is able to predict skeletal response to low-dose HRT at least at the 12-month time-point. The appropriate cut-off level for baseline PINP was found to be 40 µg/l in postmenopausal women. Only those who are classified as 'high bone turnover' individuals show statistically significant BMD increment and PINP decrease at the 12-month time-point.

Based on these results, low-dose HRT can still be regarded as a feasible option for the long-term prevention of postmenopausal bone loss.

The final results of this study from the 10-year measuring point, 1 year after discontinuing HRT, will most probably shed more light on how bone reacts to the stopping of long-term hormone therapy and decreasing the estrogen dose before ending therapy.

References

1. Writing Group for the Women's Health Initiative Investigators. Risks and benefits of estrogen plus progestin in healthy postmenopausal women. Principal results from the Women's Health Initiative randomized controlled trial. *J Am Med Assoc* 2002; 228: 321–33

2. North American Menopause Society. Estrogen and progestogen use in peri- and postmenopausal women: September 2003 position statement of the North American Menopause Society. *Menopause* 2003; 10: 497–506

3. Heikkinen J, Vaheri R, Kainulainen P, et al. Long-term continuous combined hormone replacement therapy in the prevention of postmenopausal bone loss: a comparison of high- and low-dose estrogen–progestin regimens. *Osteoporos Int* 2000; 11: 929–37

4. Heikkinen J, Vaheri R, Timonen U. Long-term safety and tolerability of continuous-combined hormone therapy in postmenopausal women: results from a seven-year randomized comparison of low and standard doses. *J Br Menopause Soc* 2004; 10: 95–102

The use of alendronate in osteoporosis treatment: 10-year experience

33

M. L. Brandi

Bisphosphonates (BPs) are pyrophosphate analogs in which the oxygen bridge has been replaced by a carbon with various side-chains (P–C–P). These compounds have been known to chemists since the 19th century, the first synthesis dating back to 1865[1]. They were first used in various industrial procedures, among other things as anticorrosive and antiscaling agents[2]. After discovering that they can effectively control calcium phosphate formation and dissolution *in vitro*, as well as mineralization and bone resorption *in vivo*[3,4], they were developed and used in the treatment of metabolic bone diseases, mostly Paget's disease, hypercalcemia of malignancy and, lately but not least, primary and secondary osteoporosis[5].

The bisphosphonate group, like pyrophosphate, binds strongly to hydroxyapatite[6]. BPs deposit where bone mineral is exposed to the surrounding fluids, thus, especially where bone is formed and resorbed. The release of bisphosphonates occurs primarily when the bone where they are deposited is resorbed again, accounting for their long *in vivo* half-life in humans[7]. The P–C–P group is resistant to enzymatic hydrolysis, which explains why bisphosphonates are not metabolized in the body and are excreted unaltered. Bisphosphonates released during bone remodeling might therefore be pharmacologically active. The amount of bisphosphonate released daily in this manner after 10 years of treatment is estimated at ~ 25% of the amount absorbed from a daily dose, and depends upon the location in the skeleton. It will be higher for cancellous, lower for compact bone. The charge and bulk of the bisphosphonate group limits penetration of cell membranes. This may account for the low absorption in the gut (between below

1 and 10%), which is probably paracellular[8], and the limited cellular uptake. Bisphosphonates are rapidly excreted by the kidney, in part by an active tubular secretion process[9].

The key pharmacological action of bisphosphonates in clinical use is inhibition of bone resorption. The mechanism of action of BPs has not been fully elucidated, and could differ among BPs. Since this is not the subject of this chapter, it is suggested that the reader refers to a very recent review[10].

Sodium alendronate has been the first agent to be developed according to US and European regulatory guidelines for marketing authorization of new agents for osteoporosis treatment. Alendronate efficacy has been demonstrated in terms of hard end-points, i.e. the reduction of both new incident vertebral fractures and non-vertebral fractures in patients with established osteoporosis. In 1995, Liberman and colleagues reported that alendronate increases bone mineral density at the spine and hip as well as the whole body, and reduces the risk of radiographically defined vertebral fractures in women with low bone mineral density (BMD)[11].

The Fracture Intervention Trial (FIT) is unanimously considered a milestone in the history of osteoporosis pharmacology; for the first time, a randomized placebo-controlled trial was specifically designed for evaluating the efficacy of an active drug, sodium alendronate, in reducing the incidence of vertebral and non-vertebral fractures in postmenopausal women with low bone mass, with ($n = 2027$, vertebral deformity arm[12]) or without ($n = 4432$, clinical fracture study[13]) prevalent vertebral fractures at baseline.

In the first arm, 3-year alendronate treatment of established osteoporosis reduced the risk of

289

new morphometric vertebral fractures by 47% and of clinical vertebral fractures by 55%. Wrist fractures and hip fractures were also reduced by alendronate treatment by 48% and 51%, respectively.

In the clinical fracture arm, 4.25 years of alendronate treatment reduced the risk of clinical fractures by 36% and of newly diagnosed vertebral deformities by 50% in those women who had a BMD T-score below -2.5, according to the third National Health and Nutrition Examination Survey reference database.

A cumulative FIT database analysis evaluated the efficacy of alendronate in osteoporosis patients (existing vertebral fracture at baseline or femoral neck T-score of 2.5 or less)[13]. Table 1 summarizes the key results.

Very recently, FIT 10-year follow-up study (FLEX, FIT long-term extension) data were publicly disclosed. FLEX is a randomized, double-blind, placebo-controlled study aimed at assessing the efficacy of continuing treatment with alendronate (ALN) 5 or 10 mg/day (combined) for an additional 5 years, versus discontinuing therapy (i.e. placebo) in osteoporotic women previously treated with alendronate for ∼5 years. The primary objective was change in total hip BMD. Secondary end-points were changes of femoral neck, trochanter, spine and total body BMD, and safety and tolerability data. As additional objectives, the study looked at the different effects of ALN 5 and 10 mg/day on total hip, femoral neck, trochanter, spine and total body BMD, and resolution of the effect of prior

alendronate treatment on bone markers. The incidence of clinical or morphometric vertebral fractures compared with placebo was also assessed as an exploratory objective.

The study enrolled 1099 postmenopausal women previously enrolled in FIT and randomized to alendronate. Prior treatment with alendronate was for 3 to ∼6 years (average 5 years). All patients had been treated for 3–4.25 years during FIT and for 1–2 years of open-label alendronate 10 mg/day after the end of FIT. Total hip BMD T-score was above -3.5, and current total hip BMD > total hip BMD at FIT baseline. Patients were randomized to three arms: 437 patients were treated with placebo for 5 years; 329 and 333 patients received alendronate either 5 mg/day or 10 mg/day, respectively; and 995 patients completed the 5-year study and 759 women (69%) completed study therapy. The baseline characteristics of the study population are summarized in Table 2.

Both alendronate 5 mg and 10 mg/day dosages were effective in maintaining total hip, femoral neck and femoral trochanter BMD, which was decreased in the placebo group ($p < 0.001$ for comparison between placebo group and pooled alendronate groups at each skeletal site). However, BMD levels were still higher in the placebo group than at FIT baseline; the latter observation allows exclusion of any 'catch-up' phenomenon loss at the hip.

Lumbar spine BMD was largely increased in both ALN groups (+5.0% and +5.6% in 5-mg and 10-mg/day groups) versus a slight increase

Table 1 Key results of alendronate efficacy in osteoporosis

Fracture class	RR (95% CI)	p Value
Radiologic vertebral	0.52 (0.42–0.66)	0.001
Multiple vertebral (radiologic)	0.13 (0.07–0.25)	0.001
Clinical vertebral	0.55 (0.36–0.82)	0.003
Any clinical	0.70 (0.59–0.82)	0.001
Non-vertebral	0.73 (0.61–0.87)	0.001
Non-vertebral (osteoporotic)	0.64 (0.51–0.80)	0.002
Hip	0.47 (0.26–0.79)	0.005
Wrist	0.70 (0.49–0.98)	0.038

RR, relative risk; CI, confidence interval

Table 2 Baseline characteristics of study population in Fracture Intervention Trial (FIT) long-term extension (FLEX)

	ALN→PBO	ALN→ALN 5 mg	ALN→ALN 10 mg
Age (years)	74	73	73
Spine BMD (g/cm^2)	0.90	0.90	0.89
T-score	−1.6	−1.6	−1.7
Total hip BMD (g/cm^2)	0.72	0.73	0.73
T-score	−1.8	−1.7	−1.7
NTx (pmol/μmol creatinine)	23.5	22.4	22.3
BSAP (ng/ml)	9.7	9.3	9.5
Prevalent vertebral fractures (%)	32.2	29.5	31.5
Prevalent vertebral fractures or hip BMD T-score < −2.5 (%)	54.2	51.2	53.6

BMD, bone mineral density; NTx, cross-linked N-telopeptides of type I collagen; BSAP, bone-specific alkaline phosphatase; ALN, alendronate; PBO, placebo

Table 3 Bone mineral density changes (%) in three study groups

Site	ALN→PBO	ALN→ALN 5 mg	ALN→ALN 10 mg
Total hip	−3.4***	−1.3***	−0.7**
Femoral neck	−1.5**	0.1	0.9*
Trochanter	−3.3***	−0.2	0.1
Lumbar spine	1.5***	5.0***	5.6***
Total body	−0.3	0.6*	1.5***
Total forearm	−3.2***	−0.9**	−1.5***

*$p \leq 0.05$ vs. baseline; **$p \leq 0.01$ vs. baseline; ***$p \leq 0.001$ vs. baseline; ALN, alendronate; PBO, placebo

which was still observed in the placebo group (+1.5%, $p < 0.001$ for comparison between placebo group and pooled treated groups).

Table 3 shows BMD changes at different measurement sites in the three groups.

According to BMD figures, bone turnover markers (urinary cross-linked N-telopeptides of type I collagen (NTx) and serum bone alkaline phosphatase) were stable in the actively treated group, but they were statistically significantly increased (∼30%) in the placebo group. As mentioned before, a pre-specified exploratory analysis was conducted in order to assess the incidence of clinical vertebral fractures in study subjects. The risk of clinical vertebral fractures was 54% lower in the alendronate than in the placebo group ($p = 0.01$): 23 women experienced clinical vertebral fractures (5.4%) in the placebo group, compared with 16 women (2.5%) in the pooled alendronate groups.

Overall safety was similar across groups. Bone safety was also assessed by two-dimensional (2-D) and 3-D evaluation of bone biopsy: no qualitative abnormalities were observed at both histologic and mineralization levels.

The FLEX data disclosure follows the recent publication[14] of the 10-year follow-up data of the alendronate phase III trial[11]. Initially, 994

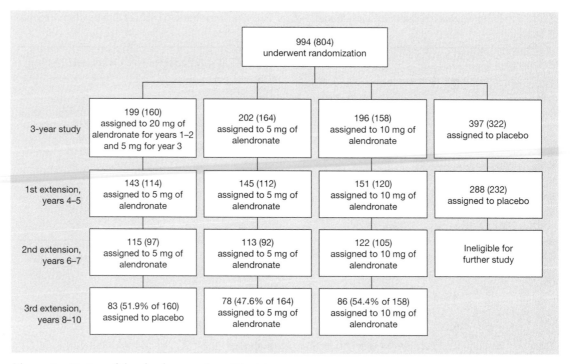

Figure 1 Design of the alendronate phase III trial

women had been randomly assigned to receive 5, 10 or 20 mg of oral alendronate or placebo daily (Figure 1). Women in the placebo group were given open-label alendronate for years 4 and 5 and then discharged from the study. The original 5-mg and 10-mg alendronate groups continued to receive the same doses in all three extensions of the study (years 4 and 5, 6 and 7 and 8–10). Those in the original 20-mg group received 5 mg for years 3–5 and placebo for years 6–10 (the discontinuation group). Their cumulative exposure to alendronate was similar to exposure in the 10-mg group after 5 years, and to that in the 5-mg group after 10 years. Both the investigators and the women were aware that all long-term participants had received alendronate for at least 5 years and that the discontinuation group had been switched to placebo, but all remained unaware of each woman's current treatment.

The primary end-point was lumbar spine BMD change. Secondary end-points were changes in BMD at the hip (femoral neck, trochanter, total proximal femur), total body and forearm regions, and changes in the levels of

urinary NTx and serum bone-specific and total alkaline phosphatase (ALP).

Lumbar spine BMD continued to increase during years 6–10 and 8–10 in both alendronate groups (Figure 2). The mean change after 10 years of the 10-mg daily dose was $+13.7\%$, compared with baseline; smaller changes were observed in the 5-mg group. During years 6–10, the alendronate groups had no significant decline in BMD. In the discontinuation group, spine BMD did not change significantly after year 5; significant decreases occurred at the total hip, femoral neck and forearm, but bone mineral density at the lumbar spine, trochanter, total hip and total body remained significantly above basal values at year 10. Almost 90% of women who took the 10-mg dose daily had an increase in total hip BMD.

The fast reduction of bone turnover back to the premenopausal range which had been observed after initial 3–6-month treatment was sustained through 10 years of treatment. NTx values declined by almost 66% at the end of year 10 (Figure 3). During years 8–10, urinary NTx

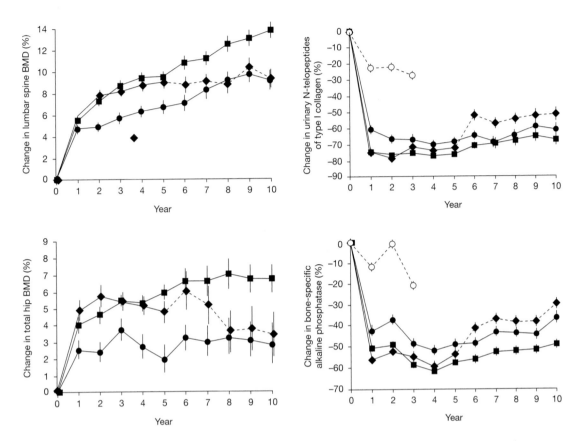

Figure 2 Changes in lumbar spine and total hip bone mineral density (BMD) in the 10-mg alendronate group (square symbols), 5-mg alendronate group (circle symbols) and discontinuation group (diamond symbols)

Figure 3 Changes in bone markers in the 10-mg alendronate group (filled squares), 5-mg alendronate group (filled circles), discontinuation group (filled diamonds) and placebo group (open circles)

remained stable in the alendronate groups. Serum bone-specific alkaline phosphatase levels declined by 49% in the 10-mg group at the end of year 10. After discontinuation of alendronate, bone markers increased within 1 year, but they still remained below baseline values.

Fracture incidence was evaluated for safety purposes. During the initial 3-year study, 6.2% of women in the placebo group had new morphometric vertebral fractures, compared with 3.2% in the pooled alendronate groups ($p = 0.03$). Proportions among the three alendronate groups were similar. For this analysis, 228 women could be evaluated for years 6–10. The incidence of new morphometric vertebral fractures did not differ significantly among the

three groups. The rate of radiologically confirmed non-vertebral fractures in the 10-mg group was similar to that in the pooled alendronate groups during the first 3 years of the study.

The latter and the FLEX trial both represent the longest follow-up that has been extended to date for assessing the long-term efficacy and safety of an osteoporosis drug, i.e. alendronate, in the treatment of postmenopausal osteoporosis.

Some concerns have been raised about the long-term bone safety of continuous BP treatment. The amount of BP retained in bone after 10 years of alendronate treatment was estimated at 75 mg per 2 kg mineral, using a pharmacokinetic model for a dose of 10 mg per day. This small fraction, which is unevenly distributed between cancellous and cortical bone, seems unlikely to change bone mechanical properties.

Since 1999, oral risedronate has also been available on the market for the treatment of postmenopausal osteoporosis. Risedronate has shown benefits for BMD and risk of fracture in the Vertebral Efficacy with Risedronate Therapy (VERT) trial and in the Hip Intervention Program (HIP) trial[15–17]. Both alendronate and risedronate are now available in once-weekly formulations approved on the basis of studies showing BMD gains comparable to those seen with daily formulations of both drugs[18,19].

The appropriate way to evaluate the relative efficacy of two drugs is to examine evidence from a head-to-head clinical comparison.

The FACT (Fosamax™ Actonel® Comparison Trial) was a randomized, double-blind, active-comparator study that evaluated 1053 postmenopausal women at 77 US sites. The patient population consisted of community-dwelling, ambulatory women who were at least 40 years of age (or at least 25 years of age if surgically menopausal) and postmenopausal for at least 6 months. Patients were required to have osteoporosis, defined as a BMD T-score of at least -2.0 at the hip trochanter, total hip, femoral neck or lumbar spine. Patients were excluded if they were taking or had recently taken any treatments that might influence bone turnover. As recommended by the prescribing information for alendronate, patients with abnormalities of the esophagus that delay emptying (i.e. stricture, achalasia) were excluded; there were no other gastrointestinal (GI) exclusions[20].

The mean age of patients was 64.5 years, and the mean time since menopause was 18.5 years. Approximately 95% of patients in each group were Caucasian, and a mean of 25% in each group had a history of an upper-GI disorder. Almost half of all randomized patients had a history of hip, spine or wrist fracture, and almost one-third had experienced a fracture after the age of 45.

Patients were randomized 1 : 1 to receive 12 months of therapy with either alendronate 70 mg once weekly plus a risedronate placebo once weekly, or risedronate 35 mg once weekly plus an alendronate placebo once weekly. Patients were instructed to take a minimum of 1000 mg of calcium and 400 IU of vitamin D daily.

The primary objective of this study was to evaluate the mean percentage change from baseline in hip trochanter BMD after 12 months of treatment. Secondary objectives included the difference between treatment groups in mean percentage change from baseline in total hip, femoral neck and lumbar spine BMD at 12 months, and the mean percentage change from baseline in biochemical markers of bone turnover (serum bone-specific alkaline phosphatase (BSAP), N-terminal propeptide of type I procollagen (PINP), serum C-telopeptide (CTx) and urinary NTx) at 3, 6 and 12 months. Other secondary objectives were the difference between treatment groups in the percentage of patients with BMD gains of at least 0% and 3%, the mean percentage change in BMD at all sites at 6 months, and overall safety and tolerability, including percentage of patients with any upper-GI adverse events at 12 months.

Table 4 shows mean BMD values at baseline in both treatment groups at the hip and the spine: baseline T-scores were similar in the two groups.

At baseline, mean BMD values at the hip trochanter were 0.571 and 0.572 g/cm^2 in the alendronate and risedronate groups, respectively. The mean percentage change from baseline was 3.4% with alendronate and 2.1% with risedronate, representing a treatment difference of 1.4% in favor of alendronate (95% confidence interval (CI) 0.8–1.9%, $p < 0.001$) (Figure 4).

Table 4 Mean bone mineral density values (T-scores) at baseline

Site	Alendronate ($n = 520$)	Risedronate ($n = 533$)	Total ($n = 1053$)
Trochanter	−1.58	−1.58	−1.58
Total hip	−1.76	−1.78	−1.77
Femoral neck	−2.12	−2.16	−2.14
Lumbar spine	−2.26	−2.23	−2.24

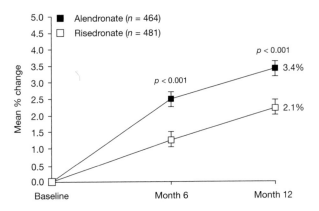

Figure 4   Mean percentage change from baseline of bone mineral density at the hip trochanter

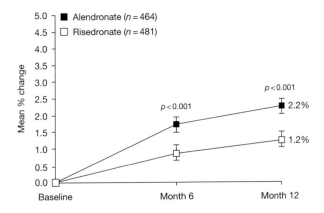

Figure 5   Mean percentage change from baseline of bone mineral density at the total hip

The effect of alendronate became evident by month 6 ($p < 0.001$ vs. risedronate).

The mean baseline total hip BMD was 0.750 (alendronate) and 0.749 g/cm^2 (risedronate), respectively. At month 12, the mean total hip BMD increased by 2.2% from baseline in the alendronate group and by 1.2% in the risedronate group. The treatment difference was 1.1% (95% CI 0.7–1.4%, $p < 0.001$ vs. risedronate) (Figure 5).

At baseline, the mean BMD at the femoral neck was 0.660 and 0.654 g/cm^2 in the alendronate and risedronate groups, respectively. The mean percentage change from baseline was 1.6% with alendronate and 0.9% with risedronate. The treatment difference at 12 months was 0.7% (95% CI 0.2–1.29%, $p = 0.005$ vs. risedronate) (Figure 6).

The mean baseline posteroanterior (PA) lumbar spine BMD was 0.839 (alendronate) and 0.837 g/cm^2 (risedronate), respectively. Lumbar spine BMD increases were 3.7% for alendronate and 2.6% for risedronate. This finding reflected a treatment difference of 1.2% (95% CI 0.7–1.6%, $p < 0.001$ vs. risedronate) (Figure 7).

The proportion of patients who experienced a PA lumbar spine BMD decrease of at least 3%

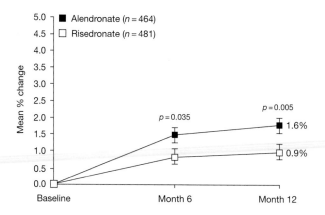

Figure 6 Mean percentage change from baseline of bone mineral density at the femoral neck

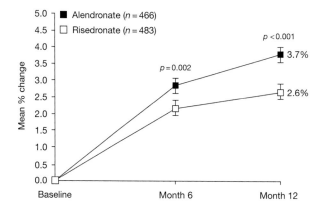

Figure 7 Mean percentage change from baseline of bone mineral density at the posteroanterior lumbar spine

was significantly higher in the risedronate group (4%) than in the alendronate group (1%) ($p = 0.008$). Conversely, the proportion of patients who experienced BMD gains of at least 0%, 3% and 5% was significantly higher in the alendronate group (all $p < 0.001$ vs. risedronate).

Hip trochanter data were similar to those at the PA lumbar spine: the proportion of patients who experienced a BMD decrease at the hip trochanter of at least 3% was significantly higher with risedronate (11%) than with alendronate (5%) ($p < 0.001$). Conversely, a significantly higher proportion of patients in the alendronate group experienced BMD gains of at least 0% ($p < 0.001$), 3% ($p = 0.002$) and 5% ($p < 0.001$).

At all time points (months 3, 6 and 12), alendronate produced significantly ($p < 0.001$) greater decreases in markers of bone resorption (NTx and CTx) than did risedronate. Differences in favor of alendronate became evident from as early as month 3 (Figure 8). NTx reductions of 53% (alendronate) and 40% (risedronate) were observed at month 12. This represented a treatment difference of 13% (95% CI −16.6 to −8.5, $p < 0.001$ vs. risedronate)[10].

At month 12, mean CTx reductions of 74% and 55% were observed with alendronate and risedronate, respectively, representing a treatment difference of 19% (95% CI −22.7 to −15.6, $p < 0.001$ vs. risedronate).

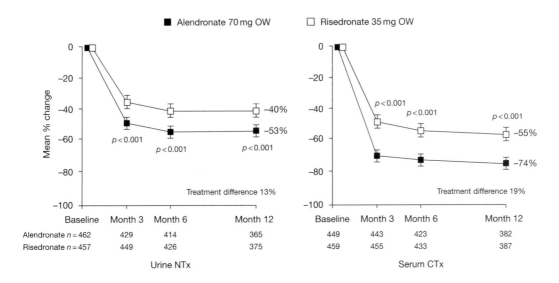

Figure 8 Mean percentage changes from baseline of markers of bone resorption. OW, once weekly; NTx, N-telopeptide; CTx, C-telopeptide

In addition to reducing markers of bone resorption, alendronate produced significantly ($p < 0.001$) greater decreases in markers of bone formation (BSAP and PINP) than risedronate at all time points (months 3, 6 and 12). Together, these results indicated an overall reduction in bone turnover from as early as month 3 (Figure 9). BSAP value decreases of 41% and 28% were observed at month 12 in the alendronate and risedronate groups, respectively. This represented a treatment difference of 13% (95% CI −15.3 to −9.6, $p < 0.001$ vs. risedronate). At month 12, PINP mean values decreased by 64% and 48% with alendronate and risedronate, respectively, representing a treatment difference of 16% (95% CI −18.9 to −12.9, $p < 0.001$ vs. risedronate).

Overall, a clinical adverse experience was reported by 76% of patients in each treatment group. However, only fewer than a third of these were drug-related; the rate of drug-related adverse experiences was 23% with alendronate and 21% with risedronate. Serious adverse experiences were uncommon, with rates of 9% in the alendronate group and 8% in the risedronate group. Thirty-three patients in each group discontinued due to an adverse experience.

There were no significant differences between treatment groups in the clinical adverse-experience profile. Upper-GI adverse experiences were reported by 22.5% of patients in the alendronate group and 20.1% of patients in the risedronate group. These events resulted in discontinuation in a minority of patients: 2.5% in the alendronate group and 3% in the risedronate group. There were no significant differences between treatment groups in the upper-GI adverse-experience profile.

Superiority of weekly alendronate versus weekly risedronate at marketed doses in reducing bone turnover and increasing BMD represents an essential finding for distinguishing the efficacies of the two drugs. Bone turnover is the major driver of fracture risk: it characterizes the relationship between bone resorption and bone formation. When bone resorption exceeds bone formation, bone is lost. The primary mechanism of action of bisphosphonates is inhibition of bone resorption, resulting in reduced bone turnover. The reduced rate of bone turnover leads to increases in BMD in postmenopausal women with osteoporosis. Although increased BMD is independently associated with a reduced risk of fracture, it is critical that the new bone formed

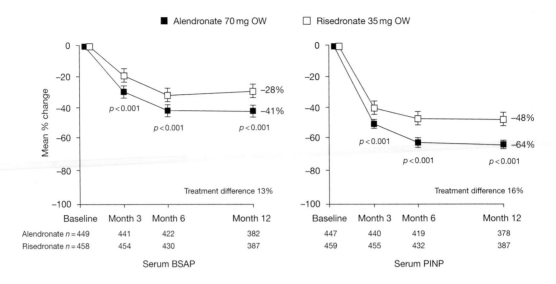

Figure 9 Mean percentage changes from baseline of markers of bone formation. OW, once weekly; BSAP, bone-specific alkaline phosphatase; PINP, N-terminal propeptide of type I procollagen

during therapy is of normal quality to effect greater strength and resistance to fracture. Histomorphometric studies have confirmed that bisphosphonate treatment produces new bone of normal quality, with normal lamellar architecture and mineralization. BPs work by decreasing bone turnover, increasing bone mineral density and strengthening bone, thus playing a vital role in the reduction of fracture risk. Although bisphosphonates may have similar mechanisms of action, the results of the FACT study show that bisphosphonates are not equally effective.

Recently, a randomized, double-blind, multicenter 12-month study has compared the efficacy and tolerability of once-weekly (OW) alendronate (ALN) 70 mg and raloxifene (RLX) 60 mg daily in the treatment of postmenopausal osteoporosis[21]. In total, 456 postmenopausal women with osteoporosis (223 ALN, 233 RLX) were enrolled at 52 sites in the United States. Efficacy measurements included lumbar spine (LS), total hip and trochanter BMD at 6 and 12 months, biochemical markers of bone turnover and percentage of women who maintained or gained BMD in response to treatment. The primary end-point was percentage change from baseline in spine BMD at 12 months. Adverse

experiences were recorded to assess treatment safety and tolerability. Over 12 months, OW ALN produced a significantly greater increase in spine BMD (4.4%, $p < 0.001$ than did RLX (1.9%). The percentages of women with $\geq 0\%$ increase in LS BMD (ALN 94%, RLX 75%; $p < 0.001$) and $\geq 3\%$ increase in LS BMD (ALN 66%, RLX 38%; $p < 0.001$) were significantly greater with ALN than with RLX. Total hip and trochanter BMD increases were also significantly greater ($p \leq 0.001$) with ALN. Greater ($p < 0.001$) reductions in N-telopeptide of type I collagen and bone-specific alkaline phosphatase were achieved with ALN compared with RLX at 6 and 12 months. No significant differences in the incidence of upper-gastrointestinal or vasomotor adverse experiences were seen.

Long-term efficacy of alendronate has also been demonstrated in the prevention of bone loss in early postmenopausal women. The Early Postmenopausal Intervention Cohort (EPIC) study[22] enrolled 1609 women across four centers. Women were 45–59 years old, in good general health and at least 6 months postmenopausal at baseline; 585 patients were randomized to receive the same dose of alendronate (2.5 or 5 mg daily) or placebo continuously for 6 years of the

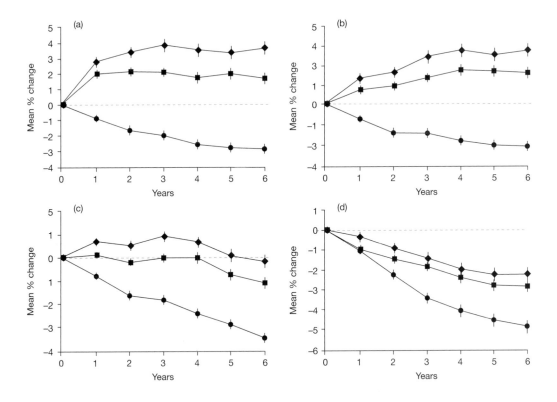

Figure 10 The Early Postmenopausal Intervention Cohort (EPIC) study. Both alendronate groups (2.5 mg ■ and 5 mg ♦) exhibited significantly larger bone mineral density (BMD) increases at the spine (a) and the hip (b) at the end of 6 years compared with the placebo group (●). Treatment with 5 mg alendronate also prevented total body bone loss (c) and attenuated BMD loss at the forearm (d) when compared with placebo. Furthermore, BMD increases were significantly larger for the 5-mg alendronate group compared with the 2.5-mg group, except for the femoral neck

study. Postmenopausal women treated with placebo for 6 years experienced significant progressive decreases in BMD of the spine, hip, forearm and total body (all p values < 0.001) (Figure 10). In contrast, women who received 6 years of treatment with alendronate (2.5 or 5 mg daily) experienced significant gains versus baseline values in mean lumbar spine, trochanter and total hip BMD ($p < 0.001$). A significant increase in BMD at the femoral neck versus baseline values ($p < 0.01$) was observed only in women who received continuous 5 mg alendronate for 6 years.

Patients who received placebo for 6 years experienced a small mean decrease in urinary NTx levels (approximately 25% at 6 months)

followed by a progressive further decline until approximately 3 years (Figure 11). The levels remained relatively stable from then to the end of 6 years, resulting in a final value 37.9% below baseline.

In the groups receiving alendronate, 2.5 mg and 5 mg daily for 6 years, there was a much greater dose-related decrease in mean urinary NTx during the first year of treatment followed by a further small decline up to year 3, and then it remained relatively stable within the normal premenopausal range. At the end of 6 years, the mean percentage changes from baseline were -63.9 and -68.0% for the 2.5-mg and 5-mg alendronate groups, respectively. The decreases in bone resorption in the two alendronate groups

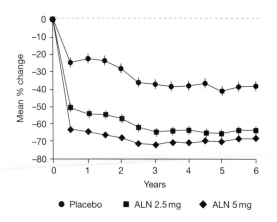

Mean % change

● Placebo   ■ ALN 2.5 mg   ◆ ALN 5 mg

Figure 11 Mean percentage change in urinary N-telopeptide (NTx) level

were significantly ($p < 0.001$) different from the placebo group at the end of year 6.

Alendronate efficacy has been elucidated also in secondary osteoporosis. In corticosteroid-induced osteoporosis, 2-year alendronate treatment has been shown to be very effective in reducing new vertebral fracture risk by 90% and

in preventing bone loss both at the spine and the hip[23].

A 2-year double-blind trial was conducted, aimed at assessing the effect of 10 mg daily of alendronate on bone mineral density in 241 men (aged 31–87 years, mean 63 years) with osteoporosis[24]. Approximately one-third had low serum free-testosterone concentrations at baseline. Men with other secondary causes of osteoporosis were excluded. Alendronate increased BMD by 7.1% at the lumbar spine, 2.5% at the femoral neck and 2.0% for the total body ($p < 0.001$ for all comparisons with baseline). Men who received placebo had an increase in spine BMD of 1.8%, and no significant changes in femoral neck or total body BMD. BMD changes in the alendronate group were greater than in the placebo group at all skeletal sites ($p < 0.001$). New vertebral fracture incidence was decreased by 89% in the alendronate group (0.8% vs. 7.1% in placebo group, $p = 0.02$).

In conclusion, alendronate efficacy and safety have been extensively verified by the longest intervention trials available to date in prevention and treatment of osteoporosis.

References

1. Menschutkin N. Ueber die Einwirkung des Chlorazetyls auf phosphorige Säure. *Ann Chem Pharm* 1865; 133: 317–20

2. Blomen LJMJ. History of bisphosphonates: discovery and history of the non-medical uses of bisphosphonates. In Bijvoet OLM, Fleisch HA, Canfield RE, Russell RGG, eds. *Bisphosphonate on Bones*. Amsterdam: Elsevier Science Publishers, 1995: 11–124

3. Fleisch H, Russell RGG, Francis MD. Diphosphonates inhibit hydroxyapatite dissolution in vitro and bone resorption in tissue culture and in vivo. *Science* 1969; 65: 1262–64

4. Francis MD, Russell RGG, Fleisch H. Diphosphonates inhibit formation of calcium phosphate crystals in vitro and pathological calcification in vivo. *Science* 1969; 165: 1264–6

5. Fleisch H. *Bisphosphonates in Bone Disease. From the Laboratory to the Patient*. London: Parthenon Publishing, 1995: 176

6. Jung A, Bisaz S, Fleisch H. The binding of pyrophosphate and two diphosphonates on hydroxyapatite crystals. *Calcif Tissue Res* 1973; 11: 269–80

7. Kasting GB, Francis MD. Retention of etidronate in human, dog, and rat. *J Bone Miner Res* 1992; 7: 513–22

8. Boulenc X, Marti E, Joyeux H, et al. Importance of the paracellular pathway for the transport of new bisphosphonate using the human CACO-2 monolayers model. *Biochem Pharmacol* 1993; 46: 1591–600

9. Troehler U, Bonjour JP, Fleisch H. Renal secretion of diphosphonates in rats. *Kidney Int* 1975; 8: 6–13

10. Reszka AA, Rodan GA. Nitrogen-containing bisphosphonate mechanism of action. *Mini Rev Med Chem* 2004; 4: 711–19

11. Liberman UA, Weiss SR, Broll J, et al. Effect of oral alendronate on bone mineral density and the incidence of fractures in postmenopausal osteoporosis. The Alendronate Phase III Osteoporosis Treatment Study Group. *N Engl J Med* 1995; 333: 1437–43

12. Black DM, Cummings SR, Karpf DB, et al. Randomised trial of effect of alendronate on risk of fracture in women with existing vertebral fractures. Fracture Intervention Trial Research Group. *Lancet* 1996; 348: 1535–41

13. Cummings SR, Black DM, Thompson DE, et al. Alendronate reduces the risk of vertebral fractures in women without pre-existing vertebral fractures: results of the Fracture Intervention Trial. *J Am Med Assoc* 1998; 280: 2077–82

14. Bone HG, Hosking D, Devogelaer JP, et al. for the Alendronate Phase III Osteoporosis Treatment Study Group. Ten years' experience with alendronate for osteoporosis in postmenopausal women. *N Engl J Med* 2004; 350: 1189–99

15. Reginster J, Minne HW, Sorensen OH, et al. Randomized trial of the effects of risedronate on vertebral fractures in women with established postmenopausal osteoporosis. Vertebral Efficacy with Risedronate Therapy (VERT) Study Group. *Osteoporos Int* 2000; 11: 83–91

16. Harris ST, Watts NB, Genant HK, et al. Effects of risedronate treatment on vertebral and nonvertebral fractures in women with postmenopausal osteoporosis: a randomized controlled trial. Vertebral Efficacy with Risedronate Therapy (VERT) Study Group. *J Am Med Assoc* 1999; 282: 1344–52

17. McClung M, Geusens P, Miller P, et al. Effect of risedronate on the risk of hip fracture in elderly women. *N Engl J Med* 2001; 344: 333–40

18. Schnitzer T, Bone, H, Crepaldi G, et al. Therapeutic equivalence of alendronate 70 mg once weekly and alendronate 10 mg daily in the treatment of osteoporosis. *Aging (Milano)* 2000; 12: 1–12

19. Brown JP, Kendler DL, McClung MR, et al. The efficacy and tolerability of risedronate once a week for the treatment of postmenopausal osteoporosis. *Calcif Tissue Int* 2002; 71: 103–11

20. Hosking D, Adami S, Felsenberg D, et al. Comparison of change in bone resorption and bone mineral density with once-weekly alendronate and daily risedronate. *Curr Med Res Opin* 2003; 19: 383–94

21. Luckey M, Kagan R, Greenspan S, et al. Once-weekly alendronate 70 mg and raloxifene 60 mg daily in the treatment of postmenopausal osteoporosis. *Menopause* 2004; 11: 405–15

22. McClung MR, Wasnich RD, Hosking D, et al. Prevention of postmenopausal bone loss: six-year results from the Early Postmenopausal Intervention Cohort study. *J Clin Endocrinol Metab* 2004; 89: 4879–85

23. Adachi JD, Saag KG, Delmas PD, et al. Two-year effects of alendronate on bone mineral density and vertebral fracture in patients receiving glucocorticoids: a randomized, double-blind, placebo-controlled extension trial *Arthritis Rheum* 2001; 44: 202–11

24. Orwoll E, Ettinger M, Weiss S, et al. Alendronate for the treatment of osteoporosis in men. *N Engl J Med* 2000; 343: 604–10

Index